Hartman's Complete Guide for the Phlebotomy Technician

Hartman Publishing, Inc.

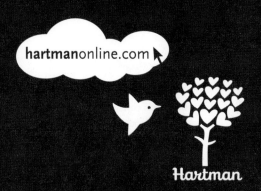

hartmanonline.com

Hartman

Credits

Managing Editor
Susan Alvare Hedman

Developmental Editor
Kristin Calderon

Designer
Kirsten Browne

Production
Elena Reznikova

Illustration
Tracy Kopsachilis and Tess Marhofer

Editorial Assistant
Angela Storey

Proofreaders
Sapna Desai, Joanna Owusu, and Barbara Winbush

Sales/Marketing
Deborah Rinker-Wildey, Kendra Robertson, Erika Walker, and Col Foley

Customer Service
Fran Desmond, Thomas Noble, Brian Fejer, Henry Bullis, and Della Torres

Information Technology
Eliza Martin

Warehouse Coordinator
Chris Midyette

Copyright Information

1313 Iron Ave SW
Albuquerque, New Mexico 87102
(505) 291-1274
web: hartmanonline.com
email: orders@hartmanonline.com
Twitter: @HartmanPub

ISBN 978-1-60425-129-6

PRINTED IN CANADA

Third Printing, 2023

Notice to Readers

Though the guidelines and procedures contained in this text are based on consultations with healthcare professionals, they should not be considered absolute recommendations. They should be used as a general guide. The instructor and readers should follow employer, local, state, and federal guidelines, as well as current standards concerning healthcare practices. These guidelines change, and it is the reader's responsibility to be aware of these changes and of the policies and procedures of her or his healthcare facility. The publisher, authors, editors, and reviewers cannot accept any responsibility for errors, omissions, injury, liability, or for any consequences from application of the information in this book and make no warranty, express or implied, with respect to the contents of the book. The publisher does not warrant or guarantee any of the products described herein or perform any analysis in connection with any of the product information contained herein.

Gender Usage

This textbook uses gender pronouns interchangeably to denote healthcare team members and patients.

Special Thanks

A very warm thank you goes to our insightful reviewers, listed in alphabetical order:

Seham Cramer, BS, MT (ASCP)
Arlington, TX

Judith Kimelman Kline, RMA (AMT), NCPT, NCEKG, NCRMA
Miami, FL

Merri Michele Knorpp, LVN
Elkhart, TX

Jamie Mirabilio, LPN, CPT
Waterbury, CT

Pamela Molnar, RN
Lynnville, TN

Susan N. Omare, MBA/HCM, MSc-HCQ, RN-BSN, BSc-IT
Overland Park, KS

Amanda Young, RN, BSN, CMA
Ashland, OH

Paula Zagel, MS
Brighton, CO

We are very appreciative of the many sources who shared their informative images with us:

- American Hospital Association
- Becton, Dickinson and Company
- Benchmark Scientific
- Centers for Disease Control and Prevention
- Dreamstime
- Globe Scientific
- Greiner Bio-One
- March of Dimes
- MarketLab
- Medline
- Nova Biomedical
- Occupational Safety and Health Administration
- Ram Scientific
- Shutterstock
- TriCore

Contents

Learning Objective *Page*

6 Overview of the Human Body

7 The Circulatory System in Depth

8 Preparing for Specimen Collection

Learning Objective *Page*

9 Collecting Blood Specimens by Venipuncture

10 Collecting Blood Specimens by Capillary (Dermal) Puncture

Procedures

Using a Hartman Textbook

Understanding how this book is organized and what its special features are will help you make the most of this resource!

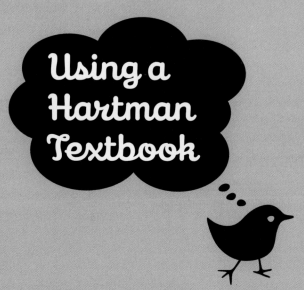

We have assigned each chapter its own colored tab. Each colored tab contains the chapter number and title, and is located on the side of every page.

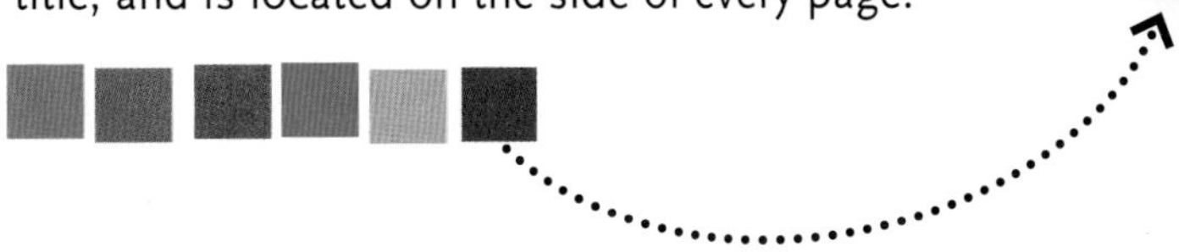

8. Describe preparations for the safe collection of blood specimens

Everything in this book and the instructor's teaching material is organized around **learning objectives.** A learning objective (LO) is a very specific piece of knowledge or a very specific skill. After reading the text, you will know you have mastered the material if you can do what the learning objective says.

hematology

Bold key terms are located throughout the text, followed by their definitions. They are also listed in the glossary at the back of this book.

Washing hands (hand hygiene)

All **care procedures** are highlighted by the same black bar for easy recognition.

Guidelines: Legal and Ethical Behavior

Guidelines lists are colored green for easy reference.

Patients' Rights

Blue Patients' Rights boxes teach important information about how to support and promote legal rights and patient-centered care.

Extra protection

Gray boxes contain extra information that will help you be an even better phlebotomy technician.

Quality Counts

Orange Quality Counts boxes highlight ways phlebotomy technicians can practice the highest standards of care in their work.

Chapter Review

Chapter-ending questions test your knowledge of the information found in the chapter. If you have trouble answering a question, you can return to the text and reread the material.

1

Healthcare Settings and the Role of the Phlebotomy Technician

Note: There are many different ways to refer to healthcare workers whose primary duty is to collect blood specimens. This book uses the terms *phlebotomy technician* and *phlebotomist* interchangeably, and uses the abbreviation *PBT*.

1. Discuss the healthcare system and describe changes in staffing trends

Health care is a growing field. *The healthcare system* refers to the different kinds of providers, facilities, and payers involved in delivering medical care. **Providers** are people or organizations that provide health care, including doctors, nurses, clinics, and agencies. **Facilities** are places where care is delivered or administered, including hospitals, doctors' offices, clinical laboratories, and treatment centers (such as for cancer). **Payers** are people or organizations paying for healthcare services. These include insurance companies, government programs such as Medicare and Medicaid, and individual patients or clients. Together, these people, places, and organizations make up the healthcare system.

Many facilities hire workers with specialized skills and build teams to care for patients, with each team member meeting a specific patient need. In the past, doctors examined patients, **diagnosed** illness, and planned treatment, while nurses did most of the other patient care tasks. Today many healthcare workers share those other duties. Specially trained technicians perform medical tests such as electrocardiograms or sonograms. Medical assistants record patients' medical histories or measure their vital signs, among other tasks (Fig. 1-1). Nursing assistants provide routine personal care such as feeding and bathing and can also measure vital signs and report their observations of patient conditions.

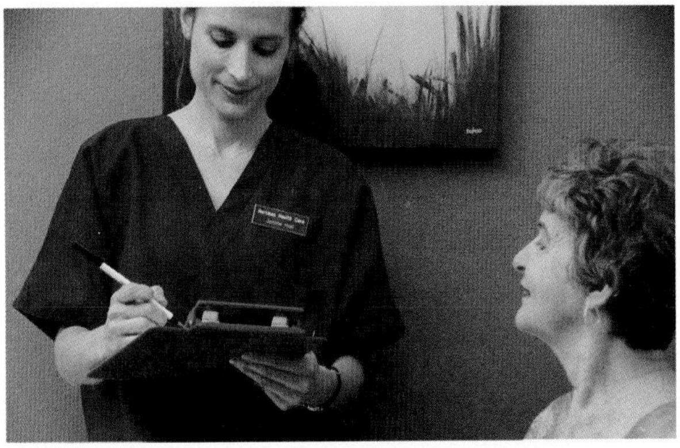

Fig. 1-1. *Many types of healthcare workers perform duties that once were mostly performed by nurses, such as taking patients' medical histories.*

Phlebotomy technicians are part of this trend toward hiring specialized healthcare workers. The Department of Labor forecasts 23% growth in the hiring of phlebotomy technicians over the next several years. Average growth for a job category is 7%, so this is a fast-growing field. Healthcare workers of all kinds will likely continue to be in high demand. People will always need to receive health care and populations in particular need of care, such as the elderly, are growing.

2. Describe common healthcare settings

Health care is provided either in an **inpatient** or **outpatient** setting. Inpatient care is provided to patients who must stay at the healthcare facility overnight. Hospitals generally provide inpatient care, and usually care for people whose illnesses are **acute**, meaning the illness is short-term and must be treated immediately. Urgent care centers, public health clinics, doctors' offices, and freestanding emergency departments (i.e., those not physically connected to a hospital) are all examples of outpatient healthcare facilities. Outpatient care (sometimes called *ambulatory care*) does not require the patient to stay overnight. Outpatient care has become common for surgery and other procedures that once required a hospital stay.

Hospitals may be public, meaning they are funded by taxes, or private. Private hospitals may be for-profit (a money-making business) or nonprofit (costs are covered but profit is not generated). What both public and private hospitals have in common is that they operate 24 hours a day to care for sick and injured patients. They are organized into different departments to care for patients with different needs. Hospitals also have emergency departments, where care is provided to patients who need immediate care for an injury or illness (Fig. 1-2). The patients are either treated and **discharged** (allowed to leave the facility), or they are **admitted** (checked in to receive inpatient care).

Urgent care centers and freestanding emergency departments are outpatient healthcare facilities where patients can be treated without an appointment. Urgent care centers usually have longer hours than a typical doctor's office but are not open 24 hours a day. Freestanding emergency departments, which may be associated with a hospital or may be independent, are usually open 24 hours a day, seven days a week. Most freestanding emergency departments are staffed at all times by an emergency physician, and most have more services and equipment available than an urgent care center has. As more freestanding emergency departments open around the country, many states are establishing rules about the services, medicines, and equipment that must be available at these facilities.

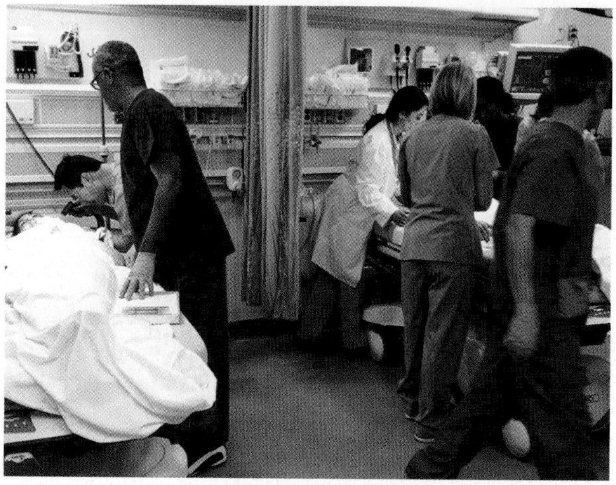

Fig. 1-2. *Emergency departments provide care for patients with immediate needs.*

Doctors may run their own private practices, with or without partners, or may have offices associated with a hospital or healthcare organization. These facilities can range from an office staffed by a small number of employees to a multi-doctor clinic with a large staff and a full range of medical services, including laboratory services. Smaller offices usually send patients to an outpatient laboratory for any necessary tests.

Public health clinics are outpatient healthcare facilities where patients with low or moderate incomes can receive medical treatment at a reduced cost. Each clinic is different, but these facilities generally receive support from federal, state, or local government and provide basic services like vaccinations, well checks for school-aged children, or women's health services and family planning. They may be operated by city or county health departments.

Long-term care facilities are businesses that provide skilled care 24 hours a day to residents who live in the facilities. These facilities may offer assisted living housing, dementia care, or subacute care, which is inpatient care for patients who require more care than can be provided in the home, but who do not need to be in a hospital (Fig. 1-3). Some facilities offer specialized care, while others care for all types of residents. The typical long-term care facility offers personal care for all residents and focused care for residents with special needs. Phlebotomy technicians and some other types of healthcare workers often visit long-term care facilities so the residents do not have to leave to receive care.

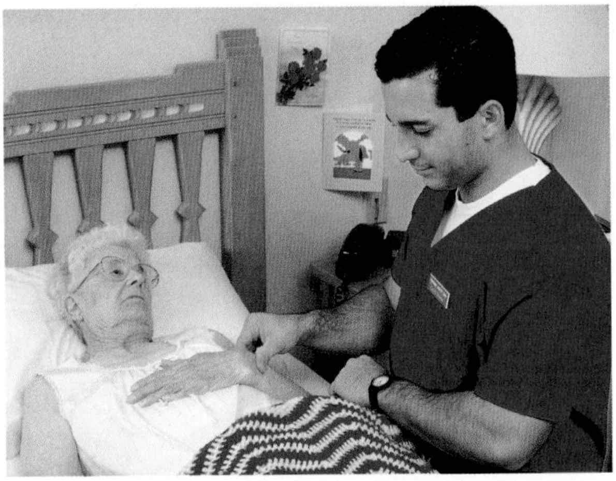

Fig. 1-3. People who live in long-term care facilities can receive care whenever it is needed.

Clinical laboratories, which may also be called *medical laboratories* or *diagnostic laboratories*, are key to both inpatient and outpatient health care. These laboratories collect and analyze specimens from patients in order to provide doctors and other healthcare professionals with information. This information may be used for routine screening, as in an annual wellness exam. It may also be used to help diagnose an illness or to gather more information about a problem the patient is experiencing. Laboratories can be located inside a hospital or other healthcare facility, or they can be separate facilities (Fig. 1-4). Some doctors' offices have limited laboratory facilities and refer patients to larger labs for certain tests.

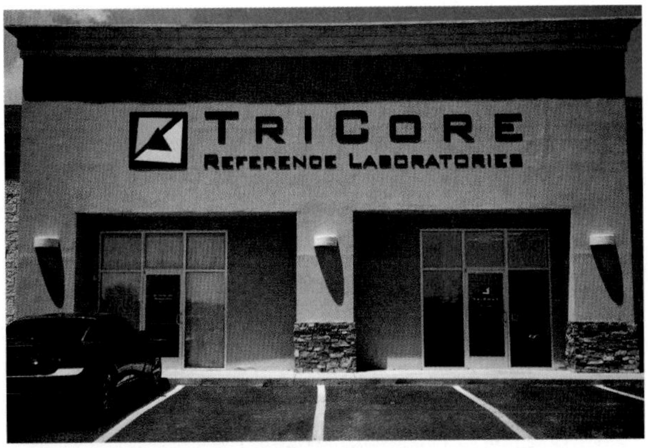

Fig. 1-4. Laboratories collect and analyze specimens to assist in diagnosis and patient care. (PHOTO COURTESY OF TRICORE REFERENCE LABORATORIES, WWW.TRICORE.ORG, 800-245-3296)

3. Discuss the organization and function of clinical laboratories

Each clinical laboratory is different, but they have some things in common. All laboratories collect and analyze **specimens**, or samples, from patients. Common specimens include blood, urine, stool (feces), and sputum (mucus coughed up from the lungs). They can also include body cells, such as a swab collecting cells from the inside of a cheek, or tissues, as in a biopsy that removes tissue to examine it for signs of disease. Not all specimens are analyzed at the same laboratory where they are collected. **Reference laboratories** do not collect specimens, but analyze specimens collected in another place. These laboratories may be far away from the laboratory or doctor's office where the specimen was collected.

Laboratories in the United States must meet standards listed in a set of regulations called the **Clinical Laboratory Improvement Amendments (CLIA)**. These include educational requirements for certain laboratory employees, as well as rules for handling patient specimens and tests and quality assurance and control practices. The goal of CLIA is to make sure patients receive the best quality care and that their laboratory tests are performed safely and accurately by qualified personnel (more information about CLIA in Chapter 2). Although they are not legally required to do so, laboratories may also be **accredited**, or officially approved, by several different independent organizations. The American Association for Laboratory Accreditation, The **Joint Commission** (formerly called the Joint Commission on Accreditation of Healthcare Organizations [JCAHO], jointcommission.org), and the College of American Pathologists are some of the most common accrediting agencies.

Figure 1-5 shows a simplified version of an organizational chart at a typical clinical laboratory.

Scientists and technologists are likely specialized in the following areas, which are departments within the laboratory:

Chemistry. This department works to analyze blood and other specimens for the presence of particular chemicals. Cholesterol, glucose, and hormone levels are examples of analyses done in the chemistry department.

Hematology. Blood, blood diseases, and **coagulation**, or the process of blood clotting, are all studied in this department (Fig. 1-6). The numbers and types of blood cells in specimens, and details about the composition of the blood, such as its capacity to carry oxygen, are part of hematology.

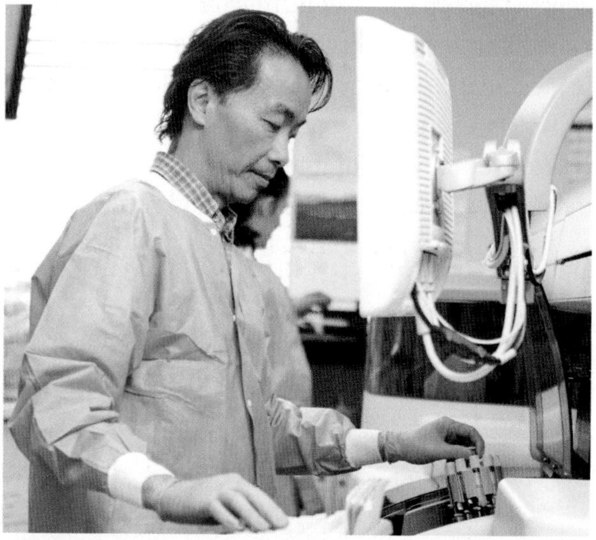

Fig. 1-6. Studies of blood and its properties and components are completed in the hematology department.

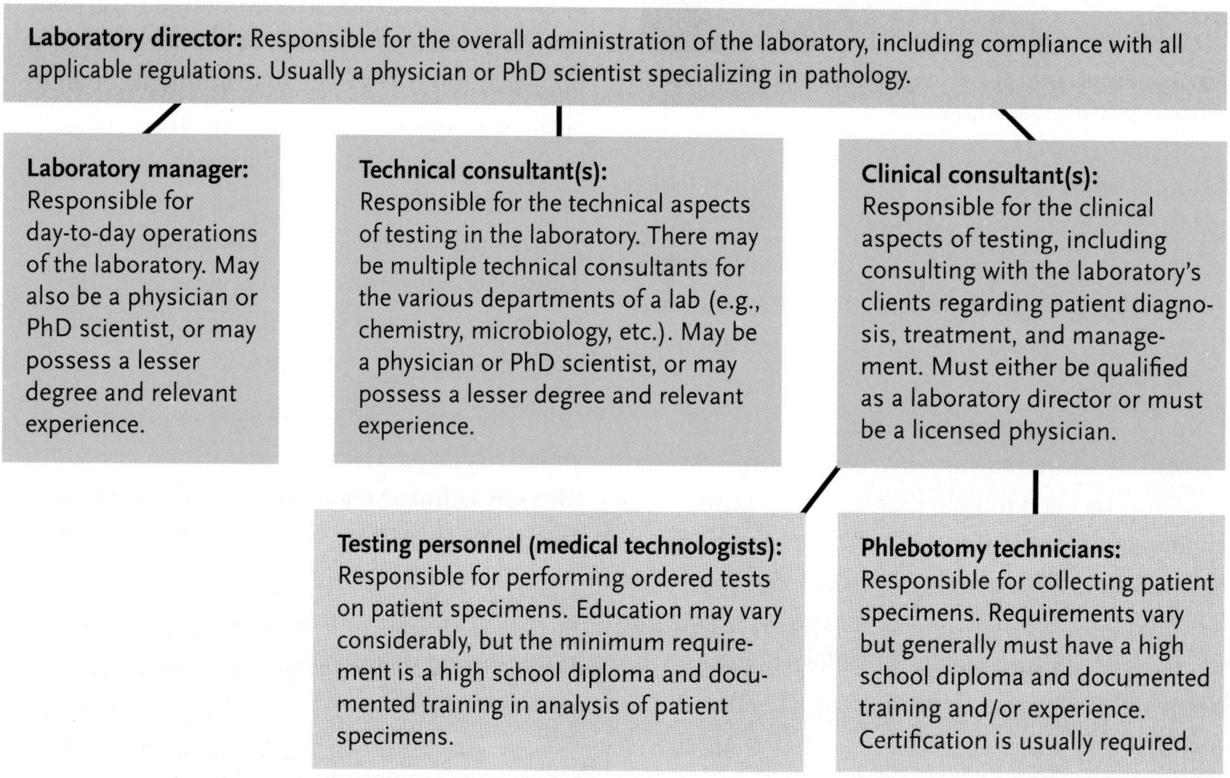
Laboratory director: Responsible for the overall administration of the laboratory, including compliance with all applicable regulations. Usually a physician or PhD scientist specializing in pathology.
Laboratory manager: Responsible for day-to-day operations of the laboratory. May also be a physician or PhD scientist, or may possess a lesser degree and relevant experience.
Technical consultant(s): Responsible for the technical aspects of testing in the laboratory. There may be multiple technical consultants for the various departments of a lab (e.g., chemistry, microbiology, etc.). May be a physician or PhD scientist, or may possess a lesser degree and relevant experience.
Clinical consultant(s): Responsible for the clinical aspects of testing, including consulting with the laboratory's clients regarding patient diagnosis, treatment, and management. Must either be qualified as a laboratory director or must be a licensed physician.
Testing personnel (medical technologists): Responsible for performing ordered tests on patient specimens. Education may vary considerably, but the minimum requirement is a high school diploma and documented training in analysis of patient specimens.
Phlebotomy technicians: Responsible for collecting patient specimens. Requirements vary but generally must have a high school diploma and documented training and/or experience. Certification is usually required.

Fig. 1-5. This simplified laboratory organizational chart shows the line of authority from the director to the medical technicians and phlebotomists.

Microbiology. In this area of the laboratory, scientists study **microorganisms**, or living things so small they can only be seen under a microscope. Bacteria and viruses are types of microorganisms, and they can sometimes cause disease. Blood and other specimens can be **cultured**, which means that any microorganisms present are caused to multiply. In this way, the microbiologist can analyze microorganisms in patients' specimens. This helps the doctor diagnose illness and plan the best treatment. In the case of a bacterial infection, culturing the blood can help the doctor understand which antibiotics might be most successful in fighting the type of bacteria present.

Immunology. In this department, blood and other body fluids are tested for different factors, such as **antibodies**, that affect the body's response to disease. Antibodies are part of the body's response to foreign materials like viruses and bacteria. These tests can help in monitoring a patient's response to cancer treatment, for instance, or in managing the body's response to an organ transplant. Allergy testing is also part of immunology.

Blood Bank or *Immunohematology*. These operations focus on collecting and preparing blood for transfusion (Fig. 1-7). Blood typing and analysis for donor/recipient compatibility are performed in this department, and blood and blood products are prepared for transfusion.

Pathology. Pathology is the study of the causes and effects of disease. This department studies body tissues and other specimens to determine the presence or progress of disease.

Cytology. The cytology department specializes in the examination of the structure and function of cells. In a clinical laboratory, cells are studied for signs of disease.

Urinalysis. This department performs various tests on urine, including visual inspection, microscopic inspection, and chemical testing. Urine may be tested to diagnose illnesses or as part of the management of various illnesses or conditions.

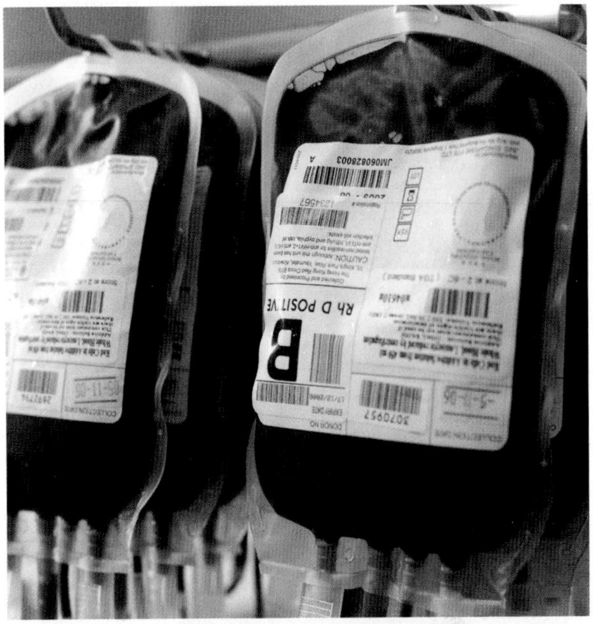

Fig. 1-7. *Donated blood and blood products are needed in times of disaster, as well as on a daily basis for patients undergoing surgery, cancer treatment, and transplants.*

Stat. A *stat* test is one that must be performed immediately, and laboratories may have a department specifically designed to handle these tests. The stat department may perform tests normally done in other departments when results are needed urgently.

4. Discuss the healthcare team

Every patient at a healthcare facility has different needs and problems. Healthcare professionals with a wide range of education and experience will help care for them. These people are considered the healthcare team, and together they provide all of the different types of care a patient might need. Members of the healthcare team include the following:

The patient: The patient is an important member of the healthcare team and is actually the reason the team exists. Providing quality care means placing the patient's well-being first and giving her the right to make decisions and choices about her own care.

Certified healthcare workers: Phlebotomy technicians, EKG technicians, and patient care technicians are examples of team members who are trained to perform specific tasks (Fig. 1-8). They do jobs like drawing blood, conducting tests, or measuring vital signs to gather information doctors need to care for the patient. They must have high school diplomas, as well as additional education, training, and certification to perform their job duties.

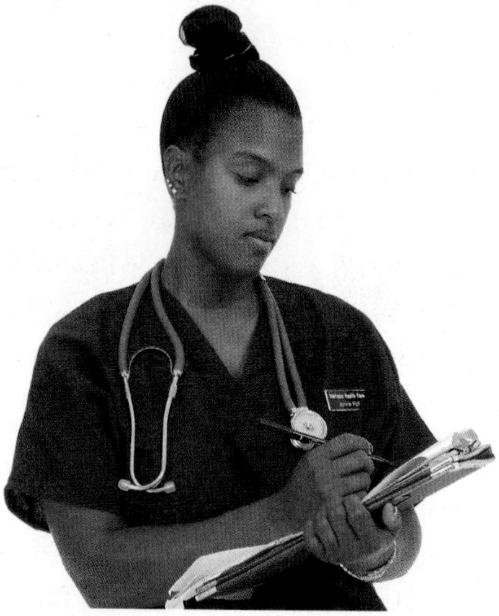

***Fig. 1-8.** Technicians do many of the tasks and make many of the observations that help ensure patients get the best possible care.*

Licensed practical nurse (LPN) or licensed vocational nurse (LVN): A licensed practical nurse or licensed vocational nurse administers medications and gives treatments. An LPN or LVN is a licensed professional who has completed one to two years of education and has passed a national licensure examination. **Licensure** is a legally required process that must be completed to practice a medical profession in a state.

Registered nurse (RN): In a hospital, long-term care facility, or clinic, a registered nurse coordinates, manages, and provides skilled nursing care. This includes administering special treatments and giving medication as prescribed by a physician. In a hospital a registered nurse also assigns tasks and supervises daily care of patients by nursing assistants or patient care technicians. An RN is a licensed professional who has graduated from a two- to four-year nursing program. RNs have diplomas or college degrees and have passed a national licensure examination. They may have additional academic degrees or education in specialty areas.

Therapists: Hospitals and other healthcare facilities employ a wide variety of therapists who help meet patient needs (Fig. 1-9). Speech-language pathologists, physical therapists, and respiratory therapists are a few examples. All of these team members have different education and clinical experience requirements for their jobs. Most physical therapists have doctoral degrees. Speech-language pathologists must have master's degrees, and respiratory therapists must have an associate's or bachelor's degree. All must meet state licensure requirements.

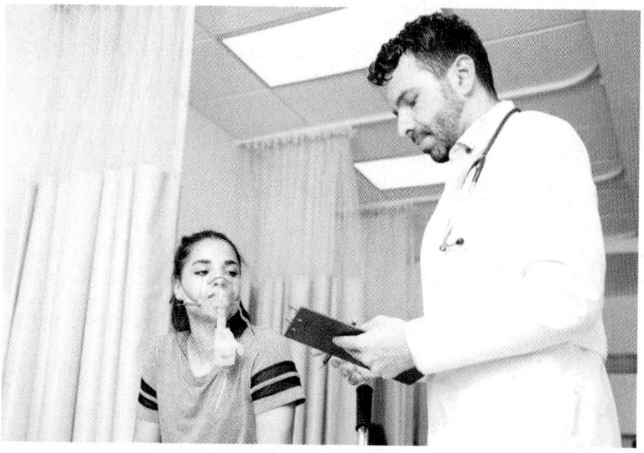

***Fig. 1-9.** Respiratory therapists assist patients with breathing treatments and perform other tasks related to the lungs and the respiratory system.*

Registered dietician (RD or RDN): A registered dietitian assesses a patient's nutritional status and creates diets to meet patients' special needs, and may also supervise the preparation of food and educate people about nutrition. Registered dietitians have completed bachelor's degrees and may also have completed postgraduate work. Most states require that registered dietitians be licensed or certified.

Pharmacist and pharmacy technician: A facility's pharmacy department maintains supplies of medications and ensures that patients receive the medications they need. Pharmacists must have doctoral degrees and are licensed to practice. Pharmacy technicians, who assist with measuring, packaging, and labeling medications, generally have a high school education and specialized training/certification.

Nurse practitioner (NP) or physician assistant (PA): These members of the healthcare team can perform many duties usually associated with doctors. In addition to the responsibilities common for RNs, nurse practitioners and physician assistants can examine patients, diagnose, and usually can prescribe medications. States have differing rules about the tasks these practitioners can perform and the level of doctor supervision they are required to have. NPs and PAs have master's or doctoral degrees and several years of experience in the healthcare field. They must also be licensed.

Physician or doctor (MD [medical doctor] or DO [doctor of osteopathy]): A doctor diagnoses disease or disability and prescribes treatment (Fig. 1-10). Doctors have graduated from four-year medical schools, which they attend after receiving bachelor's degrees. Many doctors also attend specialized training programs after medical school. Doctors must be licensed to practice medicine and may also be certified in one or more specialties.

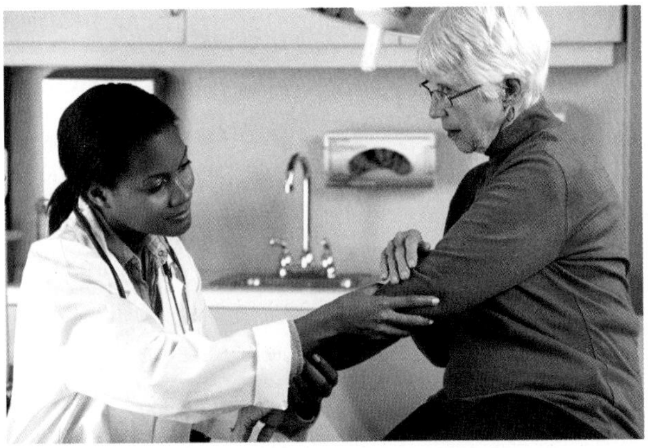

Fig. 1-10. *A doctor makes a diagnosis and prescribes treatment.*

Healthcare workers like phlebotomists carry out instructions given to them by their supervisors. The supervisors act on the instructions of a physician, laboratory director, or other member of the care team. This is called the **chain of command**. It describes the line of authority at a facility and helps to make sure that patients get proper health care. The chain of command also protects employees and employers from liability. **Liability** is a legal term that means someone can be held responsible for harming someone. For example, if a patient has a seizure during a blood draw and is injured, there may be a question of whether the phlebotomist is responsible for the injury. If the blood draw was ordered by the patient's physician, performed according to policy and procedure, and the phlebotomist responded to the patient's seizure appropriately, the phlebotomist is unlikely to be found liable. This is why it is important for team members to follow procedures carefully and for the facility to have a chain of command.

All healthcare workers must understand what they can and cannot do. This is important so that they do not harm patients or involve themselves or their employers in lawsuits. Certified healthcare workers like phlebotomy technicians are not licensed healthcare providers. Everything they do in their job is assigned to them by a licensed healthcare professional and must fall within their **scope of practice**. A scope of practice defines the tasks that healthcare workers are allowed to perform according to state or federal law or to facility policy. Laws and regulations vary from state to state. It is very important that healthcare workers follow their facility's policies regarding scope of practice.

Extra protection

Following the facility's chain of command and policies and procedures, as well as respecting scope of practice, helps protect healthcare workers from liability. Some healthcare workers take the extra step of having *liability insurance* as well. This insurance helps cover any costs associated with legal action against a healthcare worker. Some employers may provide this insurance for employees. It is also possible to purchase liability insurance independently.

5. Explain the phlebotomy technician's role

Drawing and processing blood specimens is the phlebotomy technician's primary responsibility. Specimens of a patient's blood may be required for routine screening, such as checking cholesterol levels or the number of red and white blood cells. Routine blood tests can also give doctors an idea of how well patients' organs or body systems are working. If a patient is experiencing symptoms, a blood draw might be necessary to investigate possible illnesses or disorders. Cancer, heart disease, and diabetes are some of the illnesses that cause changes a blood test can detect. Blood tests can also measure the effectiveness of an ongoing medical treatment, such as whether a blood thinner is causing the patient's blood to clot more slowly.

PBTs are most commonly employed in hospitals, doctors' offices, clinical laboratories, and blood donor centers. They may also work at care centers for specific populations, such as cancer patients, or they may work at urgent care centers or freestanding emergency rooms. Some phlebotomists work for insurance companies, dialysis facilities, or for employers providing mobile phlebotomy services at nursing homes, assisted living centers, and other locations (Fig. 1-11).

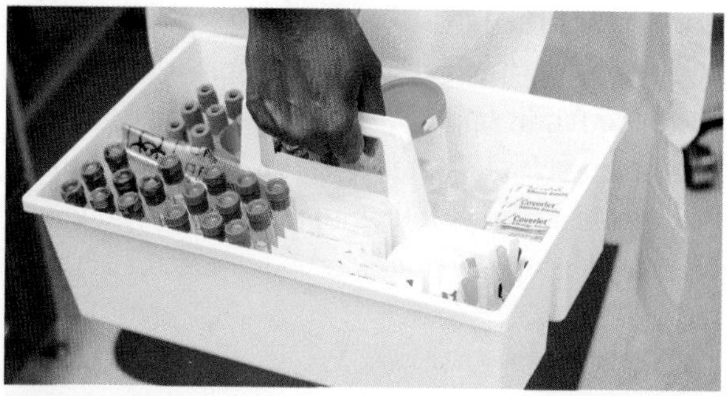

Fig. 1-11. *Mobile phlebotomists work at a number of different sites over the course of a day, carrying their supplies with them.*

Most blood specimens a PBT collects are collected through **venipuncture**, or the puncture of a **vein** with a hollow needle. Veins are the blood vessels that carry blood toward the heart.

Some blood specimens are not collected from a vein, but from the tiny blood vessels just beneath the skin called **capillaries**. **Capillary puncture**, or *dermal puncture*, specimens are collected by puncturing the patient's skin, usually on a fingertip for adults and children, or on a heel for infants.

Phlebotomy technicians are responsible for making sure the blood specimens used to perform tests are of the highest quality. This involves several key tasks:

- Working professionally with all patients, some of whom might be anxious about needles or blood, or fearful about a possible diagnosis (Fig. 1-12)

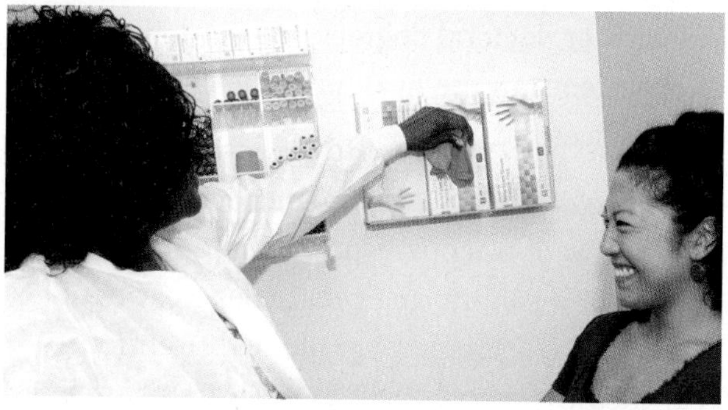

Fig. 1-12. *From the beginning of an interaction with a patient the phlebotomy technician can help put the patient at ease. This results in a higher quality specimen and better patient care.*

- Creating a calming atmosphere
- Ensuring accurate patient identification
- Carefully explaining the specimen collection procedure
- Answering patient questions about the procedure as appropriate, referring questions about results or diagnosis to the patient's doctor
- Closely following the correct collection procedures for each type of test
- Observing infection prevention precautions and procedures
- Protecting patients' confidential health information

- Keeping patients safe during the collection process
- Correctly labeling and transporting specimens

The scope of practice for phlebotomy technicians may vary from facility to facility. Usually it is limited to the collection of blood specimens through venipuncture and capillary (dermal) puncture. In some cases PBTs may also collect nonblood specimens such as urine, stool, or cells from the cheek or throat. They may perform some very simple tests on blood or nonblood specimens. PBTs should not discuss why a doctor has ordered a test or what diagnosis might be associated with particular results. For these questions the patient should be referred to the person who ordered the test. Phlebotomists should not offer opinions about a patient's health and should refer any questions or concerns of this sort to a doctor.

In some facilities technicians are trained in broader skills such as taking a patient's medical history or measuring vital signs. These duties should only be performed if a PBT is trained and authorized to perform them.

Tasks that are usually considered to be outside the scope of practice for a phlebotomy technician include the following:

- Providing test results
- Discussing or interpreting results
- Offering medical advice of any kind, including provider recommendations
- Performing tests on specimens (other than certain simple tests, as ordered and as allowed by the facility; more on this topic in later chapters)
- Drawing blood from arteries or performing arterial blood gas tests
- Drawing blood from an indwelling port or an intravenous line (IV)
- Any type of injection
- Inserting or removing IVs

An instructor or an employer may provide a list of other tasks outside the phlebotomy technician's scope of practice. In some cases a PBT may have the training to perform a task that her employer considers outside the PBT's scope of practice. PBTs must follow employer policy on which tasks they may perform.

6. Explain policies and procedures

All facilities have policies and procedures developed specifically for their organizations. A **policy** is a course of action that should be taken every time a certain situation occurs. For example, a very basic policy is that healthcare information must remain confidential. A **procedure** is a method, or way, of doing something. For example, a facility will have a procedure for reporting any incidents that occur with patients, like a patient fainting during a blood draw. The procedure explains how to respond, what form to complete to document the incident, when to fill it out, and to whom it is given.

Employers will have policies and procedures for every patient care situation. New employees will be told where to find a list of policies and procedures that all staff are expected to follow. These have been developed to give quality care and protect patient safety. Procedures may seem long and complicated, but each step is important. Phlebotomists must become familiar with and always follow policies and procedures. Common policies at hospitals and clinical laboratories include the following:

- All patient information must remain confidential. This is not only a facility rule; it is also the law. More information about confidentiality, including the Health Insurance Portability and Accountability Act (HIPAA), can be found in Chapter 2.

- The **requisition**, or testing order form, must always be followed. Phlebotomy technicians only collect specimens assigned through the requisition form. Collection of specimens for tests that are not listed or approved by the practitioner who completed the requisition should not be performed (Fig. 1-13).
- Healthcare workers should not do tasks that are not included in their job description (i.e., they must stay within their scope of practice).
- Healthcare workers must report important events or problems with patients to a supervisor.
- All employees must be on time for work and must be dependable.

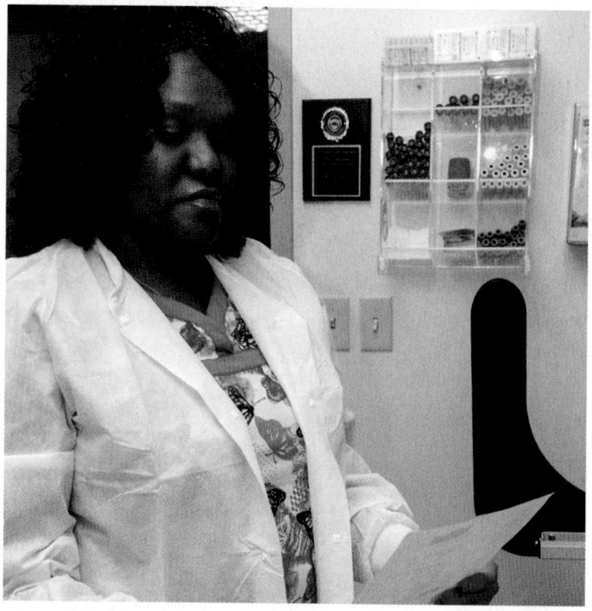

Fig. 1-13. Every task a phlebotomy technician performs must be assigned. Following requisition forms carefully is essential.

7. Discuss the importance of quality assurance and quality improvement in healthcare organizations

Quality assurance and **quality improvement** are both important ideas in healthcare settings. Quality assurance practices make sure care is being provided according to facility policy and procedures, with results that meet expectations. **Quality control** measures are part of quality assurance. They are processes put in place to document that standards are being met. Quality improvement practices seek to make care better in a way that can be measured. There are many ways in which facilities put quality assurance and quality improvement practices into action. Continuous quality improvement (CQI) is a goal of all healthcare providers.

Organizations like The Joint Commission conduct regular surveys, or inspections, of hospitals, laboratories, and other healthcare facilities. These are quality assurance reviews designed to measure a facility's success in providing safe and effective care. Although participation in these surveys is not required, facilities that receive federal money for care must meet specific quality standards. Joint Commission surveys are one way to prove that a facility meets these standards. The **Clinical & Laboratory Standards Institute** (**CLSI**, clsi.org) is a nonprofit organization that works with government agencies and healthcare providers and institutions to develop standards of practice for laboratories worldwide. Although CLSI does not perform reviews or accredit laboratories, following CLSI standards is an important part of providing quality care.

Quality Counts

The Joint Commission works with healthcare practitioners, providers, and consumers to identify issues related to patient safety. Based on these collaborations the Joint Commission issues National Patient Safety Goals: areas of particular importance to providing the best and safest possible care. National Patient Safety Goals are established for a wide variety of different facilities. For laboratories, the goals are to *identify patients correctly*, *improve staff communication*, and *prevent infection*. All facilities have policies and procedures that relate to these goals. When phlebotomists carefully follow policies and procedures, they help keep patients safe.

Different states have different requirements for quality assurance and improvement in healthcare facilities. Each facility may have its own policies and procedures regarding quality assurance and improvement. In 2011, the US Department of Health and Human Services established the National Strategy for Quality Improvement in Health Care (also called the *National Quality Strategy*). The National Quality Strategy has three aims:

Better Care: Improve the overall quality of care by making health care more patient centered, reliable, accessible, and safe.

Healthy People/Healthy Communities: Improve health outcomes by addressing behavioral, social, and environmental factors related to health.

Affordable Care: Reduce the cost of quality health care for individuals, families, employers, and government.

Healthcare workers at hospitals, laboratories, and other facilities are trained in the practices their facility has adopted to meet these goals and achieve continuous quality improvement. For phlebotomy technicians, CQI centers on following procedures carefully to reduce the risk of patient harm, getting high-quality samples, and processing specimens appropriately.

8. Describe certification, recertification, and continuing education for the phlebotomy technician

Many healthcare workers are required to have a certificate or license in the state where they practice. **Certification** is a process used in healthcare to ensure skills are mastered for particular positions. A school or organization offers a training program designed to enable students to meet certain standards in that healthcare field. The school, organization, or a state government agency may maintain a registry that can be checked by potential employers to verify certification.

Nursing assistants (NAs), patient care technicians (PCTs), and phlebotomists are examples of healthcare workers who may need to be certified. Laws addressing certification for these positions are different from one state to another. There are no national laws addressing phlebotomy certification, but some states require it. Many facilities require certification, and having it is definitely an advantage when looking for a job.

Several organizations certify phlebotomy technicians. Some of the most widely recognized certifications are from the American Society for Clinical Pathology, the National Center for Competency Testing, and the National Healthcareer Association. Before taking a certification test, students must complete a recognized training course and/or must already have clinical experience working as a phlebotomy technician.

Phlebotomy programs should include **clinical experience** to give students hands-on practice with patients. *Clinicals*, as this training is sometimes called, may be arranged by the instructor and take place under the supervision of healthcare professionals (Fig. 1-14). If it is not possible to do clinicals at a healthcare facility, the instructor may set up a lab area for volunteers to have phlebotomy procedures performed. Certification agencies require that students perform a set number of venipunctures and capillary punctures before receiving certification. The number varies widely from one agency to another.

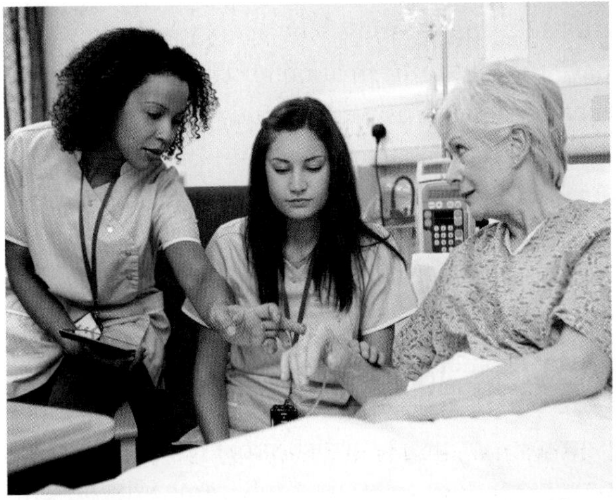

Fig. 1-14. *Phlebotomists in training may gain clinical experience at diagnostic laboratories, hospitals, or other healthcare facilities.*

Certification options

Many organizations offer certification for phlebotomy technicians. Students should take steps to make sure the organization or agency offers a widely accepted, legitimate certificate. Certificates granted without proof of clinical experience are not likely to be respected or recognized. The same is true for certificates granted with entirely internet-based instruction. Instructors and potential employers are good sources of information about certification. Not all states require certification, but those that do may only accept certificates from particular agencies. Before seeking to work as a phlebotomist, a student should research his state's requirements. This is a partial list of well-known and reputable organizations:

- American Medical Technologists (AMT, americanmedtech.org)
- American Society for Clinical Pathology (ASCP, ascp.org/content)
- American Society of Phlebotomy Technicians (ASPT, aspt.org)
- National Center for Competency Testing (NCCT, ncctinc.com)
- National Healthcareer Association (NHA, nhanow.com)
- National Phlebotomy Association (NPA, nationalphlebotomy.org)

Many certifying agencies feature test plans or lists of information students should have mastered before taking their tests.

A student seeking certification as a phlebotomy technician should check the certifying agency's website at the beginning of training and several times during training. The agency website will have the latest information about testing requirements and fees, as well as study and review materials available for purchase. In most cases certification tests are computer-based and timed, and results are received immediately after testing is complete. The tests are given at special testing centers and must be scheduled in advance. A phlebotomy technician must either receive a high school diploma before certification is granted or must furnish proof of receiving a diploma within a certain time frame after receiving the certificate. Some testing agencies award temporary certificates to high school students until they submit copies of their high school diplomas, but facilities are unlikely to employ a PBT who has not completed high school.

Once a phlebotomy technician is certified, she will need to maintain her certification. Most certificates must be renewed every few years and require proof of ongoing work in the field as well as a set number of hours of **continuing education**. Continuing education, also called *in-service education*, keeps healthcare workers up to date on changes in medicine that affect their jobs. It may also address new equipment, new procedures, or an employer's policy changes. The phlebotomy technician is responsible for meeting deadlines and fulfilling the requirements for recertification.

9. Explain professionalism and list examples of professional behavior

Professional means having to do with a work or a job. **Personal** refers to life outside a job, such as family, friends, and home life. **Professionalism** is behaving properly when on the job. It includes dressing appropriately and speaking well. It also includes being on time, completing tasks, and reporting to supervisors as needed. For a phlebotomy technician, professionalism means performing assigned duties carefully and efficiently, interacting appropriately with patients and coworkers, and assuring that specimens collected are the highest possible quality (Fig. 1-15).

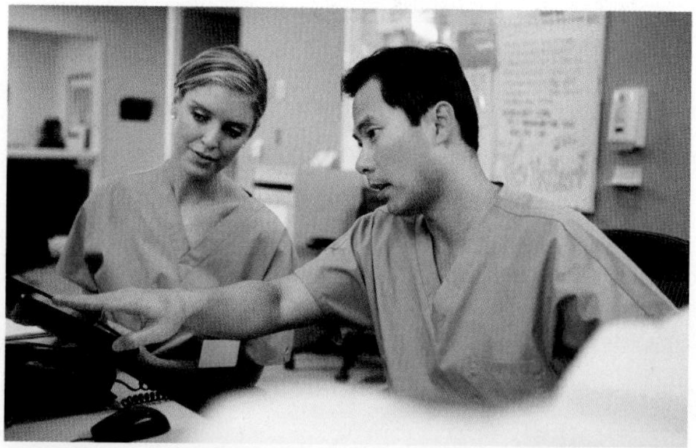

Fig. 1-15. *Behaving professionally on the job includes communicating well with colleagues and supervisors.*

Following policies and procedures is an important part of professionalism. Patients, coworkers, and supervisors respect employees who behave professionally. Professionalism helps people keep their jobs and may also help them earn promotions and raises.

Professional interactions with patients include the following:

- Providing care appropriate to each patient (for example, adjusting communication as needed based on the age or condition of the patient)
- Performing only assigned tasks and not discussing information that is beyond a phlebotomy technician's scope of practice
- Keeping all patients' information confidential
- Always being polite and keeping a positive attitude
- Not discussing personal subjects with patients
- Not discussing possibly controversial subjects like politics or religion with patients
- Not using personal phones in patient care areas
- Not using profanity
- Listening to patients' concerns and taking them seriously
- Calling a patient *Mr., Mrs., Ms.,* or *Miss* and his or her last name, or by the name he or she prefers; terms such as *sweetie, honey,* and *dearie* are unprofessional and should not be used
- Always explaining procedures before beginning
- Using correct terms rather than slang (e.g., "I'm going to perform your blood draw now" rather than "I'm going to stick you now")
- Following infection control practices, such as handwashing, to protect oneself and patients

A professional relationship with an employer includes the following:

- Completing tasks efficiently
- Always following policies and procedures
- Documenting and reporting carefully and correctly
- Reporting problems with patients or tasks
- Reporting anything that keeps a PBT from completing duties
- Asking questions when the PBT does not know or understand something
- Taking directions or feedback without becoming upset
- Being clean and neatly dressed or groomed (see Learning Objective 10)
- Always being on time
- Communicating with the employer if unable to report for work
- Following the chain of command
- Participating in education programs
- Being a positive role model for the facility

In order to do their jobs well, phlebotomists must have or develop certain qualities. Phlebotomy technicians must be

Empathetic: Showing **empathy** means identifying with the feelings of others. People who are empathetic work to understand other people's problems (Fig. 1-16). They care about them. Many people find needles and medical settings in general to be frightening. Patients may also be fearful about possible diagnoses. Approaching patients with empathy is a key part of a phlebotomist's job.

Honest: An honest person tells the truth and can be trusted. Patients need to feel that they can trust the people who care for them. Employers count on truthful records of care provided.

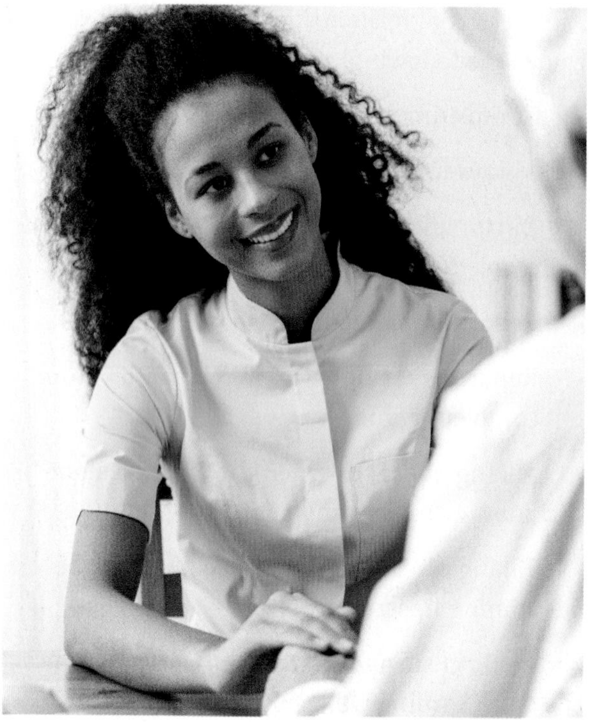

Fig. 1-16. Patients are more comfortable and more confident in the care they receive when healthcare workers are empathetic.

Tactful: Being **tactful** means showing sensitivity and having a sense of what is appropriate when dealing with others. It is the ability to speak and act without offending others. There is an important balance between honesty and tact. For example, a phlebotomy technician should not lie and tell a patient that a needlestick will not hurt. However, she should be tactful about the way she explains the feeling. Tact and empathy are also connected. Tact is required when a PBT is caring for a patient who is very anxious.

Conscientious: People who are **conscientious** try to do to their best. They are guided by a sense of right and wrong. They are alert, observant, accurate, and responsible. Giving conscientious care means taking responsibility for one's actions during each patient interaction. Accuracy in performing procedures, care with infection prevention and safety, and appropriate interaction with patients are all aspects of providing conscientious care. Without it, a patient's health can be endangered.

Dependable: Phlebotomy technicians must be able to make and keep commitments. They must report to work on time. They must skillfully perform assigned tasks, avoid absences, and help their peers when needed.

Patient: People who are patient do not lose their tempers easily. They do not act irritated or complain when things are hard. Patients may be anxious, sick, or in pain. They may be hesitant about having their blood drawn. It is important that technicians not rush patients or act annoyed.

Respectful: Being respectful means valuing other people's individuality, including their age, religion, culture, feelings, practices, and beliefs. People who are respectful treat others politely and kindly. They avoid negative conversations and gossip.

Unprejudiced: Phlebotomy technicians work with people from many different backgrounds (Fig. 1-17). They must give each patient the same quality care regardless of age, gender or gender identity, sexual orientation, religion, race, ethnicity, or condition.

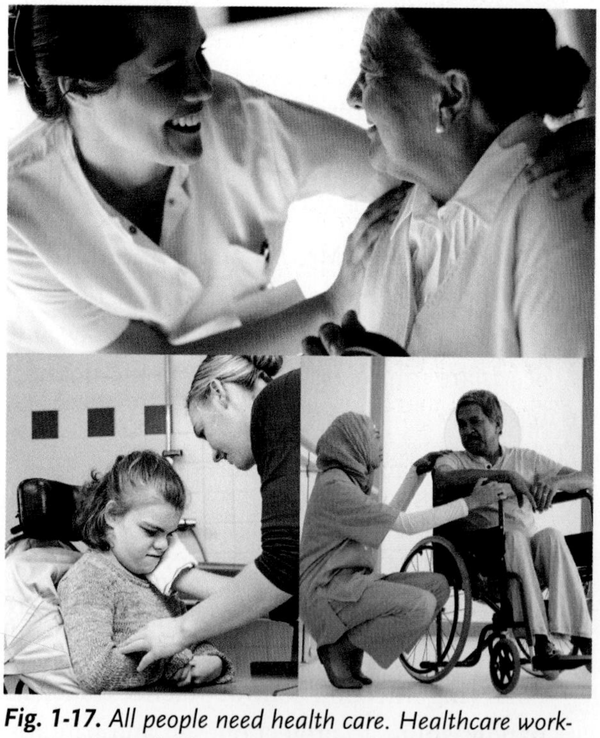

Fig. 1-17. All people need health care. Healthcare workers must provide the same excellent care to every patient.

10. Describe proper personal grooming habits

Regular grooming makes people feel good about themselves, and it makes a positive impression on others. A phlebotomy technician's grooming habits affect how confident patients feel about the care given. Professional PBTs have the following personal grooming habits:

- Bathing or showering daily and using deodorant (perfume, cologne, aftershave, and scented body creams or lotions should not be used, as patients and coworkers may not like scents or may have illnesses that are worsened by scents)
- Brushing teeth frequently and using mouthwash when necessary
- Keeping hair clean and neatly brushed or combed and tying long hair back in a bun or ponytail
- Keeping facial hair short, clean, and neat
- Dressing neatly in a clean, wrinkle-free uniform (Fig. 1-18)
- Not wearing clothes that are too tight or too baggy, torn or stained, or too revealing (short skirts, low-cut blouses, see-through fabrics)
- Not wearing large jewelry (the main exception to this rule is a simple watch that may be used for timing certain procedures)
- Wearing an identification badge as required by the facility
- Following facility policy regarding visible tattoos and piercings
- Wearing comfortable, clean, high-quality, closed-toe shoes
- Keeping fingernails short, smooth, and clean
- Not wearing artificial nails (acrylic, gel, sculptured, or wraps) because they harbor bacteria
- Wearing little or no makeup

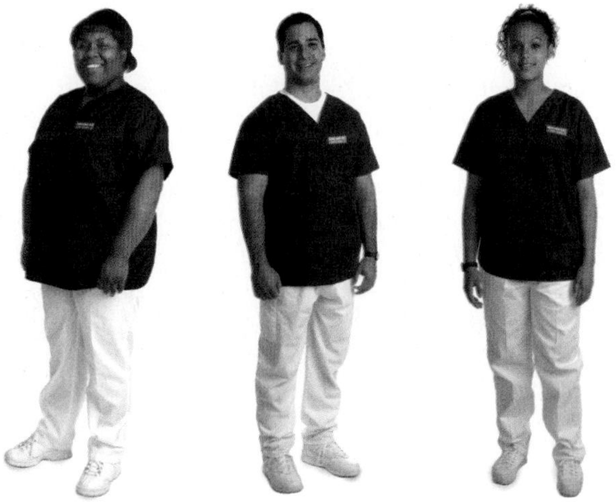

Fig. 1-18. *Wearing a clean, wrinkle-free uniform, keeping long hair tied back, and wearing clean, closed-toe shoes are all parts of proper grooming.*

Phlebotomy technicians should follow facility rules regarding their appearance.

11. Demonstrate how to manage time and assignments

Phlebotomy technicians must manage their time well. There are many tasks that must be done during their shifts, and each patient will require different tests and individual attention. Managing time properly helps phlebotomy technicians complete their tasks efficiently.

Planning is the single best way to manage time better. Sometimes it is hard to find time to plan, but it is essential. Patients who need blood drawn are prioritized differently based on the tests ordered. Multiple tests are often needed, and there is a specific sequence required for filling the specimen tubes so that each test is as accurate as possible. Phlebotomy technicians must take time to check to make sure they have all the supplies needed for each patient. Supplies should be organized to make it easy to collect specimens in the correct order. Taking the time to organize and then recheck can improve focus, decrease stress, and prevent errors.

Quality Counts

A time management skill that is often overlooked is asking for help when it is needed. A patient may ask questions the PBT is not able to answer, or a patient might be especially challenging in some way. A requisition form may be unclear or require a test the PBT has never seen before. Asking for help when it is needed ensures patient safety and saves time for everyone involved.

12. List appropriate ways to deal with stress

Stress is the state of being overwhelmed by mental or emotional demands. It can cause a person to feel frightened, excited, confused, in danger, or irritated. It is often thought that only bad things cause stress, but positive situations cause stress, too. For example, graduating from school or getting a new job are usually positive situations. However, both can cause enormous stress because of the changes they bring to a person's life.

Learning how to recognize stress and what causes it is helpful. A **stressor** is something that causes stress. Any change or situation, positive or negative, can be a stressor.

Some examples include the following:

- Life changes like graduating or moving
- Feeling unprepared for a task
- Starting a new job
- Problems at work
- New responsibilities at work
- Feeling unsupported at work (not enough guidance or resources)
- Losing a job
- Difficulties with supervisors
- Difficulties with coworkers
- Challenging patients
- Illness
- Finances

Stress is not only an emotional response. When a person experiences stress, changes occur in the body (Fig. 1-19). Heart rate, breathing rate, and blood pressure rise. This is why, in very stressful situations, a person's heart beats fast and he may breathe quickly and feel warm or perspire. Each person has a different tolerance level for stress. What one person would find overwhelming might not bother another person. A person's tolerance for stress depends on his personality, life experiences, and physical health.

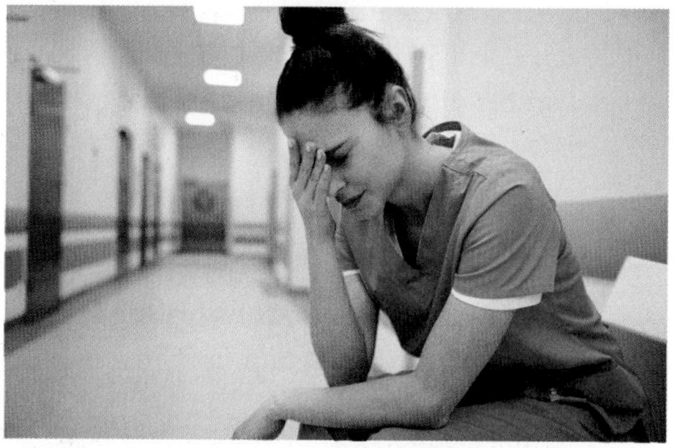

Fig. 1-19. *Stress can cause physical changes that may damage health and have a negative impact on a person's life.*

The job of a phlebotomist can be a stressful one. Some facilities where PBTs work, such as hospitals or emergency departments, can be hectic. There may be pressure to complete tasks on a tight schedule. Patients are not always pleasant or helpful, and may be anxious or hesitant, which can add to the stress of the job. These factors are simply part of the job of the phlebotomy technician. Learning to manage stress in all areas of life can help work-related stress feel less overwhelming.

Developing a plan for managing stress can be very helpful. The plan can include things to do every day and things to do in stressful situations. Before a person builds a plan, it is important to answer these questions:

- What are the sources of stress in my life?
- When do I most often feel stress?
- What effects of stress do I see in my life?

- What can I change to decrease the stress I feel?
- What do I have to learn to cope with because I cannot change it?

After answering these questions, a person will have a clearer picture of the challenges he faces. Then he can try to come up with strategies specific to his situation. The following guidelines are general and could be helpful to anyone.

Guidelines: Managing Stress

G To manage stress, develop healthy dietary, exercise, and lifestyle habits:

- Eat nutritious foods.
- Exercise regularly, alone or with partners (Fig. 1-20).
- Get enough sleep.
- Drink alcohol only in moderation.
- Do not smoke.

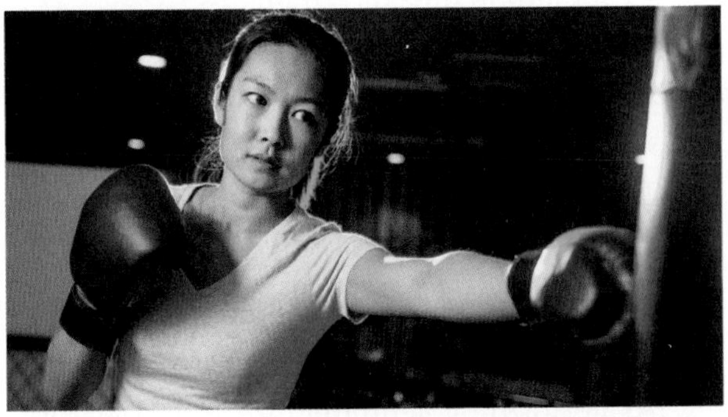

Fig. 1-20. *Regular exercise is a healthy way to decrease stress.*

G Find time at least a few times a week to do something relaxing, such as reading a book, watching a movie, sewing, or any of the following:

- Being outdoors
- Doing something artistic (painting, drawing, writing, singing, etc.)
- Doing yoga
- Getting a massage
- Listening to music
- Meditating

Not managing stress can cause many problems. Some of these problems can affect the quality of a person's work. Signs of not managing stress well include the following:

- Showing anger or being abusive to patients
- Arguing with supervisors
- Having poor relationships with coworkers
- Complaining frequently about one's job and responsibilities
- Feeling work-related burnout (burnout is a state of mental or physical exhaustion caused by prolonged stress)
- Feeling tired even when rested
- Having a difficult time focusing on patients and procedures

Stress can seem overwhelming when a person tries to handle it alone. Often just talking about stress can improve the situation. Sometimes another person can offer helpful suggestions for managing stress.

These resources can be helpful when managing stress:

- A supervisor or another member of the care team for work-related stress
- Family members
- Friends
- A support group
- A place of worship
- A primary care doctor or a mental health specialist
- A local mental health agency
- Any phone hotline that deals with related problems (check online)

It is not appropriate to talk to patients about personal or job-related stress.

Chapter Review

Multiple Choice

1. Medicare and Medicaid are considered
   (A) Healthcare payers
   (B) Healthcare providers
   (C) Healthcare facilities
   (D) Healthcare enablers

2. Which of the following is true of freestanding emergency rooms?
   (A) They are usually staffed by nurses, with a physician available on call.
   (B) They are not subject to regulation by state or federal governments.
   (C) They are required to operate as satellites of established hospitals.
   (D) They usually have more medical equipment and services available than urgent care centers.

3. This laboratory department would be responsible for testing how quickly a patient's blood clots:
   (A) Immunology
   (B) Cytology
   (C) Hematology
   (D) Pathology

4. Which of the following is a task only a doctor, physician assistant, or nurse practitioner can perform?
   (A) Measuring vital signs
   (B) Recording a patient's medical history
   (C) Making a diagnosis
   (D) Performing an electrocardiogram

5. Which of the following is true about employers who hire phlebotomists?
   (A) Only hospitals hire phlebotomists.
   (B) Only diagnostic laboratories hire phlebotomists.
   (C) Only doctors' offices hire phlebotomists.
   (D) Healthcare facilities, laboratories, and insurance companies hire phlebotomists.

6. ____________________ is beyond the scope of practice for a phlebotomist.
   (A) Collecting a urine sample
   (B) Swabbing a patient's cheek to collect a cell specimen
   (C) Drawing blood from an intravenous port
   (D) Answering patient questions about a blood draw such as "How many tubes of blood will you be collecting?" or "Where will you draw the blood from?"

7. What is the term for a course of action that should be taken every time a certain situation occurs?
   (A) Policy
   (B) Best practice
   (C) Procedure
   (D) Official guidance

8. Which of the following exemplifies continuous quality improvement for a PBT?
   (A) Accurately guessing a patient's diagnosis based on the tests ordered
   (B) Following procedures carefully to obtain a high-quality specimen
   (C) Saving time for supervisors by performing tests on patient specimens without being asked to do so
   (D) Streamlining facility procedures by eliminating time-consuming steps

9. Clinical experience for a phlebotomist in training must include
   (A) Performing venipuncture and capillary puncture procedures
   (B) Observing venipuncture and dermal puncture procedures, but not performing them
   (C) Taking written or computer-based tests
   (D) Observing surgeries

10. Which of the following is true about certification for phlebotomy technicians?
    (A) There is one national certification agency.
    (B) The federal government regulates phlebotomy technician certification.
    (C) Costs and requirements for certification are the same across all agencies.
    (D) Different certification agencies have different requirements for clinical experience.

11. A phlebotomy technician notices that a patient is biting her lip and breathing deeply. He tells the patient, "Having blood drawn can be nerve-wracking. Would it help if we took a few minutes to relax?" He is demonstrating
    (A) Dependability
    (B) Lack of prejudice
    (C) Empathy
    (D) Honesty

12. Which of these professional behaviors is also a legal requirement for phlebotomy technicians?
    (A) Not discussing personal subjects with patients
    (B) Keeping all patients' information confidential
    (C) Not using personal phones in patient care areas
    (D) Not discussing possibly controversial subjects like politics or religion with patients

13. Why should phlebotomists not wear artificial nails or nail wraps?
    (A) Because they make it difficult to feel for a patient's veins
    (B) Because they are distracting to patients
    (C) Because they interfere with computer use
    (D) Because they can harbor bacteria

14. One reason a phlebotomist should organize his supplies before beginning a blood draw is that
    (A) Specimens must be collected in a particular order
    (B) Patients find this reassuring
    (C) Supervisors might be watching and want to see that the phlebotomist is organized
    (D) This prevents other phlebotomists from taking needed supplies during the course of the draw

15. Causes of stress
    (A) Are the same for all people
    (B) Are always negative situations
    (C) Are different for different people
    (D) Are situations that cannot be changed or managed

2
Legal and Ethical Issues

1. Define the terms *law* and *ethics* and list examples of legal and ethical behavior

Ethics and laws guide behavior. **Ethics** are the knowledge of right and wrong. An ethical person has a sense of duty and responsibility toward others. He tries to do what is right. If ethics tell people what they should do, **laws** tell them what they must do. Laws are usually based on ethics. Governments establish laws to help people live peacefully together and to ensure order and safety. When someone breaks the law, he may be punished by having to pay a fine or spend time in prison. Ethics and laws are extremely important in health care (Fig. 2-1).

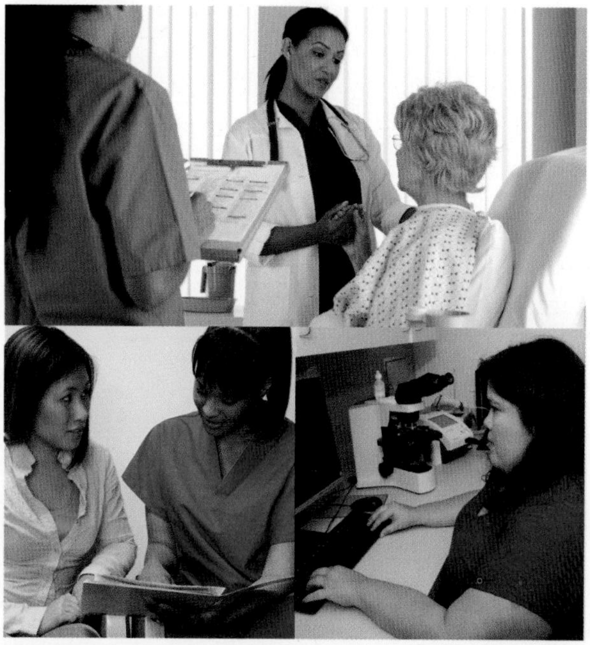

Fig. 2-1. *All healthcare providers must behave ethically and follow the law.*

They protect people receiving care and guide people giving care. Phlebotomy technicians and other healthcare providers should be guided by a code of ethics. They must also know the laws that apply to their jobs.

Guidelines: Legal and Ethical Behavior

- **G** Be honest at all times. Stealing or lying about the care you provided are examples of dishonesty. Communicate honestly with all team members.
- **G** Protect patients' privacy. Do not discuss their cases except with other members of the care team. Keeping patient information confidential is one of the rights protected in the Patient Care Partnership, which is covered later in this chapter. All team members must keep patient information confidential.
- **G** Keep staff information confidential. Do not share information about your coworkers at home or anywhere else.
- **G** Report abuse or suspected abuse of patients. Help patients report abuse if they wish to make a complaint of abuse. This guideline is especially important to phlebotomy technicians who work in long-term care settings.
- **G** Follow the requisition and your assignments. Report any mistakes you make promptly. This helps prevent any further problems. Reporting mistakes promotes the safety and well-being of all patients.

- Do not perform any task outside your scope of practice.
- Report all patient incidents to the appropriate person, according to facility policy. An incident is any unexpected event during the course of care (e.g., a patient fainting).
- Document accurately and promptly.
- Follow rules about safety and infection prevention. Chapters 4 and 5 contain information about these rules.
- Do not accept gifts or tips.
- Keep interactions with patients professional and do not share or exchange personal information.

Many organizations and companies have created a code of ethics for their members or employees to follow. These codes vary, but generally focus on promoting proper conduct and high standards of practice. If a facility has its own code of ethics, all staff members will be given a copy and expected to follow it.

Crimes in healthcare settings

Most of the crimes that occur in communities can also occur in healthcare settings. Theft is frequently reported. Physical abuse, including hitting, punching, shoving, and rough handling can occur. Abuse of patients can be prosecuted as a crime. It is important for phlebotomy technicians to know what to observe for and how to report any illegal activity. Being vigilant can help prevent crimes and promote legal and ethical behavior in the workplace.

2. Explain HIPAA and discuss ways to protect patients' privacy

To respect **confidentiality** means to keep private things private. Phlebotomy technicians will learn confidential (private) information about patients. They may learn about a patient's state of health and will also view information such as address, date of birth, and telephone number. Ethically and legally, they must protect this information. This means that PBTs should not share information about patients with anyone other than the patients themselves, the care team, or the patients' legal representatives (such as parents or guardians of children under 18).

Congress passed the **Health Insurance Portability and Accountability Act** (**HIPAA**, hhs.gov/hipaa) in 1996. It has been further defined and revised since then. One reason this law was passed was to help keep health information private and secure. All healthcare organizations must take special steps to protect health information. They and their employees can be fined and/or imprisoned if they do not follow special rules to protect patient privacy.

Under this law, a person's health information must be kept private. **Protected health information** (**PHI**) is information that can be used to identify a person and that relates to the patient's physical or mental condition, any health care the person has had, and payment for that health care. Examples of PHI include a person's name, address, telephone number, social security number, email address, and medical record number. Only people who must have information to provide care or to process records should know a person's private health information. They must make sure they protect the information so that it does not become known or used by anyone else. It must be kept confidential.

The Health Information Technology for Economic and Clinical Health (HITECH) Act became law at the end of 2009. It was enacted as a part of the American Recovery and Reinvestment Act of 2009. HITECH was created to expand the protection and security of consumers' electronic health records (EHR). HITECH increases civil and criminal penalties for sharing or accessing PHI and expands the ability to enforce these penalties. HITECH also offers incentives to providers and organizations to adopt the use of electronic health records.

HIPAA applies to all healthcare providers, including doctors, nurses, phlebotomy technicians, and any other members of the care team. PBTs cannot give out any information about a patient to anyone who is not directly involved in the patient's care unless the patient gives official consent or unless the law requires it.

Guidelines: Protecting Privacy

- **G** Make sure you are in a private area when you are listening to or reading your messages.
- **G** Know with whom you are speaking on the phone. If you are not sure, get a name and number to call back after you find out it is all right to share information with this person.
- **G** Do not talk about patients in public (Fig. 2-2). Public areas include elevators, grocery stores, lounges, waiting rooms, parking garages, schools, restaurants, etc.
- **G** Ensure privacy when discussing patient information with other care team members. Keep your voice low when discussing patient information with other care team members.
- **G** Make sure nobody can see private and protected health or personal information on your computer screen while you are working. Log out and/or exit the browser when you are finished with any computer work.
- **G** Do not give confidential information in emails; you do not know who has access to your messages.
- **G** Make sure fax numbers are correct before faxing healthcare information. Use a cover sheet with a confidentiality statement.
- **G** Do not leave documents where others may see them.
- **G** Store, file, or shred documents according to your facility's policy. If you find documents with a patient's information, give them to a nurse.

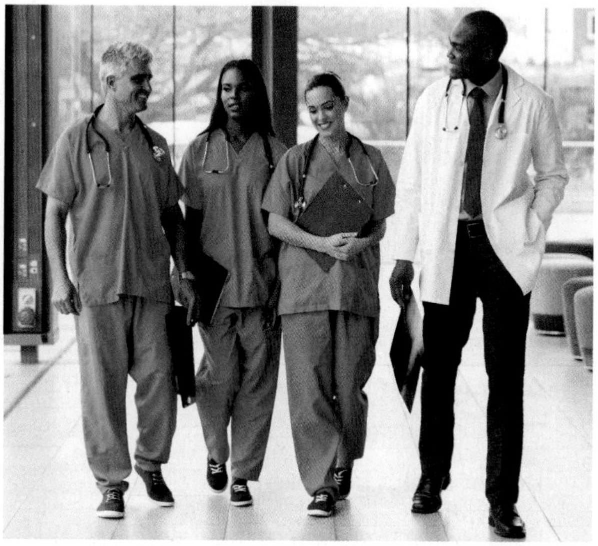

Fig. 2-2. *Patient care should only be discussed in private settings and not in lobbies or other areas open to the public.*

All healthcare workers must comply with HIPAA regulations, no matter where they are or what they are doing. There are serious penalties for violating these regulations, including the following:

- Fines ranging from $100 to $1.5 million
- Prison sentences of up to 10 years

Maintaining confidentiality is a legal and ethical obligation. It is part of respecting patients and their rights. Discussing a patient's care or personal affairs with anyone other than members of the care team violates the law.

3. Explain the Clinical Laboratory Improvement Amendments (CLIA) and laboratory certification

The **Centers for Medicare & Medicaid Services** (**CMS**, cms.gov) is a federal agency within the United States Department of Health and Human Services. CMS runs two national healthcare programs: Medicare and Medicaid. They both help pay for health care and health insurance for millions of Americans. CMS has many other responsibilities as well. One of those responsibilities is to oversee the regulation of laboratory testing in the United States. Passed in 1988, the Clinical Laboratory Improvement Amendments outline the standards required of clinical laboratories testing human specimens, not including laboratories conducting research. The goal of CLIA is to improve patient outcomes by ensuring that laboratory tests are performed by qualified personnel and follow proven, effective procedures.

CMS certifies laboratories at a number of different levels based on CLIA requirements. The most basic level is the *Certificate of Waiver* for facilities offering only simple, easy-to-perform tests that involve little risk of error. Tests such as pregnancy tests and blood glucose tests may be performed quickly and accurately even by individuals who have limited medical training. CMS maintains a list of tests granted waived status under CLIA, and these tests are commonly known as **CLIA waived tests** or simply *waived tests* (Fig. 2-3). Phlebotomy technicians may perform these tests at some facilities. Many CLIA waived tests are **point-of-care tests**, meaning the testing is done near or in the presence of the patient, but not all point-of-care tests are CLIA waived, and not all can be performed by phlebotomy technicians.

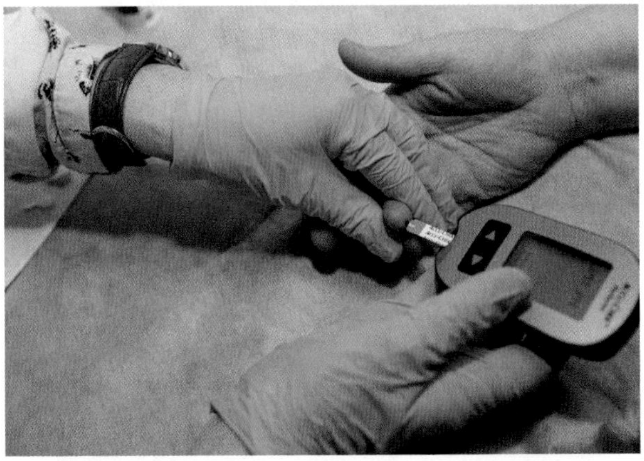

Fig. 2-3. *Tests with very little risk of error are known as CLIA waived tests. PBTs sometimes perform these tests.*

The highest level of CLIA certification is the *Certificate of Accreditation* for facilities performing moderate- to high-complexity tests (Fig. 2-4). Organizations such as The Joint Commission can certify that a laboratory meets CLIA standards for this level, and CMS then performs a validation survey within 90 days. This process must be repeated every two years for a facility to maintain its accreditation.

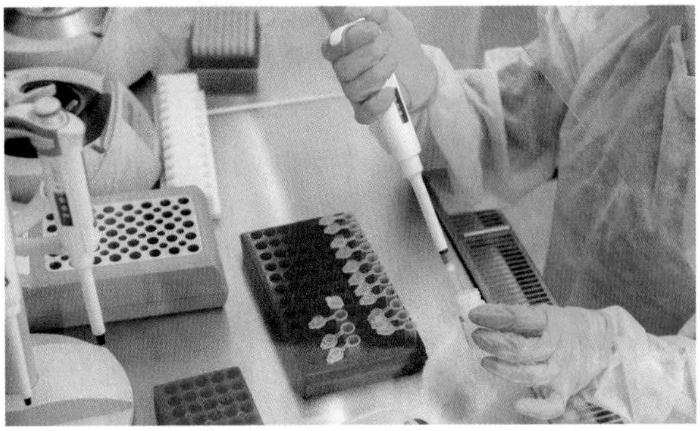

Fig. 2-4. *Laboratories performing complex tests must receive a Certificate of Accreditation from CMS.*

The American Society for Clinical Laboratory Science, a professional organization, summarizes the goals of quality laboratory testing in this way:

- Perform the correct test
- Perform the test on the right person
- Perform the test at the right time
- Produce accurate test results
- Achieve the best outcome
- Perform the test in the most cost-effective manner

CLIA is intended to ensure that these goals are met. Phlebotomy technicians do their part by respecting their scope of practice, not performing tasks for which they are not trained, and following their facility's policies and procedures at all times.

4. Discuss common legal considerations in health care, including negligence, abuse, and consent

There are two types of law that deal with wrongdoing. **Criminal law** deals with offenses considered to harm all of society. Even though the victims may be individuals, the public is thought to be harmed by acts that violate criminal law. These acts are called *crimes*. **Civil law** deals with disputes between individuals, and violations of civil law are called **torts**. As described in Learning Objective 2, failing to keep a patient's protected health information confidential can have both criminal and civil consequences.

Civil offenses (torts) deal with wrongdoing between individuals. Torts may be intentional or they may occur as a result of negligence or inattentiveness. They can result in lawsuits against a healthcare worker or facility. Healthcare workers who speak or write defamatory or untrue comments about a patient, for example, are guilty of the civil offenses of *slander* (for spoken statements) or *libel* (for written statements). Such comments should never be documented in a patient's chart or spoken to coworkers, patients, or family members. Healthcare workers can be taken to court for such actions.

Negligence and **abuse** are other possible causes of legal action against healthcare workers. *Negligence* is a civil offense describing actions, or the failure to act, that result in injury to a patient. An example of negligence is a phlebotomist unintentionally damaging a patient's nerves during a blood draw due to improper technique. *Abuse* is purposeful mistreatment that causes physical, mental, or emotional pain or injury to someone. Rough handling of a patient is considered abuse. PBTs must never abuse patients and must follow all applicable policies and procedures to avoid possible harm to patients, as well as to protect against charges of negligence. All healthcare workers are **mandated reporters**, which means they are legally required to report suspected or observed abuse or neglect.

The concept of **consent** is a very important legal issue for healthcare workers. Before a patient is treated at a doctor's office or hospital, she must provide *consent*, which means she must agree to be treated. In most cases, a facility requires that a patient sign a general consent form before receiving any kind of treatment. This general consent is considered valid for routine procedures, including laboratory tests and blood draws. The patient will not need to sign a new consent form for each routine service provided. General consent forms are usually valid for one year unless a patient takes action to revoke, or take back, the consent.

This type of consent is known as **informed consent**. It may also be called **express consent**, but these phrases have slightly different meanings. When a patient gives *informed consent*, she is acknowledging that she understands the treatment she will receive and agrees to receive it. Informed consent is a form of *express consent*, which means that the patient is able to actively, consciously acknowledge her agreement to treatment. A signed general consent form provides legal proof of the patient's informed, express consent to routine care (Fig. 2-5). More detailed consent forms are required for surgeries or other treatments that are not considered routine care.

Hartman

HARTMAN PHYSICIANS' GROUP
1313 IRON AVENUE SW
ALBUQUERQUE, NM 87102
505-291-1274 | HARTMANONLINE.COM

GENERAL CONSENT FOR TREATMENT

Date: ____________

Patient Name: ____________ Phone #: ____________

DOB: ____________ Medical Record #: ____________

CONSENT TO TREATMENT
I consent to receive medical and healthcare services, including diagnostic procedures, examinations, X-rays, and medical treatment provided under the instructions of the Hartman Physicians' Group physician(s), employees, and other healthcare providers as they deem reasonable and necessary. I acknowledge that no warranty or guarantee has been made to me as to result or cure.

I understand that this consent to treatment will be valid and remain in effect as long as I attend or receive services from Hartman Physicians' Group, unless revoked by me in writing. Any revocation will not be effective until received by Hartman Physicians' Group.

I certify that I have read and understand this information and that all of my questions have been answered to my satisfaction.

PATIENT 18 YEARS OF AGE OR OLDER:

PATIENT	**OR**	**LEGAL REPRESENTATIVE**
SIGNATURE: ____________		SIGNATURE: ____________
PRINT NAME: ____________		PRINT NAME: ____________
DATE: ____________		DATE: ____________

PATIENT UNDER 18 YEARS OF AGE:

PARENT, GUARDIAN OR LEGAL REPRESENTATIVE

SIGNATURE: ____________ DATE: ____________

PRINT NAME: ____________

RELATIONSHIP TO PATIENT: ____________

NOTE: POA (copy of legal document(s) required for placement in patient medical record)

Fig. 2-5. *General consent forms ensure that healthcare providers receive patient permission for routine medical care.*

Even though a patient who sees a phlebotomy technician with orders for blood tests will likely have signed a general consent form, the technician should not draw blood or provide any care if the patient does not agree. Before providing any care, the PBT must describe what will happen and answer any patient questions within his scope of practice. Any further questions should be referred to the appropriate care provider. Blood should never be drawn against a patient's wishes, even if that patient has signed a general consent form. Using words to threaten or coerce a patient to consent could be considered **assault**, which is the use of words or actions to cause another person to feel fearful of being harmed. Actually drawing blood from a patient who does not consent constitutes **battery**, which is the intentional touching of another person without permission. Assault and battery are crimes. A healthcare worker who even touches a patient who has not signed a consent form could also be committing battery.

Patients' Rights

Patient consent and HIV testing

Some states have specific laws about the way in which healthcare workers must get consent for HIV testing. Each facility will have a policy that reflects its state's regulations. Testing for HIV can have complex emotional, ethical, and health implications. It is very important that PBTs know and understand how to apply their facilities' policies related to HIV testing. Patients always have the right to decline tests, including HIV tests. While PBTs can emphasize that a test is recommended by a patient's doctor, they cannot perform a test without patient consent.

Sometimes a patient may seem to consent to a procedure but not really understand it. This can create a situation in which the healthcare worker performing the procedure may be considered negligent. The patient has provided express consent, but the consent was not truly informed. Negligence is a civil violation. A healthcare worker or his facility can be sued in such cases. Always following facility policy, providing full information about procedures, and making sure the patient understands will help protect a PBT from charges of negligence. If a patient expresses doubts or concerns, the PBT must address those concerns before continuing, involving a supervisor when necessary.

Understanding consent is especially important when working with patients who speak a language other than English. Patients have a right to receive medical information in a language they understand. True informed consent requires that the patient fully understands what he is consenting to. Friends and relatives who speak the patient's language are not a substitute for a professional interpreter or interpretation service. If a phlebotomy technician is unsure whether a patient understands her explanation of a procedure, she should contact her supervisor.

There are some situations that make patient consent more difficult to obtain. A patient who is a **minor**, or less than 18 years of age, cannot consent to treatment. A parent or guardian must provide consent. Procedures should never be performed on minors without an appropriate adult present who has provided consent (Fig. 2-6).

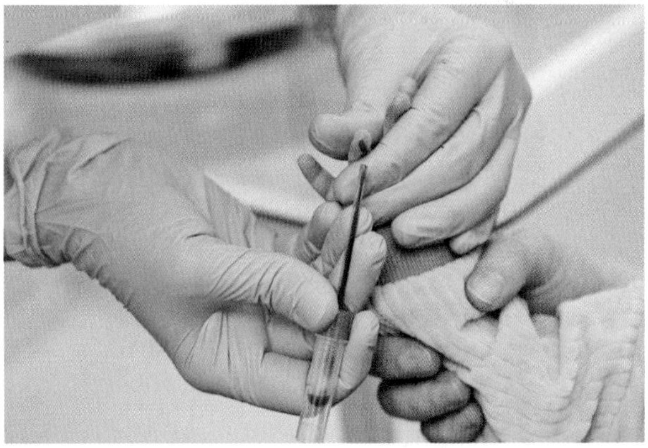

Fig. 2-6. *Parents or legal guardians must consent to medical procedures on behalf of minors.*

Some adults may also require the consent of a guardian or designated caretaker. Adults who have intellectual disabilities or who have illnesses that affect their **cognitive** ability (ability to think and process information) may be unable to consent. An adult who is considered unable to provide consent will have a legal representative who can do so. If a technician has doubts about a patient's ability to consent, she should contact her supervisor.

In emergency situations involving minors and adults it can be difficult to get informed or express consent. The patient may be unconscious, in shock, or otherwise unable to give express consent, or a child's parent may not be available to provide consent. In these cases patients may be treated with **implied consent**. Although laws vary from state to state, the common idea is that when a person is temporarily unable to provide express consent, healthcare workers can provide care that a "reasonable person" would consent to in order to protect his life and well-being. In situations like this it is very important for PBTs to follow the chain of command and provide services only as directed.

Patients' Rights

Implied consent

Implied consent can be complicated. If a patient has not provided express, informed consent by signing a consent form, her actions may still communicate, or imply, consent. If she voluntarily sits at a phlebotomist's station, extends her arm, and rolls up her sleeve, she is communicating consent by her actions. The act of entering a healthcare facility for consultation or treatment could be seen as a form of implied consent. Even so, getting informed consent is a far more reliable way of ensuring that a patient understands and agrees to treatment. A signed consent form provides the facility with clear proof of consent. Facility policies require signed consent whenever it is possible to receive it. It is the best way to respect patients' rights and provide high-quality care. It is also the best way to avoid possible criminal or civil penalties.

Implied consent may also become important when a driver is suspected of being under the influence of alcohol or other substances. Most states have laws allowing police officers to require drivers to submit to some form of test for intoxicating substances when there is reason to believe the driver is intoxicated. In some cases this means blood may be drawn. In states with certain types of implied consent laws, blood may be drawn even if the patient does not provide express consent.

5. Explain the American Hospital Association's Patient Care Partnership and discuss why patient rights are important

The **American Hospital Association** (**AHA**, aha.org) was founded in 1898. Its goals include educating healthcare leaders and providing information both to the healthcare industry and to the public about healthcare issues and trends. It is a membership organization designed to serve hospitals of all kinds, healthcare networks, patients, and the communities in which healthcare facilities operate. The AHA also advocates with all levels of government, which means it expresses its opinion about laws that affect healthcare facilities and providers and their patients.

In 1973 the AHA introduced a document called the *Statement on a Patient's Bill of Rights* and encouraged all healthcare facilities to use it, adapting it as needed to the patients they serve. This document outlined 15 rights to which all patients are entitled when receiving care and addressed issues such as informed consent, the expectation of privacy, and understanding of caregivers' identities and roles. The Patient's Bill of Rights was updated and revised in 1992. In 2003 the Patient's Bill of Rights was replaced by the Patient Care Partnership, which outlines what patients can expect during the course of a hospital stay (Fig. 2-7).

According to the Patient Care Partnership, patients can expect the following:

High quality hospital care. This includes the patient's right to know the title and identity of any person providing care, and to know if that person is a student, medical resident, or trainee of any kind.

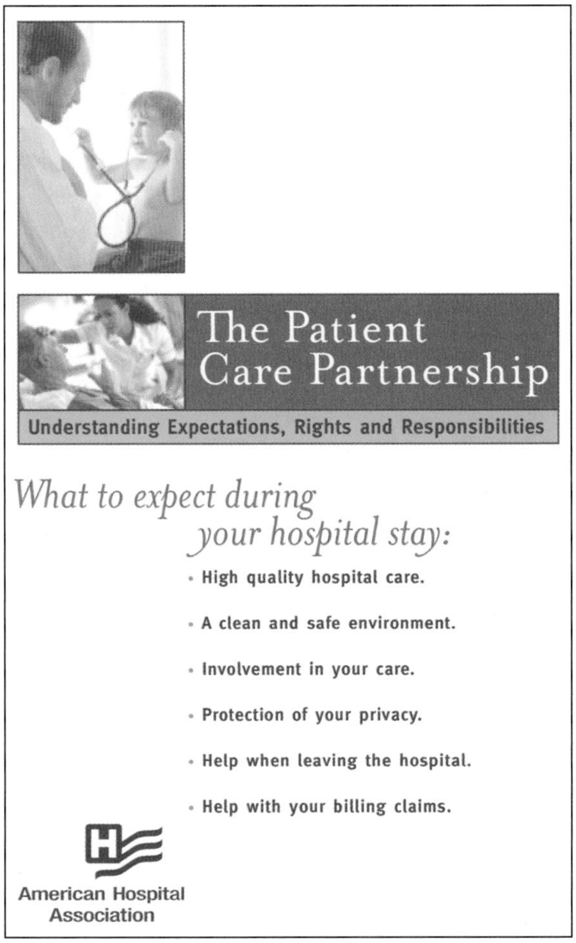
The Patient
Care Partnership
Understanding Expectations, Rights and Responsibilities
What to expect during
your hospital stay:
• High quality hospital care.
• A clean and safe environment.
• Involvement in your care.
• Protection of your privacy.
• Help when leaving the hospital.
• Help with your billing claims.
American Hospital
Association

Fig. 2-7. *Many inpatient facilities provide printed copies of the Patient Care Partnership in their admission packets.* (USED WITH PERMISSION. ©AMERICAN HOSPITAL ASSOCIATION. 2019. HTTPS://WWW.AHA.ORG/SYSTEM/FILES/2018-01/AHA-PATIENT-CARE-PARTNERSHIP.PDF)

A clean and safe environment. This addresses the importance of infection prevention and control for patients (covered in Chapter 4). It also emphasizes the importance of communicating with the patient about any incident that might have an impact on her care or outcome. For instance, if a phlebotomy technician does not draw enough blood to accurately perform a test ordered for a patient, the patient should be informed of the error and its possible effects, which could include a delayed diagnosis.

Involvement in your care. Informed consent falls into this category. Doctors and other healthcare providers must thoroughly explain care, including risks and benefits. They must also tell patients if a treatment is experimental or part of a research study. Patients must agree to participate in these studies based on a thorough explanation. Doctors are also required to inform patients what might happen if they refuse a particular treatment or type of care. Patients also have the right to be informed about the likely cost of care. Patients have responsibilities related to their involvement in care as well. They must provide their caregivers with accurate information about their condition, symptoms, history, and insurance coverage.

Patients have the right to have—and the responsibility to communicate—**advance directives**. Advance directives are legal documents that allow people to decide what kind of medical care they wish to have in the event they are unable to make those decisions themselves. One type of advance directive is known as a **living will**, also known by various other names such as *directive to physicians* and *health care directive*. This document outlines specific medical care a person wants or does not want to receive. A **do-not-resuscitate** (**DNR**) order is another type of advance directive and indicates that the patient does not wish for medical professionals to perform cardiopulmonary resuscitation (CPR) in the event of cardiac or respiratory arrest. An advance directive can also designate a person other than the patient to make medical decisions if the patient becomes ill or disabled. This is called **durable power of attorney for health care**.

Protection of your privacy. Hospitals must follow HIPAA regulations and any other federal, state, and local laws about patient privacy. They also must let patients know about their privacy policies. Patients are required to sign documents acknowledging that they have received this notification. If a patient wishes for his health information to be shared with someone outside the facility, he will have to sign a release allowing it.

Help when leaving the hospital. When a patient leaves a hospital or other healthcare facility after treatment, the facility will provide information about any follow-up care needed. This may include training the patient, family member, or other caregiver about particular care procedures or about the use of prescribed medications (Fig. 2-8). If there are follow-up appointments the patient must keep, the facility will inform the patient.

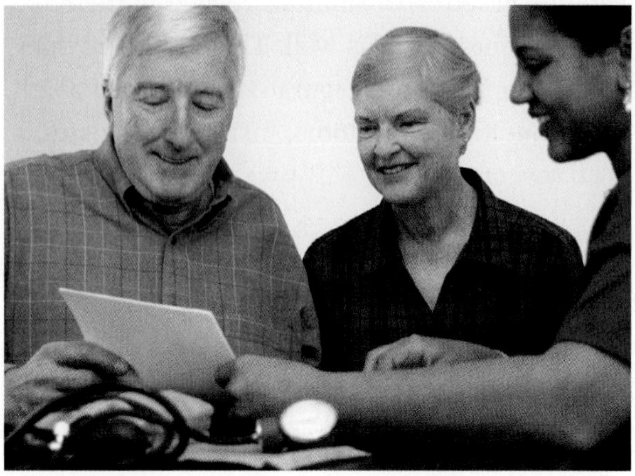

Fig. 2-8. When a patient leaves a facility he will receive instructions about how to continue his care at home.

Help with your billing claims. This category relates to insurance and payment of hospital bills. Hospital staff will file claims with a patient's insurance provider. If a patient does not have insurance, the hospital will direct him to possible sources of assistance. Hospitals employ **medical social workers** who are available to help with financial issues and other assistance a patient may require.

Phlebotomy technicians can help protect patients' legal rights by following these guidelines:

Guidelines: Protecting Patients' Rights

- G Never abuse a patient. Abuse can include rough handling of a patient during a procedure. It can also be verbal. Speaking abusively to a patient is a violation of her rights.
- G Call the patient by the name the patient prefers. Use pronouns the patient prefers (he/him, she/her, or they/them).
- G Allow the patient to make as many choices as possible about how care is performed. For example, a patient may prefer that blood be drawn in a particular arm.
- G Always explain a procedure to a patient before performing it.
- G Follow all facility procedures regarding infection prevention.
- G Respect a patient's refusal of care. Patients have a legal right to refuse treatment and care. Report the refusal to a supervisor immediately.
- G Tell the nurse if a patient has questions, concerns, or complaints about a procedure.
- G Be truthful when documenting care.
- G Do not talk or gossip about patients. Keep all patient information confidential.

Chapter Review

Multiple Choice

1. How are laws and ethics related?
   (A) Ethics are usually based on laws.
   (B) Laws are usually based on ethics.
   (C) Laws existed before ethics, and ethics were developed to enhance laws.
   (D) There is no relationship between laws and ethics.
2. Which of the following details would be considered protected health information?
   (A) A patient's hair color
   (B) A patient's nationality
   (C) A patient's political party
   (D) A patient's email address
3. HIPAA applies to
   (A) All healthcare workers
   (B) Only licensed healthcare workers
   (C) Only healthcare workers in public facilities
   (D) Only healthcare workers in facilities that receive Medicare or Medicaid funds

4. Which of the following best describes a CLIA waived test?
   (A) A test of moderate complexity that can be performed by a medical technician in a laboratory
   (B) A test of high complexity that requires specific machinery
   (C) A test of low complexity that can be performed with little risk of error
   (D) A test of high complexity that must be performed by a doctor or PhD scientist

5. Which of the following is true of implied consent?
   (A) A patient gives implied consent by directly affirming that he understands and consents to treatment.
   (B) Implied consent can never apply when a patient is conscious.
   (C) Implied consent is communicated by signing a consent document.
   (D) Implied consent can be more difficult to document or prove than informed, express consent.

6. This is a circumstance in which blood might be legally drawn from a patient without the patient's informed, express consent:
   (A) When an officer of the law suspects a driver to be under the influence of alcohol
   (B) When a patient is refusing a blood test that relates to a life-or-death diagnosis
   (C) When a patient who is cognitively impaired but judged legally competent to make her own decisions refuses a test the PBT thinks she needs
   (D) When a healthcare worker may have been exposed to an illness but refuses a test to determine infection status

7. The Patient Care Partnership
   (A) Is a set of federal guidelines designed to ensure high-quality patient care
   (B) Is a proposal made by medical schools to guarantee the rights of patients in teaching hospitals
   (C) Is a set of principles hospitals must follow in order to be reimbursed by insurance companies
   (D) Is the most recent version of the American Hospital Association's Patient's Bill of Rights

8. Which of the following is a type of advance directive?
   (A) An acknowledgement of privacy policies
   (B) A do-not-resuscitate order
   (C) An informed consent document
   (D) An authorization to release records

3 Communication and Patient Diversity

1. Define *communication* and understand the importance of both verbal and nonverbal communication

Communication is the process of exchanging information with others. It is a process of sending and receiving messages. People communicate by using signs and symbols, such as words, drawings, pictures, and emojis. They also communicate through their behavior.

The simplest form of communication is a three-step process that takes place between two people (Fig. 3-1). In the first step, the sender (the person who communicates first) sends a message. In the second step, the receiver receives the message. The receiver and sender constantly switch roles as they communicate. The third step involves providing feedback. The receiver repeats the message or responds to it in some way. This lets the sender know that the message was received and understood. Feedback is especially important when working in a healthcare setting. Phlebotomists must take time to make sure patients understand messages.

All three steps must occur before the communication process is complete. During a conversation, this process is repeated over and over.

Effective communication is a critical part of any healthcare worker's job. Phlebotomy technicians must communicate with supervisors, the care team, patients, and family members. A patient's health is affected by the quality of communication among the healthcare workers who care for her. PBTs may also need to communicate clearly and respectfully in stressful or confusing situations.

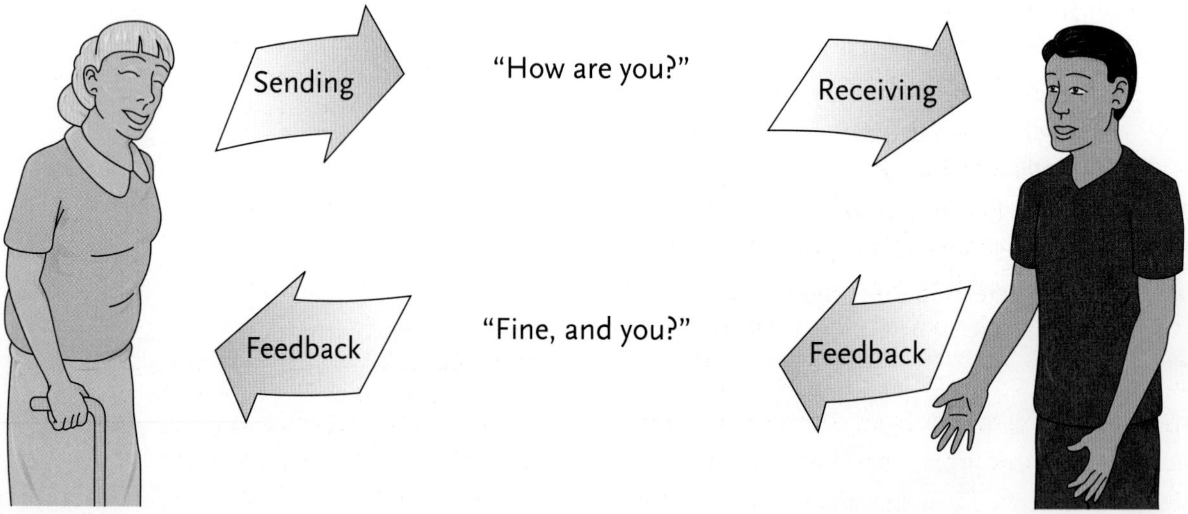

Fig. 3-1. *The communication process consists of sending a message, receiving a message, and providing feedback.*

Communication is either verbal or nonverbal. **Verbal communication** involves the use of words, spoken or written. When communicating verbally, it is important to use words that have the same meaning to both the sender and the receiver. Misunderstandings may occur if each person interprets the same words differently. For example, if a PBT asks a patient if his veins roll, the patient might not understand the question.

Nonverbal communication is communicating without using words. An example of nonverbal communication is a person extending his arm and rolling up his sleeve. This communicates that the patient is ready to have his blood drawn (although it is still important to explain the procedure and confirm consent before touching the patient). Nonverbal communication also includes how a person says something. For example, a phlebotomist says cheerfully, "I'll be right with you, Mrs. Gonzales." This communicates that the technician is ready and willing to work with a patient, but is delayed at the moment. Saying the same phrase in a different tone or emphasizing different words can communicate frustration and annoyance: "I'll be right *with* you, Mrs. Gonzales!"

Body language is another form of nonverbal communication. Movements, facial expressions, and posture can express different attitudes or emotions. Just as with speaking, body language sends messages. Other people receive and interpret them. For example, slouching in a chair and sitting erect send two different messages (Fig. 3-2). Slouching says that a person is bored, tired, or hostile. Sitting up straight says that the person is interested and respectful. Other examples of positive nonverbal communication include smiling, nodding one's head, and making eye contact with the person who is speaking.

Sometimes people send one message verbally and a very different message nonverbally. Nonverbal communication often illustrates how someone is feeling. This message may be quite different from what he is saying. For example, a patient who says, "I'm not nervous at all," but is clenching the armrest of his chair and biting his lip is sending two very different messages. Paying attention to nonverbal communication helps phlebotomists give better care. In this example, the technician should be aware that the patient is likely experiencing anxiety about the procedure, despite what he says.

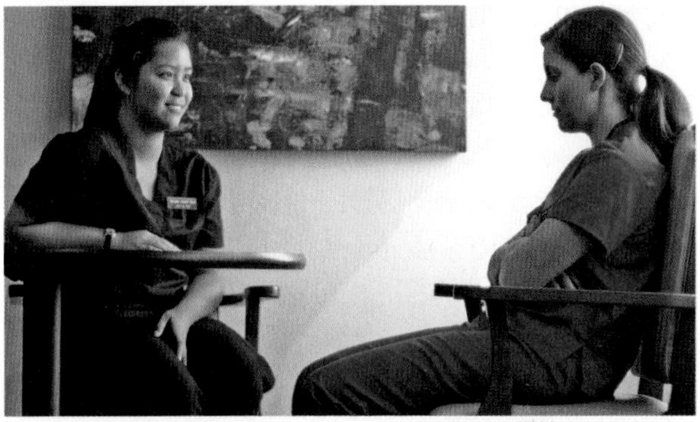

Fig. 3-2. *Body language sends messages just as words do. Which of these people seems more interested in their conversation—the person on the right who is looking down with her arms crossed or the person on the left who is sitting up straight and smiling?*

Telephone communication

Phlebotomists will sometimes use telephones to communicate while working. When communicating by phone, it is very important to identify oneself by name and title, using a pleasant, professional tone of voice. Although the person on the other end of the line cannot see the PBT, using positive body language while speaking—smiling, for example—can convey a positive tone.

When taking messages over the phone, it is important to get the name of the caller, a phone number, and a message. The time of the call should also be noted. If there is any doubt about what the caller is asking, the phlebotomist should repeat the message and ask for confirmation. It is important to ask for the proper spelling of names. Confidentiality laws apply to telephone communication as well. PBTs should never provide information about a patient over the phone to someone who is not authorized to receive it. PBTs should never give test results, whether on the phone or in person. This is beyond their scope of practice. If there is any doubt about the identity of the person on the other end of the line, or any doubt about whether the person is legally authorized to discuss the details of a patient's care, the phlebotomist should refer the call to a supervisor.

2. Identify barriers to communication and understand different communication styles and preferences

Communication can be blocked or disrupted in many ways (Fig. 3-3). The following are some communication barriers and ways for a phlebotomist to avoid them:

Patient does not hear PBT, does not hear correctly, or does not understand. The PBT should stand directly facing the patient. He should speak slowly and clearly. He should not shout, whisper, or mumble. The PBT should speak in a low voice, using a pleasant tone. Learning Objective 5 includes information on communicating with a patient who has a hearing impairment.

Patient is difficult to understand. The PBT should be patient and take time to listen. He can ask the patient to repeat or explain the message, and then state the message in his own words to make sure he has understood.

PBT, patient, or others use words that are not understood. A PBT should not use medical terminology with patients. He should speak in simple, everyday words and ask what a word means if he is not sure.

PBT uses slang or profanity. The PBT should avoid using slang words and expressions. They are unprofessional and may not be understood. He should not use profanity, even if the patient does.

PBT uses clichés. Clichés are phrases that are used over and over again and do not really mean anything. For example, "Everything will be fine" is a cliché. Instead of using a cliché, the PBT should listen to what the patient is really saying and respond with a meaningful message. For example, if a patient is afraid of needles, the PBT can say "I understand that this may be scary. What can I do to make you feel more at ease?" instead of saying "Oh, it'll be over before you know it."

PBT responds with "Why?" The PBT should avoid asking "Why?" when a patient makes a statement. "Why" questions make people feel defensive. For example, a patient may say she has changed her mind and does not want her blood drawn. If the PBT asks "Why not?" he may receive an angry response. Instead, he can ask "Do you have questions about the procedure that I can answer?" The patient may then be willing to discuss the issue. Specific questions about

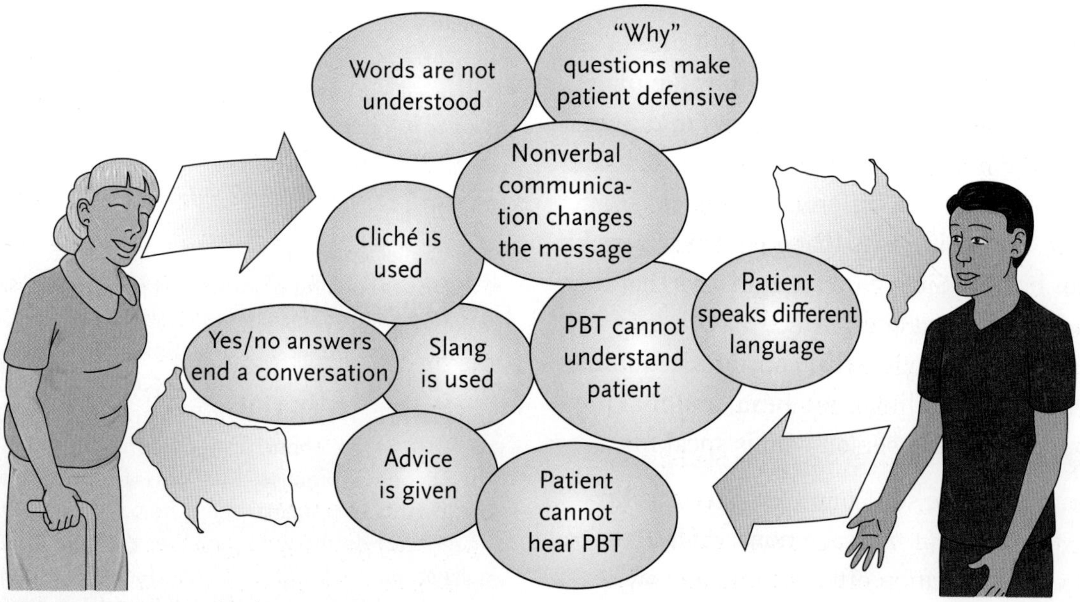

Fig. 3-3. Barriers to communication.

the reasons for the test should be referred to the healthcare professional who ordered it, as should any questions the PBT cannot answer.

PBT gives advice. The PBT should not offer his opinion or give advice. Giving medical advice is not within a PBT's scope of practice. It could be dangerous, causing both ethical and legal difficulties.

PBT asks questions that only require yes/no answers. The PBT should ask open-ended questions that need more than a "yes" or "no" answer. Yes or no answers end conversation. For example, instead of asking the patient "Are you nervous about this?" a PBT can say "How have blood draws gone for you in the past?"

Patient speaks a different language. If a patient speaks a different language than the PBT does, the PBT should speak slowly and clearly. He should keep his messages short and simple. He should be alert for words the patient understands and also be alert for signs that the patient is only pretending to understand. If the patient does not understand, or if the patient prefers to communicate in his native language, an interpreter or interpretation service should be used. Communication boards with pictures can also be helpful in these situations. Phlebotomists should follow facility policies when dealing with language barriers.

PBT or patient uses nonverbal communication. Nonverbal communication can change a message. The PBT should be aware of his body language and gestures. He can look for nonverbal messages from patients and clarify them. For example, "Mr. Feldman, you say you're feeling fine but your muscles are very tense. Would you like to take a minute to relax before we begin?"

In addition to avoiding these possible barriers to communication, phlebotomists need to be aware that communication can be influenced by factors such as personality, culture, and mood. Some people are naturally talkative and open, even with strangers. Others are quieter and more reserved. Similarly, some cultures value and encourage different styles of communication. For some people talking to strangers, being touched by strangers, or even making eye contact with strangers is very uncomfortable. This may be due to cultural, religious, or personal preferences. Additionally, people in healthcare settings may be worried about their state of health, and this concern can cause them to behave and communicate differently.

No matter how patients behave and communicate, it is always the responsibility of the PBT to follow these steps to ensure accurate communication:

Be a good listener. The PBT should allow the other person to express her ideas completely. He should concentrate on what the patient is saying and not interrupt. The PBT should not finish the patient's sentences even if he knows what she is going to say. When the patient is finished, the PBT should restate the message in his own words to make sure he has understood.

Provide feedback. Active listening means focusing on the person sending the message and giving feedback. Feedback might be an acknowledgment, a question, or repeating the sender's message. The PBT should offer general but leading responses, such as "Oh?" or "Go on," or "Hmm." By doing this, he is actively listening, providing feedback, and encouraging the sender to expand the message.

Bring up topics of concern. If the PBT knows of a topic that might concern a patient, he can raise the issue in a general, nonthreatening way. This lets the patient decide whether to discuss it. For example, if the PBT observes that a patient is fidgeting or acting nervous, he could say, "Mrs. Jones, you seem a little unsure about this."

English is the rule

When working, and especially in front of patients, it is important for healthcare workers to speak English, no matter what other languages they may speak. Patients who do not understand the language being spoken might feel that they are being talked about or might just be uncomfortable that they cannot understand. In situations in which a healthcare worker and a patient share a language that is not English, the worker can use the patient's language to determine understanding, but should not act as an interpreter unless trained or approved by the facility to do so.

Understand the importance of touch. Softly patting an anxious patient's hand or shoulder or holding her hand may communicate caring (Fig. 3-4). Some people's backgrounds may make them less comfortable being touched. The PBT should ask permission before touching a patient and should be sensitive to her feelings. PBTs must touch patients in order to do their jobs. However, they should recognize that some patients feel more comfortable when there is as little physical contact as possible. The PBT should adjust care to each patient's needs whenever possible.

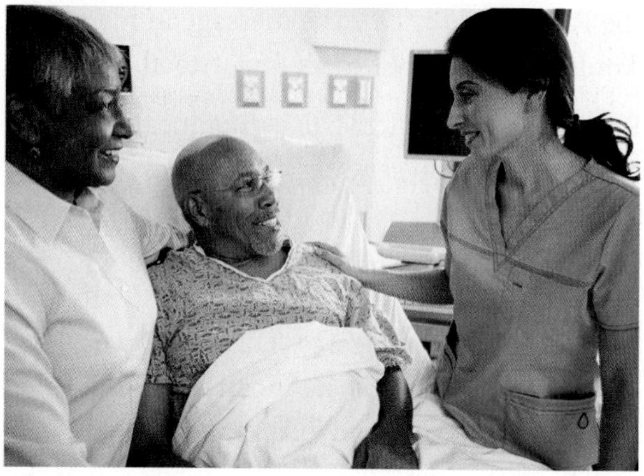

Fig. 3-4. *For many patients a gentle touch can be reassuring. PBTs should watch patient body language to ensure the touch is being received positively.*

Ask for more. When a patient reports concerns or anxiety, the PBT should have him repeat what he has said and ask him for more information. Anything the patient reports should be documented word for word.

Do not ignore a patient's concerns. Ignoring concerns can be considered negligent behavior. The phlebotomy technician should work to understand the patient's concerns and address them if they are within her scope of practice. Patient concerns should always be reported to the nurse if the PBT is unable to address them, or if they are beyond the PBT's scope of practice.

Do not talk down to any patient. A PBT should talk to patients as they would talk to any person. It is also important to not talk down or act as if the patient cannot be trusted to understand. Guidelines for communicating with patients whose situations might require a special approach are found in Learning Objective 5.

Be empathetic. The PBT should try to understand and identify with what the patient is going through. This is called empathy. She can imagine how it might feel to have a strong fear of needles or blood, or to be experiencing symptoms that might indicate a serious illness. The PBT should not tell the patient she knows how he feels, because she does not know exactly how the patient feels. She can say things like, "I know this may be difficult."

3. Understand common medical terminology and abbreviations

Throughout a phlebotomy technician's training, he will learn medical terms for specific conditions. For example, the medical term for fainting is **syncope**; skin that is blue or gray is called **cyanotic**. Medical terms are often made up of roots, prefixes, and suffixes. A root is a part of a word that contains its basic meaning or definition. The prefix is the word part that precedes the root to help form a new word. The suffix is the word part added to the end of a root that helps form a new word. Prefixes and suffixes are called *affixes* because they are attached, or affixed, to a root. Here are some examples:

- The root *phleb* or *phlebo* means vein. The suffix *itis* means inflammation. *Phlebitis* is the inflammation of a vein.

- The prefix *anti* means against. The root *coagulate* means to clot. An **anticoagulant** is a substance that stops blood from clotting.
- The root *hemo* means blood. The suffix *stasis* means slowing or stopping. **Hemostasis** is the stopping of a flow of blood.

When speaking with patients, PBTs should use simple, nonmedical terms. Medical terms should not be used because they may not be understood. But when speaking with the care team, using medical terminology will help give more complete and accurate information.

Abbreviations are another way to communicate more efficiently with care team members. For example, the abbreviation *CBC* means *complete blood count,* a common blood test. *Hgb* means **hemoglobin**, an oxygen-carrying protein in red blood cells. The word *stat,* which is a shortened version of the Latin word *statim,* means *right away.* A patient who has been ordered to not consume any food or liquids is *NPO,* an abbreviation for *nil per os,* Latin for *nothing by mouth.*

Phlebotomy technicians should learn their facility's standard medical abbreviations. They can use them to report information briefly and accurately. They may also need to know these abbreviations to read requisitions (testing orders). Important medical terms, abbreviations, and symbols will be introduced throughout this book, and a comprehensive list is also included in the instructor's guide. There may be other terms in use at a facility as well, so it is important for PBTs to follow facility policy.

4. Explain documentation and describe related terms and forms

Documentation is the creation of a record of care given to a patient. It is an essential form of communication in health care. Depending on the facility, documentation might be done using computers or tablets (electronically) or on paper (manually). There are legal aspects to careful documentation that are important to remember:

- It is the only way to guarantee clear and complete communication among all the members of the care team.
- Documentation is a legal record of every part of a patient's treatment. Medical charts can be used in court as legal evidence.
- Documentation helps protect healthcare workers and their employers from liability by proving what they did when caring for patients.
- Documentation gives an up-to-date record of the status and care of each patient.

Guidelines: Careful Documentation

G Document procedures immediately after they are performed. This makes details easier to remember. Always wait to document until after a procedure has been completed. Do not record any care before it has been done. Collection tubes should not be labeled and initialed until a blood draw has been successfully completed and the patient has confirmed that the label is accurate (Fig. 3-5).

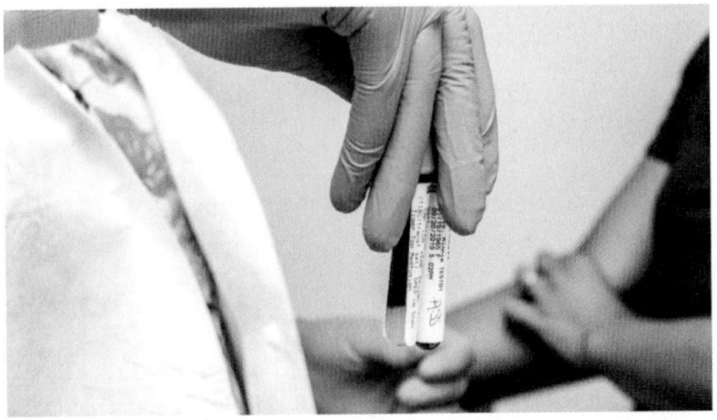

Fig. 3-5. *Careful documentation includes labeling and initialing collection tubes after a specimen has been taken.*

G Use blue or black ink when documenting by hand. Write as neatly as you can.

G If you make a mistake, draw one line through it, and write the correct information. Write your initials and the date. Do not erase what you have written. Do not use correction fluid. Documentation done on a computer is time-stamped; it can be changed only by entering another notation.

- Sign your full name and title (for example, Sara Martinez, PBT) and write the correct date.
- Document as specified by your facility. Ensure that patient identification, specimen labels, and requisitions match.
- Documentation may need to be done using the 24-hour clock, or military time (Fig. 3-6). Regular time uses the numbers 1 to 12 to show each of the 24 hours in a day. In military time, the hours are numbered from 00 to 23. Midnight is expressed as 0000 (or 2400), 1:00 a.m. is 0100, 1:00 p.m. is 1300, and so on.

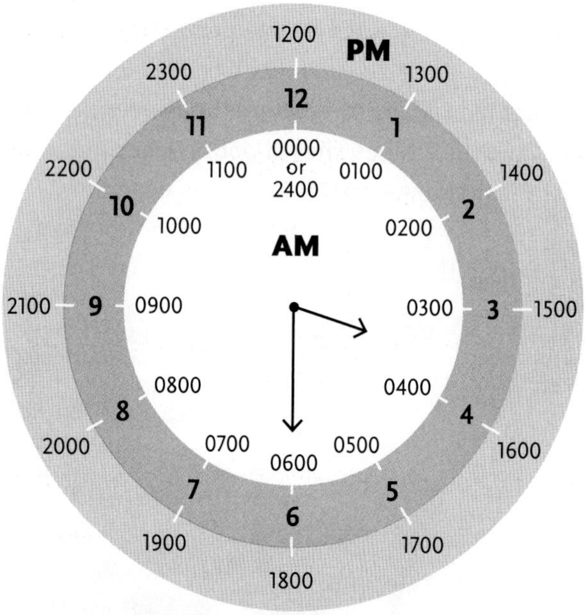

Fig. 3-6. Illustration showing the divisions in the 24-hour clock.

Both regular and military time list minutes and seconds the same way. The minutes and seconds do not change when converting from regular to military time. The abbreviations a.m. and p.m. are used in regular time to show what time of day it is. However, these are not used in military time, since specific numbers show each hour of the day. For example, to change 4:22 p.m. to military time, add 4 + 12. The minutes do not change. The time is expressed as 1622 hours.

To change the hours between 1:00 p.m. and 11:59 p.m. to military time, add 12 to the regular time. For example, to change 3:00 p.m. to military time, add 3 + 12. The time is expressed as 1500 (fifteen hundred) hours.

Midnight is the only time that differs. Midnight can be written as 0000, or it can be written as 2400. This follows the rule of adding 12 to the regular time. Follow your facility's policy on how to express midnight.

To change from military time to regular time, subtract 12. The minutes do not change. For example, to change 2200 hours to standard time, subtract 12 from 22. The answer is 10:00 p.m. To change 1610 hours to standard time, subtract 12 from 16. The answer is 4:10 p.m.

- At some facilities, computers or tablets are used to document patient care. A computer may remain in a patient's room for care team members to input information each time they provide care. A computer may be in the hallway for staff members to use. A computer or tablet may also be carried from room to room for documentation. Computers record and store information that can be retrieved when it is needed. This is faster and more accurate than writing information by hand. If your facility uses computers for documentation, you will be trained to use them. HIPAA privacy guidelines apply to computer use. Make sure nobody can see private and protected health information on your computer screen. Confidential information should not be shared with anyone except the care team.

The care a phlebotomist provides is always ordered by a physician or other licensed medical practitioner. A requisition, or order for laboratory tests, can be created in electronic or paper form. Increasingly these orders are made electronically and include bar codes that can be printed and affixed to the specimen tubes. These bar codes can be scanned to identify the patient and the test to be performed. Manual (paper) requisitions are usually in the form of a preprinted list of tests that the practitioner has marked to indicate which tests should be performed (Fig. 3-7). In emergency situations, a doctor may order a test orally (by speaking the request), but this must be followed up with documentation in electronic or paper form. More information about requisitions is found in Chapter 9.

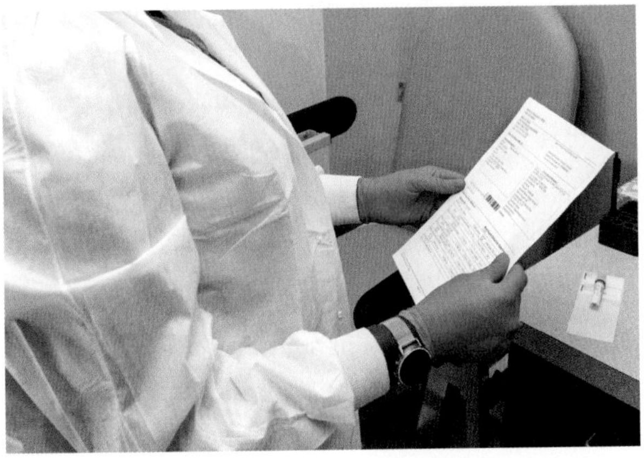

Fig. 3-7. *This requisition form was printed from an electronic order sent by the patient's doctor.*

Incident reports are also essential documents for phlebotomists to understand. An **incident** is an accident, problem, or unexpected event during the course of care. It is something that is not part of the normal routine. An accidental needlestick or a patient losing consciousness and hitting her head is an incident. Other issues that must be reported include problems with specimens, containers, patient identification, or incorrect orders. More detail about these types of incidents is found in Chapters 9 and 10.

State and federal guidelines require that incidents be recorded in an incident report. An incident report (also called an *occurrence, accident, accident/incident,* or *event report*) is a report that documents the incident and the response to it. The report is a factual, **objective** account of what happened. Objective information is based on what a person sees, hears, touches, or smells. It is collected by using the senses. It does not include opinions or assumptions about causes. If a patient falls, for instance, and the PBT did not see it, she should not write, "Mr. Quraishi passed out and fell." Instead, she should write "Found Mr. Quraishi unconscious on the floor" or "Mr. Quraishi states that he passed out and fell." Phlebotomy technicians should write brief and accurate descriptions of the events as they happened without placing blame or liability within the report.

The information in an incident report is confidential and is intended for internal use to help prevent future incidents. Incident reports should be filed when any of the following occur:

- A patient falls
- A healthcare worker makes a mistake in care, including collecting an incorrect specimen or collecting a specimen from the wrong patient or the wrong site (area on the patient's body)
- A patient or coworker makes sexual advances or remarks
- Anything happens that makes a healthcare worker feel uncomfortable, threatened, or unsafe
- A healthcare worker gets injured on the job
- A healthcare worker is exposed to blood or body fluids
- A healthcare worker or patient receives an accidental needlestick
- A patient is injured in some way during the course of a blood draw

Reporting and documenting incidents is done to protect everyone involved. This includes the patient, the employer, and the phlebotomist. When documenting incidents, PBTs should complete the report as soon as possible and give it to a supervisor. This ensures details are not forgotten.

Guidelines: Incident Reporting

- G Tell what happened. State the time and the mental and physical condition of the person.
- G Describe the person's reaction to the incident.
- G State the facts; do not give opinions.
- G Do not write anything from the incident report on the patient's medical record.
- G Describe the action taken to give care.
- G Describe notification of appropriate supervisors.

Sentinel events

A sentinel event is an unexpected occurrence that results in serious physical or psychological injury or death. A sentinel is a soldier who stands guard. Sentinel events are called *sentinel* because they signal the need for an immediate investigation and response. An example of this type of event is a blood transfusion error that results in a patient's death. A sentinel event must be reported to the proper agency.

5. List guidelines for communicating with different populations

One of the benefits of working as a phlebotomist is the opportunity to meet and help people of all different backgrounds and ages. Communication is more effective when differences are recognized and respected. Certain adjustments in communication can help PBTs when dealing with patients who have distinct needs.

Due to illness or impairments, some patients need special techniques to aid communication. An **impairment** is a loss of function or ability; it can be a partial or complete loss. Special techniques for different conditions follow.

Hearing Impairment

There are many different kinds of hearing loss. A person may be born with hearing impairment or it may happen gradually. Deafness is a partial or complete loss of hearing. It can occur as the result of heredity, disease, or injury. In the elderly, aging commonly causes loss of hearing.

People who have hearing impairment may use a hearing aid, read lips, or use sign language. People with impaired hearing also closely observe the facial expressions and body language of others to add to their knowledge of what is being said.

Guidelines: Hearing Impairment

- G If the person has a hearing aid, make sure that it is turned on and working properly.
- G Reduce or remove background noise, such as televisions, music, and loud speech.
- G Get the patient's attention before speaking. Do not startle the patient by approaching from behind. Walk in front of her or touch her lightly on the arm to let her know you are near.
- G Speak clearly, slowly, and in good lighting. Directly face the person (Fig. 3-8). Ask if she can hear what you are saying.

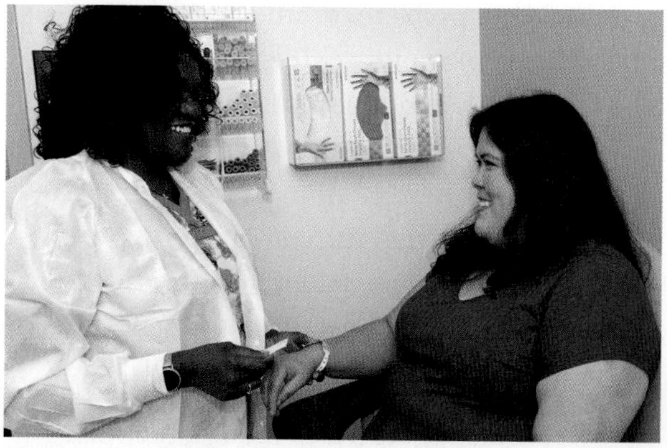

Fig. 3-8. *Speak face-to-face in good light.*

- G Do not shout or mouth words in an exaggerated way.

G Keep the pitch of your voice low.

G Patients may read lips, so keep your hands away from your face while talking.

G If the patient hears better out of one ear, try to speak and stand on that side.

G Use short sentences and simple words. Avoid sudden topic changes.

G Repeat what you have said using different words when needed. Some people who are hearing impaired want you to repeat exactly what was said because they miss only a few words.

G Use picture cards or a notepad as needed.

G Some patients who are hearing impaired have speech problems and may be difficult to understand. Do not pretend you understand if you do not. Ask the patient to repeat what was said. Observe the lips, facial expressions, and body language. Then tell the patient what you think you heard. You can also request that the patient write down words.

Vision Impairment

Vision impairment can affect people of all ages. Some vision impairment causes people to wear corrective lenses, such as contact lenses or eyeglasses.

Guidelines: Vision Impairment

G Identify yourself immediately when you approach the patient.

G Do not touch the patient until you have said your name. Explain why you are there and what procedure you will perform.

G Let the patient know if you need to step away at any time and when you have completed the blood draw. Do not simply walk away.

G Make sure there is proper lighting in the room. Face the patient when speaking.

G Always tell the patient what you are doing as you are performing procedures. Give specific directions, such as "on your right" or "in front of you."

G Talk directly to the patient whom you are assisting. Do not talk to other patients or staff members at the same time.

Cognitive Impairment

Cognitive impairment affects a person's ability to think logically and clearly. A certain amount of cognitive impairment is a normal change of aging. Illnesses such as Alzheimer's disease can cause a more dramatic form of cognitive impairment. Patients with advanced forms of cognitive impairment are likely to have family members or other caregivers assisting them as they receive medical care, but these communication guidelines are still important to remember.

Guidelines: Cognitive Impairment

G Always approach from the front, and do not startle the patient.

G Smile and look happy to see the patient. Be friendly (Fig. 3-9).

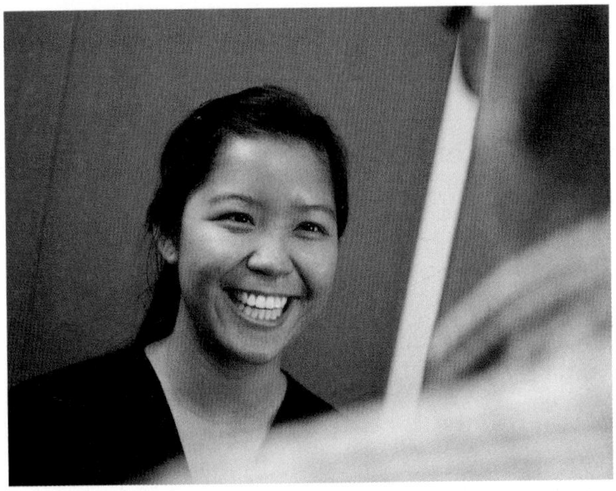

Fig. 3-9. *Smiling can communicate positivity and a willingness to help.*

G Try to minimize background noise and distraction.

- Always identify yourself and use the patient's name. Continue to use the patient's name as you provide care.
- Speak slowly, using a lower tone of voice than normal. This is calming and easier to understand.
- Repeat yourself, using the same words and phrases, as often as needed.
- Use signs, pictures, gestures, or written words to help communicate as needed.
- Phlebotomists must touch patients in order to do their job, but be aware that patients may prefer being given more personal space whenever possible.
- Check your body language; make sure you are not tense or hurried.
- Watch for nonverbal cues from the patient. Observe body language—eyes, hands, and face.
- Ask any family member or caregiver accompanying the patient for advice about communication with the patient, as appropriate.

Some **populations**, or particular groups of patients, may require special attention. With all patients, maintaining a professional but welcoming approach is an excellent start to effective communication. Following are suggestions for communicating with specific populations PBTs are likely to encounter.

Children

Pediatrics is the branch of medicine dealing with people under the age of 18. Children who are old enough to understand that having blood drawn will mean being stuck with a needle may be fearful of the experience. It is important to be reassuring and take the time necessary with young patients to help manage their anxiety. Young children should be allowed to sit in a parent or guardian's lap (Fig. 3-10).

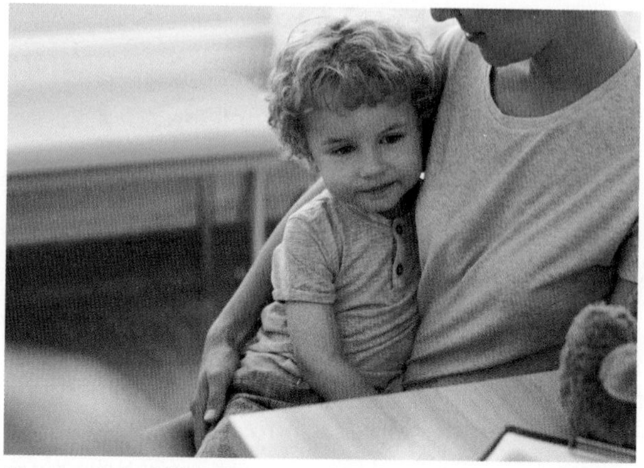

Fig. 3-10. *Small children usually feel most comfortable in a parent or guardian's lap.*

Guidelines: Pediatric Patients

- As with adult patients, introduce yourself by name and title.
- Children can find adults they do not know intimidating, especially in a medical setting. Give the child as much personal space as possible. Lower yourself physically to be on the child's eye level while speaking.
- Allow the parent/guardian to hold or soothe the child. The parent may also need to help stabilize the child during the blood draw.
- Explain to the child, in a way that is appropriate to her age, what you will do and the equipment you will use. Speak directly to the child, rather than to the accompanying parent or guardian.
- Emphasize that it is normal even for adults to be nervous about a blood draw, but that it will not take long to complete the procedure.
- It can be helpful to give the child a job during the procedure, such as holding or handing you something.
- Provide or allow distractions for the child if possible. Watching a video on the parent's electronic device or looking at pictures in a book might help calm the child.

- G Do not lie to the child about the procedure (e.g., do not say it will not hurt at all).
- G Take any questions the child has seriously. Answer them if they are within your scope of practice.
- G Do not tell the child he will get a reward if he does not cry. If your facility offers rewards to children, do not make "brave" behavior a condition of the reward. It is normal for the child to be frightened.

Elderly Patients

Geriatrics is the branch of medicine dealing with elderly patients. Older patients may have hearing, vision, or cognitive impairments, or they may not have any impairments at all. It is important not to make assumptions about this group of patients.

Guidelines: Geriatric Patients

- G Treat older patients with the same respect you give all patients. Do not talk down to them or treat them like children.
- G If an adult child or other caregiver is accompanying the patient, it is appropriate to answer any questions he may have, but it is important to communicate directly with the patient. Speaking only to the child or caregiver is disrespectful and suggests that you do not believe the elderly patient is able to understand or communicate for herself.
- G Call elderly patients by their proper names. Do not use terms like *sweetie* or *dearie*.
- G If the patient indicates that he has an impairment of some kind, follow the appropriate guidelines listed above.

Patients with Intellectual Disabilities

Developmental disabilities refer to disabilities that are present at birth or emerge during childhood, up to age 22. Intellectual disability is the most common developmental disability. An intellectual disability is neither a disease nor a mental health disorder. People with an intellectual disability develop at a below-average rate. They have below-average mental functioning. There are four different degrees of this disability: mild, moderate, severe, and profound. Depending on the level of disability, a person may have a legally designated representative for issues such as medical consent.

Guidelines: Intellectual Disability

- G Introduce yourself by name and title.
- G Describe the procedure you will perform, watching for indications that the patient understands.
- G Treat adult patients as adults, regardless of their intellectual abilities.
- G Give the patient the opportunity to ask questions. Answer questions within your scope of practice.
- G Remain calm and patient even if there are repeated questions.
- G Watch closely for nonverbal cues that the patient is confused, unsure, or anxious. Slow down and reassure as necessary.

Autism spectrum disorder (ASD) is a type of developmental disability that can result in differences in how people relate to others and communicate. Patients with ASD may seem withdrawn, and may find communication challenging. They may not be comfortable making eye contact or speaking to unfamiliar people. New situations can be overwhelming for patients with ASD, so it is essential to treat them with empathy, patience, and respect.

People Who Speak Limited or No English

According to the US Census Bureau, over 15% of adults in the United States speak a language other than English in their homes. In some communities this number is higher. As noted in Chapter 2, patients have a right to receive information about their medical care in a language they understand. Healthcare settings can be difficult to understand and even frightening, no matter the language a person speaks. This is especially true for patients whose first language is not English.

Guidelines: Patients Who Are Non-Native Speakers of English

- **G** Be familiar with the interpretation services available at your facility and use them when they are needed (Fig. 3-11).

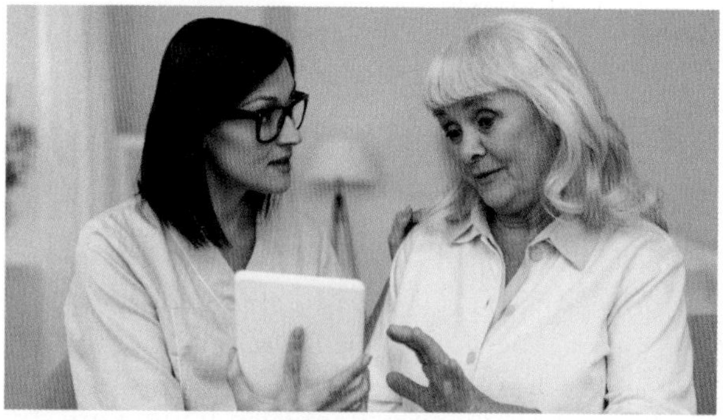

Fig. 3-11. Facilities may use computer-based interpretation services.

- **G** Watch for signs that a patient does not understand what you are saying. Sometimes people are afraid to ask for help when they do not understand.
- **G** Do not rely on a patient's friend or family member to translate medical information.
- **G** If you live in an area in which a particular language is spoken, learning some simple phrases in that language can help put a patient at ease.

Most patients a phlebotomist works with are likely to be polite and easy to work with. Occasionally patients might pose more of a challenge. Whether due to illness, anxiety, frustration, or personality, patients may display combative (meaning angry or hostile) or inappropriate behavior. The way a PBT communicates in these situations can determine whether the situation improves or worsens. Sometimes the best choice is to get help from a supervisor. If a phlebotomist ever feels threatened or unsafe, he should contact a supervisor immediately.

Guidelines: Combative, Angry, or Inappropriate Behavior

- **G** Stay calm. Do not argue or respond to verbal attacks.
- **G** Allow the patient time to calm down.
- **G** Lower the tone of your voice.
- **G** Be flexible and patient.
- **G** Try to find out what is causing the patient's behavior. Using silence may help the patient explain. Listen attentively as the patient speaks.
- **G** Stay at a safe distance if the patient becomes combative.
- **G** If a patient makes an inappropriate or sexual comment, address the behavior directly, saying something like, "That makes me uncomfortable." If the patient persists, call for help immediately.
- **G** If a patient attempts to physically strike you, block the blow or step out of the way, but never hit back. Get help immediately (Fig. 3-12).

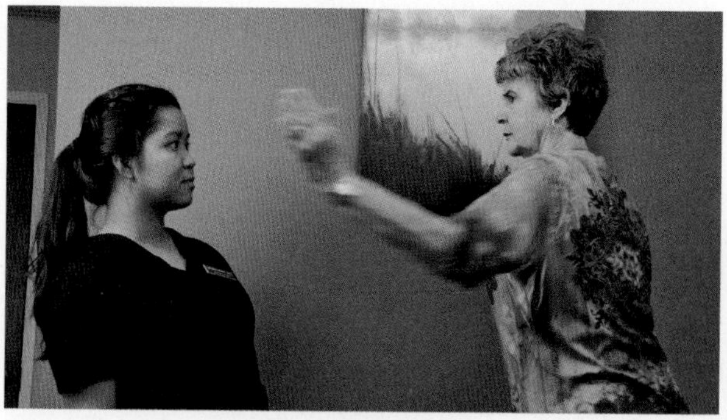

Fig. 3-12. When dealing with combative patients, step out of the way, but never hit back.

G Always report inappropriate behavior to a supervisor, even if you think it was harmless.

Chapter Review

Multiple Choice

1. Which of these describes the correct order of the 3-step form of communication?
   (A) Sender sends a message; receiver receives a message; receiver responds
   (B) Sender sends a message; receiver sends a message; sender responds
   (C) Sender receives a message; sender responds; receiver responds
   (D) Receiver receives a message; receiver responds; sender receives response

2. This is an example of nonverbal communication:
   (A) A doctor writes an order for a blood test on a piece of paper
   (B) A patient paces back and forth and does not sit down at the drawing station
   (C) A patient speaks to the phlebotomy technician through the hospital's tablet-based translation program
   (D) A patient gives one-word answers

3. A phlebotomy technician tells a patient, "Depending on what your results are from these tests, I'd get a second opinion." Which of the following is true?
   (A) This fulfills the PBT's professional responsibility to be honest with all patients.
   (B) This is standard language that should be used with all patients to ensure they get the best care.
   (C) The PBT is not giving the patient enough information to act on and should be more specific.
   (D) The PBT should not offer this or any other advice to a patient.

4. Which of these phrases best indicates that a PBT is engaging in active listening?
   (A) "Is that all?"
   (B) "Let's go ahead and do the draw, then."
   (C) "Tell me more about that."
   (D) "Oh, I've heard it all before!"

5. "The doctor ordered a CBC, stat." This sentence would be most appropriate when spoken by the
   (A) Clinic coordinator to a phlebotomist
   (B) Phlebotomist to a minor patient's parent
   (C) Phlebotomist to an adult patient
   (D) Clinic coordinator to an adult patient

6. The military time notation *2135* can also be expressed as
   (A) 9:35 p.m.
   (B) 9:35 a.m.
   (C) 11:35 p.m.
   (D) 11:35 a.m.

7. What must happen after a doctor orders a blood test orally in an emergency situation?
   (A) The phlebotomy technician must wait until the order is placed electronically or in writing before performing the blood draw.
   (B) A nurse or other licensed medical professional must confirm the order before the phlebotomy technician draws blood.
   (C) The phlebotomy technician draws the blood right away, but a written or electronic order must be created at some point.
   (D) The phlebotomy technician draws the blood right away; doctors' orders do not need to be documented in emergency situations.

8. Which of the following is the most appropriate statement to put in an incident report?
   (A) "Mrs. Johnson is scared of needles and the sight of the needle made her pass out and bump her head."
   (B) "Mrs. Johnson lost consciousness as the phlebotomy technician was preparing the needle to perform a blood draw. Her head struck the supply cart. She did not bleed and there was no bruising."
   (C) "Mrs. Johnson passed out and knocked her head. It's my fault because she told me the sight of needles makes her light-headed and I didn't really listen."
   (D) "Mrs. Johnson passed out when she saw the needle before a blood draw. Her head struck the supply cart but I don't think she has a concussion. There was no blood or bruising."

9. How should a phlebotomy technician approach a patient known to have a hearing impairment?
   (A) From the front, making sure the patient sees her
   (B) From the back, with a tap on the shoulder
   (C) Exactly as she would approach any patient
   (D) From the side, checking as she approaches that the patient's hearing aid is in

10. Which of the following is true of patients with cognitive impairment?
   (A) They will always have a legal representative accompanying them.
   (B) Because they cannot understand the procedure, there is no need to explain or seek consent.
   (C) Limiting smiling and nonverbal communication will reduce misunderstandings.
   (D) Nonverbal cues from patients with cognitive impairment can be especially important.

11. A phlebotomy technician is preparing to perform a blood draw on a patient who looks confused and unsettled. He asks the patient if she has any questions. She leans forward as if to listen closely, then shrugs and says, "I don't understand." Which of the following is the best response?
   (A) "I can see you're a bit nervous. Just let me know if you have questions or need me to explain something."
   (B) "It's OK, I'll talk slowly."
   (C) "Wait a moment while I call our interpreter."
   (D) "I won't talk, then. I'll just show you what to do."

12. Which of the following is true about sexual comments from a patient?
   (A) They should be reported even if the phlebotomy technician considers them harmless.
   (B) They should be reported only if the phlebotomy technician finds them threatening.
   (C) They should be reported only if they continue after the phlebotomy technician asks the patient to stop.
   (D) They should be reported only if there is any chance the patient will return to the facility and make similar comments again.

4

Infection Prevention and Control

1. Define *infection prevention* and discuss types of infections

Infection prevention is the set of methods practiced in healthcare facilities to prevent and control the spread of disease. Preventing the spread of infection is very important and is the responsibility of all care team members. Phlebotomy technicians must know and follow their facility's policies relating to infection prevention; these policies help protect staff members, patients, visitors, and others from disease.

A microorganism, also called a *microbe*, is a living thing that is so small it is only visible under a microscope. Microorganisms are always present in the environment (Fig. 4-1).

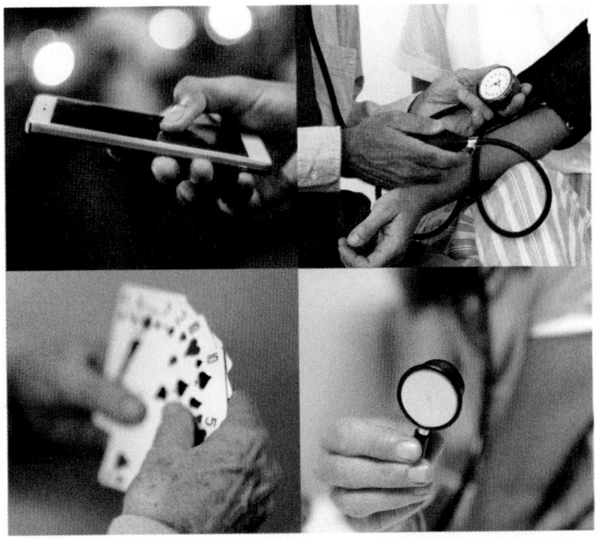

Fig. 4-1. *Microorganisms are always present in the environment. They are on almost everything a person touches.*

Microorganisms are always on and in the human body. **Infections** occur when harmful microorganisms, called **pathogens**, invade the body and multiply. The bacteria that normally exist in the body are called *normal flora*. These bacteria can become pathogens and cause infection if they invade an area outside of their normal range. Bacteria such as *Escherichia coli* (*E. coli*) and *Staphylococcus aureus* are part of the normal human flora but can also cause illness.

There are two main types of infections: localized and systemic. A **localized infection** is an infection that is limited to a specific location in the body. It has local symptoms, which means the symptoms are near the site of infection. For example, if a wound becomes infected, the area around it may become red, swollen, warm, and painful. A **systemic infection** affects the entire body. This type of infection travels through the bloodstream and is spread throughout the body. It causes general symptoms, such as fever, chills, or mental confusion.

A **healthcare-associated infection** (**HAI**), formerly called *nosocomial infection*, is an infection acquired in a healthcare setting during the delivery of medical care. It can be either localized or systemic. Healthcare settings include hospitals, outpatient surgery centers, and long-term care facilities, among others. HAIs can be transmitted from healthcare workers to patients or through equipment at the facility.

Some of the most common HAIs include urinary tract infections (often associated with the use of catheters), bloodstream infections associated with central lines (intravenous lines used to quickly provide fluids, blood, or medicines), and diarrhea or nausea caused by *Clostridioides difficile* (*C. diff* or *C. difficile*), formerly *Clostridium difficile. C. diff* can be extremely difficult to eliminate because the bacteria are spread by spores that are not killed by alcohol-based hand rubs. These spores can live on surfaces for months or even years. This illustrates clearly how improper or insufficient cleaning can contribute to the spread of HAIs. HAIs are a serious issue for patient health and well-being. It is essential for all healthcare workers to follow their facilities' policies to prevent the spread of illnesses.

Quality Counts

Every healthcare worker has a responsibility for preventing infection. PBTs can do their part by following all facility policies related to infection prevention. Performing proper handwashing, handling specimens carefully, maintaining high standards of cleanliness, and taking care not to expose patients to illnesses are some ways PBTs can reduce the spread of infection. Pediatric patients and patients with compromised immune systems are especially vulnerable to infectious illnesses. Special precautions may be necessary when caring for these patients. It is vital that PBTs exercise extreme care in these situations.

Although phlebotomy technicians usually have only brief contact with any one patient, they should be able to recognize the signs and symptoms of localized and systemic infections. Signs and symptoms of a localized infection include the following:

- Pain
- Redness
- Swelling
- Pus
- Drainage (fluid from a wound or cavity)
- Heat

Signs and symptoms of a systemic infection include the following:

- Fever
- Body aches
- Chills
- Nausea
- Vomiting
- Weakness
- Headache
- Mental confusion

It is often not possible to tell from looking at a person or even by reading her medical chart whether or not she is ill or has an infection. Because of this, PBTs should take precautions in dealing with every patient. (These precautions are outlined in Learning Objective 3.)

2. Describe the chain of infection

To understand how to prevent disease, it is helpful to first understand how it is spread. The **chain of infection** is a way of describing how disease is transmitted from one human being to another (Fig. 4-2). Definitions and examples of each of the six links in the chain of infection follow.

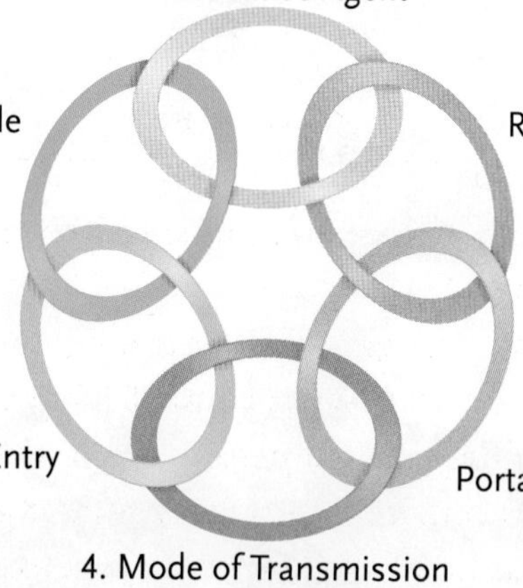

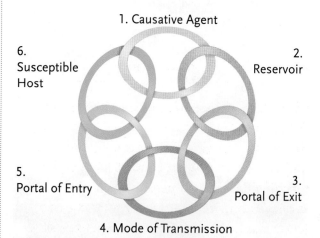

Fig. 4-2. *The chain of infection.*

Chain Link 1: The **causative agent** is a pathogenic microorganism that causes disease.

Microorganisms are small living bodies that cannot be seen without a microscope. They are everywhere—on skin, in food, in the air, and in water. Causative agents include bacteria, viruses, fungi, and parasites.

Chain Link 2: A **reservoir** is where the pathogen lives and multiplies. A reservoir can be a human, animal, plant, soil, or substance. Warm, dark, and moist places are the ideal environments for microorganisms to live, grow, and multiply. Some microorganisms need oxygen to survive, while others do not. Examples of reservoirs include the lungs, blood, and the large intestine.

Chain Link 3: The **portal of exit** is any body opening on an infected person that allows pathogens to leave (Fig. 4-3). These include the nose, mouth, eyes, or nonintact skin.

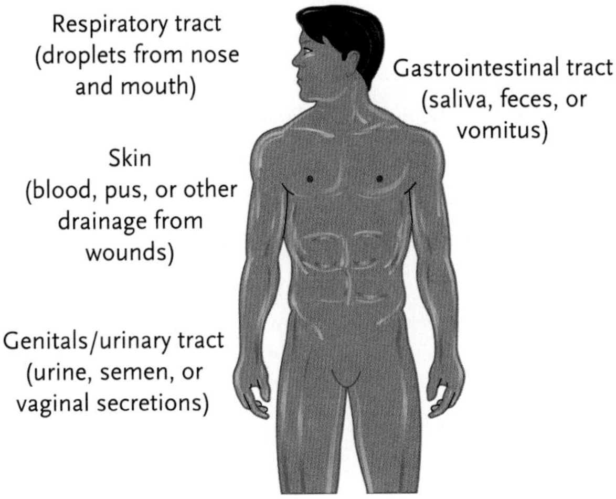

Fig. 4-3. Portals of exit.

Chain Link 4: The **mode of transmission** describes how the pathogen travels. Transmission can occur through the air or through direct or indirect contact. **Direct contact** happens by touching the infected person or his secretions. **Indirect contact** results from touching an object contaminated by the infected person, such as a needle, dressing, tissue, or bed linen. The primary route of disease transmission within the healthcare setting is via the hands of healthcare workers.

Chain Link 5: The **portal of entry** is any body opening on an uninfected person that allows pathogens to enter (Fig. 4-4). These include the nose, mouth, eyes, and other mucous membranes, cuts in the skin, and cracked skin. **Mucous membranes** are the membranes that line body cavities that open to the outside of the body. These include the linings of the mouth, nose, eyes, rectum, and genitals.

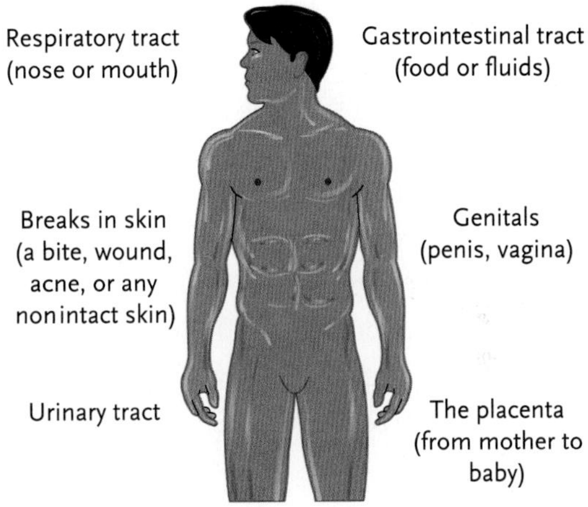

Fig. 4-4. Portals of entry.

Chain Link 6: A **susceptible host** is an uninfected person who could become ill. Examples include all healthcare workers and anyone in their care who is not already infected with that particular disease.

If one of the links in the chain of infection is broken, then the spread of infection is stopped. Infection prevention practices help stop pathogens from traveling (Link 4) and from getting on a person's hands, nose, eyes, mouth, skin, etc. (Link 5). Immunizations (Link 6) reduce a person's chances of getting sick from diseases such as hepatitis B and influenza.

Transmission (passage or transfer) of most **infectious** diseases can be blocked by using proper infection prevention practices, such as handwashing. Handwashing is the most important way to stop the spread of infection. All caregivers should wash their hands often.

Handwashing is a part of medical asepsis. **Medical asepsis** refers to measures used to reduce and prevent the spread of pathogens. Medical asepsis is used in all healthcare settings. In addition to washing hands regularly, phlebotomy technicians take measures like wearing gloves and disinfecting the blood draw site. These are also forms of medical asepsis.

Surgical asepsis makes an object or area completely free of all microorganisms (not just pathogens). Procedures requiring this level of precautions are said to be performed using *sterile technique*. Such procedures are generally considered beyond the scope of practice for entry-level phlebotomy technicians, but it is important that PBTs understand the concepts involved. Sterile technique requires sterile gloves (and any other necessary personal protective equipment, such as a mask, gown, and shoe or hair cover), sterile equipment, and the creation of a *sterile field*, or microorganism-free work area.

3. Explain Standard Precautions

State and federal agencies have guidelines and laws concerning infection prevention. The **Occupational Safety and Health Administration** (**OSHA**, osha.gov) is a federal government agency that makes rules to protect workers from hazards on the job. The **Centers for Disease Control and Prevention** (**CDC**, cdc.gov) is a federal government agency that issues guidelines to protect and improve the health of individuals and communities. Through education, the CDC aims to prevent and control disease, injury, and disability, as well as to promote public health.

The CDC created an infection prevention system to reduce the risk of contracting infectious diseases in healthcare settings. There are two levels of precautions within the CDC's infection prevention system: Standard Precautions and Transmission-Based Precautions.

Following **Standard Precautions** means treating blood, body fluids, nonintact skin (like abrasions, pimples, or open sores), and mucous membranes as if they were infected. Body fluids include tears, saliva, sputum (mucus coughed up), urine, feces, semen, vaginal secretions, pus or other wound drainage, and vomit. They do not include sweat because the concentration of potential pathogens in sweat is too low to be considered a risk.

Standard Precautions must be used with every patient; this promotes safety. A phlebotomy technician cannot tell by looking at patients or even by viewing their medical charts whether patients have a contagious disease such as tuberculosis, hepatitis, or influenza. Many diseases can be spread even before the infected person shows signs or has been diagnosed.

Standard Precautions and Transmission-Based Precautions (see Learning Objective 6) are ways to stop the spread of infection by interrupting the mode of transmission. In other words, these guidelines do not stop an infected person from giving off pathogens. However, by following these guidelines, the phlebotomy technician helps prevent those pathogens from infecting her or her patients.

Guidelines: Standard Precautions

- **Wash your hands** before putting on gloves and immediately after removing gloves. Be careful not to touch clean objects with your used gloves.
- **Wear gloves** if you may come into contact with any of the following: blood; body fluids or secretions; broken or open skin, such as abrasions, acne, cuts, stitches, or staples; or mucous membranes. Phlebotomy technicians must wear gloves every time they perform a blood draw.
- **Remove gloves** immediately when finished with a procedure and wash or sanitize your hands using an alcohol-based hand rub.

G **Immediately wash all skin surfaces that have been contaminated** with blood and body fluids.

G **Wear a disposable gown** that is resistant to body fluids if you may come into contact with blood or body fluids or when splashing or spraying of blood or body fluids is likely. If a patient has a contagious illness, wear a gown even if it is not likely you will come into contact with blood or body fluids. Phlebotomy technicians working in outpatient settings may rarely or never need to take these precautions, but in other settings they might be necessary.

G **Wear a mask and protective goggles and/or a face shield** if you may come into contact with blood or body fluids or when splashing or spraying of blood or body fluids is likely.

G **Use caution with needles, devices for capillary punctures (known as lancets), and other sharp objects**. Place sharps carefully in a puncture-proof biohazard container, sometimes called a *sharps container*. **Sharps** are needles or other sharp objects. Biohazard containers used for sharps are puncture-resistant, leakproof containers. They are color coded, clearly labeled, and warn of the danger of the contents inside (Figs. 4-5 and 4-6). They must be closable and kept in an upright position to keep items inside from spilling out. They should not be filled past the line indicating that the container is full. Biohazard bags are used for biomedical waste that is not sharp, such as soiled dressings, contaminated tubing, and other items. OSHA recommends that biomedical/ biohazard waste be disposed of at the *point of origin*, or where the waste occurs.

G **Never attempt to recap needles** or sharps after use. You might stick yourself. Most equipment used in blood draws includes safety mechanisms to reduce the risk of accidental needlesticks. Always engage these safety devices before disposing of the sharps in the appropriate biohazard container. Some newer devices can be engaged while the needle is still in the patient's arm, further reducing the phlebotomist's risk of accidental needlesticks.

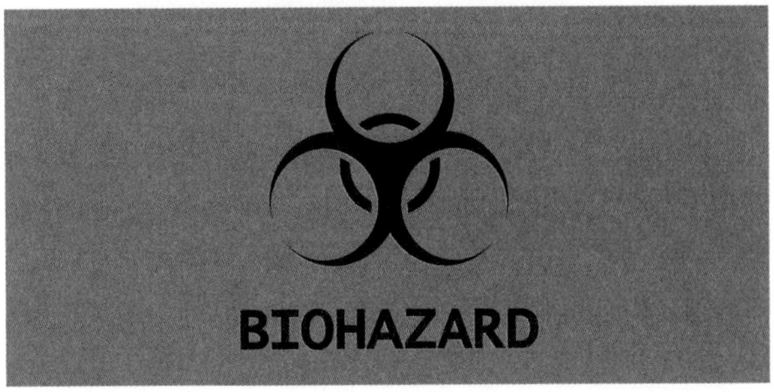

Fig. 4-5. This label indicates that the material is potentially infectious.

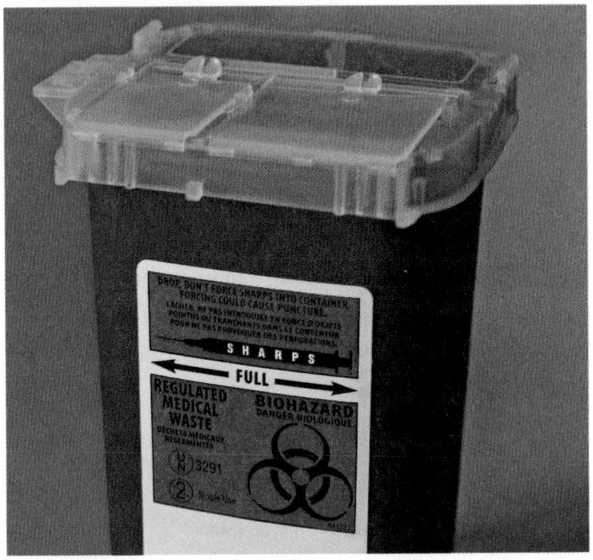

Fig. 4-6. One type of container for sharps.

G **Carefully bag all contaminated supplies**. Depending on policy, you may need to double bag some items. This means putting the contaminated bag into another bag. Discard contaminated items according to policy.

G **Clearly label body fluids that are being saved for a specimen** according to facility policy. Labeling must be on the specimen container itself and not on the lid or cap. Keep specimens in the appropriate container and place them in a biohazard specimen bag for transportation if required. More details regarding handling and transportation of blood and nonblood specimens is found in Chapters 9, 10, and 11.

G **Discard contaminated wastes according to your facility's policy**. Waste containing blood or body fluids is considered biohazardous waste. Wear proper personal protective equipment, then remove it when care is done and wash your hands.

Standard Precautions should always be practiced with all patients, regardless of their infection status. This greatly reduces the risk of transmitting infection. There is more information about Standard Precautions in the next several learning objectives.

4. Explain hand hygiene and identify when to wash hands

Phlebotomy technicians use their hands constantly while they work. Microorganisms are on everything they touch. The single most common way for HAIs to be spread is via the hands of healthcare workers. Handwashing is the most important thing PBTs can do to prevent the spread of disease (Fig. 4-7).

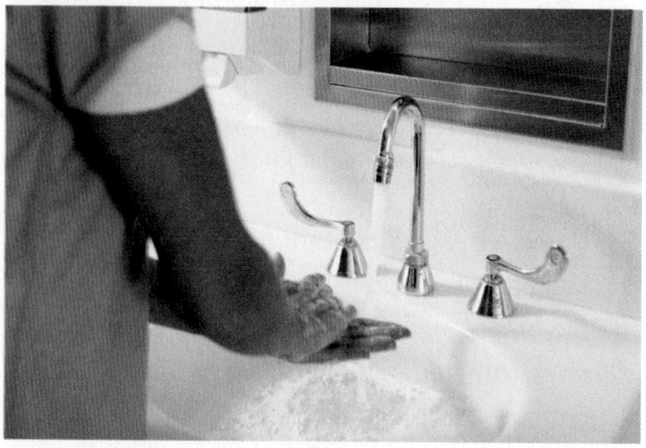

Fig. 4-7. *All people working in health care must wash their hands often. Handwashing is the most effective way to prevent the spread of disease.*

The CDC has defined **hand hygiene** as washing hands with soap and water or using alcohol-based hand rubs. Alcohol-based hand rubs (often referred to as *hand sanitizer*) include gels, rinses, and foams that do not require the use of water. Alcohol-based hand rubs have proven effective in reducing bacteria on the skin. However, they are not a substitute for frequent, proper handwashing. Some pathogens are not eliminated by hand rubs. When hands are visibly soiled, they should be washed using soap and water. Hand rubs can be used in addition to handwashing any time hands are not visibly soiled, though hands should still be washed with soap and water periodically throughout the day. Some facilities will have policies regarding the frequency of handwashing (e.g., PBTs can use hand rubs no more than twice in a row before washing hands with soap and water). When using a hand rub, the hands must be rubbed together until the product has completely dried. Hand lotion can help prevent dry, cracked skin.

Phlebotomy technicians should avoid wearing rings or bracelets while working because the jewelry may increase the risk of contamination. (Smooth, plain bands may be acceptable at some facilities.) Fingernails should be short, smooth, and clean. Artificial nails (acrylic, gel, or wraps) should not be worn, because they harbor bacteria and increase the risk of contamination even if hands are washed often. Standard nail polish may be allowed, but because chipped polish can also harbor bacteria, healthcare workers should avoid wearing it. Phlebotomists should wash their hands at these times:

- When first arriving at work
- Whenever hands are visibly soiled (must always wash with soap and water in this situation)
- Before, between, and after all contact with patients
- Before putting on gloves and after removing gloves
- After contact with any body fluids, mucous membranes, nonintact skin, or wound dressings

- After handling contaminated items
- After contact with any object in a patient's room (care environment)
- Before and after using the toilet
- After touching garbage or trash
- After picking up anything from the floor
- After blowing the nose, wiping the nose, or coughing or sneezing into the hands
- Before and after eating
- After smoking
- After touching areas on the body, such as the mouth, face, eyes, hair, ears, or nose
- Before and after applying makeup
- After any contact with pets (in the case of mobile phlebotomists who perform procedures in a patient's home)
- Before leaving the facility

Washing hands (hand hygiene)

Equipment: soap, paper towels

1. Turn on the water at the sink. Keep your clothes dry because moisture breeds bacteria. Do not let your clothing touch the outside portion of the sink or counter.
2. Wet your hands and wrists thoroughly (Fig. 4-8).

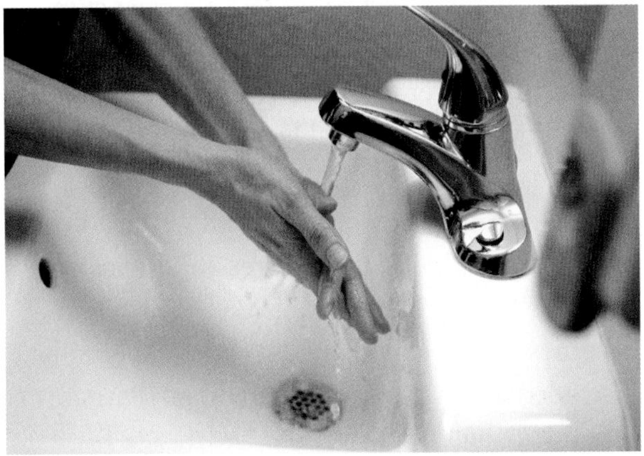

Fig. 4-8. *Keeping arms angled downward, wet hands and wrists thoroughly.*

3. Apply soap to your hands.
4. Keep your hands lower than your elbows and your fingertips down. Rub your hands together and fingers between each other to create a lather. Lather all surfaces of your wrists, hands, and fingers, using friction for at least 20 seconds. Friction helps clean (Fig. 4-9).

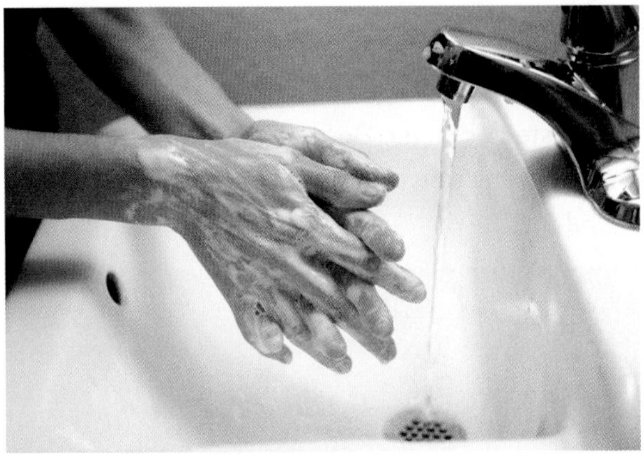

Fig. 4-9. *Using friction for at least 20 seconds, lather all surfaces of wrists, hands, and fingers.*

5. Clean your fingernails by rubbing them in the palm of your other hand.
6. Keep your hands lower than your elbows and your fingertips down. Being careful not to touch the sink, rinse thoroughly under running water. Rinse all surfaces of your wrists and hands. Run water down from your wrists to your fingertips (Fig. 4-10). Do not run water over unwashed arms down to clean hands.

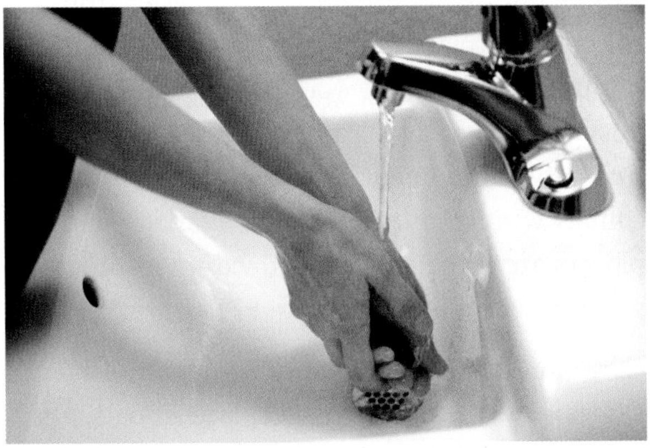

Fig. 4-10. *Rinse your wrists and hands thoroughly without touching the sink. Let water run down from wrists to fingertips.*

7. Use a clean, dry paper towel to dry all surfaces of your fingers, hands, and wrists, starting at the fingertips. Do not wipe the towel on your unwashed forearms and then wipe your clean hands. Discard the towel in the waste container without touching the container. If your hands touch the sink or wastebasket, start over.
8. Use a clean, dry paper towel to turn off the faucet (Fig. 4-11). Discard the towel in the waste container. Do not contaminate your hands by touching the surface of the sink or faucet.

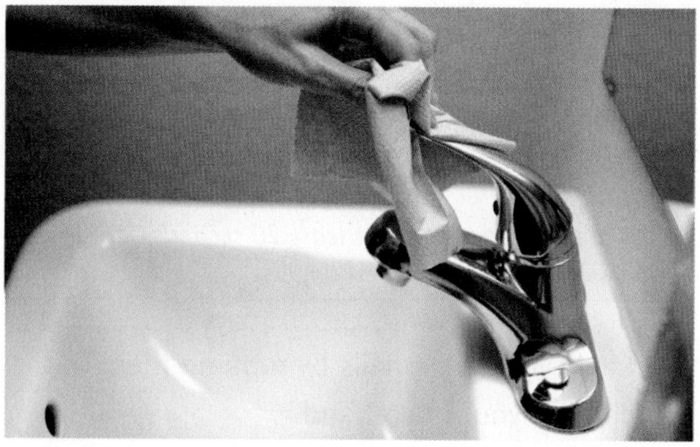

Fig. 4-11. *Use a clean, dry paper towel to turn off the faucet, so that you do not contaminate your hands.*

5. Discuss the use of personal protective equipment (PPE)

Personal protective equipment (**PPE**) is equipment that helps protect employees from serious workplace injuries or illnesses resulting from contact with workplace hazards. In hospitals, laboratories, and other healthcare settings, this equipment helps protect workers from contact with potentially infectious material. Employers are responsible for providing healthcare workers with the appropriate PPE to wear.

Common personal protective equipment includes gowns, masks, goggles, face shields, and gloves. Gowns protect the skin and/or clothing. Masks protect the mouth and nose. Goggles protect the eyes. Face shields protect the entire face—the eyes, nose, and mouth. Gloves protect the hands. Gloves are used most often by all healthcare workers. Although they are not generally considered PPE, phlebotomy technicians often wear lab coats or jackets during their work, and these garments also provide some amount of protection.

Phlebotomy technicians work with blood and are performing an **invasive procedure**, meaning a procedure that involves inserting a foreign object into the patient's body. The skin is a natural barrier to infection, and any procedure that breaks the skin poses a risk of infection. Blood is a body fluid that can transmit disease. (Learning Objective 7 contains more information.) This means a PBT must take special care with PPE to protect both the patient and himself from exposure to pathogens. In most situations, gloves are the only PPE a phlebotomy technician will use (with a new pair of gloves being used for each patient). In some cases, however, PBTs might need to wear, or **don**, gowns, masks, goggles, or face shields. This PPE is used when splashing or spraying of body fluids or blood could occur. Gowns and masks may also be used when performing procedures on patients with certain diagnoses. Hand hygiene should be performed before donning PPE and after removing and discarding PPE.

Gowns

Clean, nonsterile gowns protect exposed skin. They also prevent the soiling of clothing. Gowns should fully cover the torso from neck to knees. They should fit comfortably over the body, and have long sleeves that fit snugly at the wrists. Gowns can only be worn once before they need to be discarded. OSHA requires fluid-resistant gowns if fluid penetration is likely. If a gown becomes wet or soiled during care, it should be discarded and a new gown should be donned. When finished with a procedure, the PBT should remove, or **doff**, the gown as soon as possible and wash her hands.

Putting on (donning) and removing (doffing) a gown

1. Wash your hands.
2. Open the gown. Hold it out in front of you and allow the gown to open/unfold (Fig. 4-12). Do not shake the gown or touch it to the floor. Facing the back opening of the gown, place an arm through each sleeve.

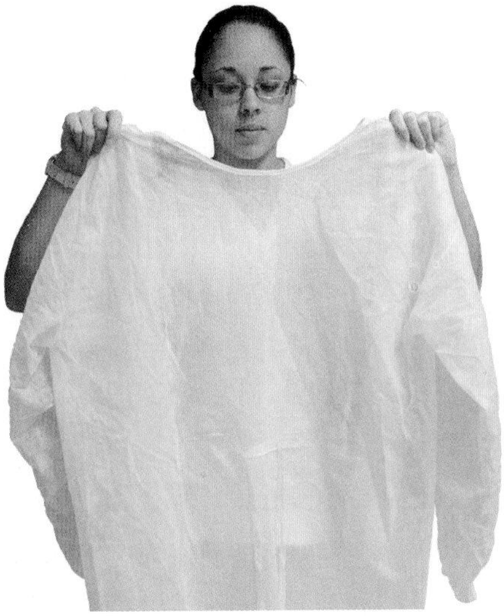

Fig. 4-12. *Let the gown unfold without shaking it.*

3. Fasten the neck opening.
4. Reaching behind you, pull the gown until it completely covers your clothing. Secure the gown at your waist (Fig. 4-13).

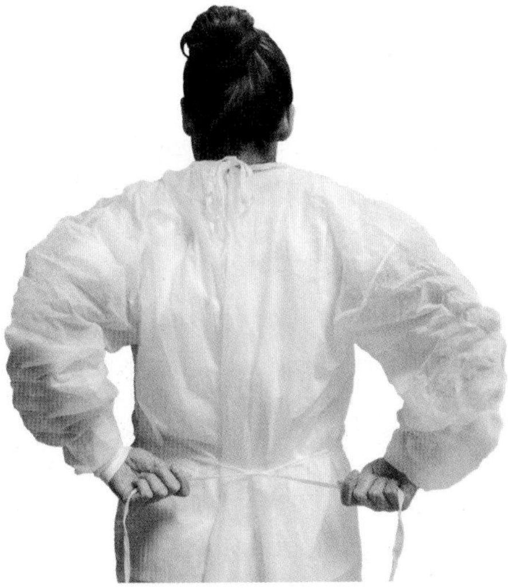

Fig. 4-13. *Reaching behind you, secure the gown at the waist.*

5. Put on your gloves after putting on the gown. The cuffs of the gloves should overlap the cuffs of the gown (Fig. 4-14).

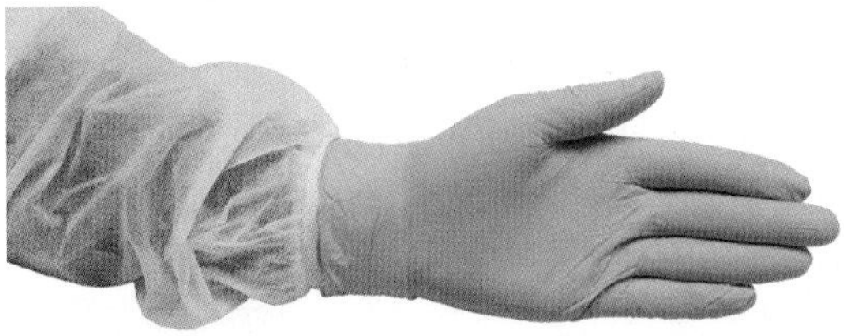

Fig. 4-14. *The cuffs of the gloves should overlap the cuffs of the gown.*

6. When removing a gown, first remove and discard gloves properly (see procedure later in the chapter). Then unfasten the gown at the waist and neck. Remove the gown without touching the outside of the gown. Roll the dirty side in, while holding the gown away from your body. Discard the gown properly and wash your hands.

Masks and Goggles

Masks can prevent inhalation of microorganisms through the nose or mouth. Masks should be worn when caring for patients with respiratory illnesses. They should also be worn when it is likely that contact with blood or body fluids may occur. Sometimes special masks called *respirators* are required for certain diseases, such as tuberculosis (TB). Masks should fully cover the nose and mouth and prevent fluid penetration. Masks should fit snugly over the nose and mouth.

Masks can be worn only once before they need to be discarded. Masks that become wet or soiled must be changed immediately without touching the outside of the soiled mask. If a phlebotomy technician cares for more than one patient who requires the use of a mask, she must change masks between patients.

Goggles provide protection for the eyes. Goggles are worn with a mask and are used whenever it is likely that blood or body fluids may be splashed or sprayed into the eye area or into the eyes. Only in very rare circumstances would a PBT need to don goggles for a blood draw (e.g., drawing blood from a trauma victim in the emergency room). Eyeglasses alone do not provide proper eye protection. Goggles should fit snugly over and around the eyes or eyeglasses.

Putting on (donning) a mask and goggles

1. Wash your hands.
2. Pick up the mask by the top strings or the elastic strap. Do not touch the mask where it touches your face.
3. Pull the elastic strap over your head, or if the mask has strings, tie the top strings first, then the bottom strings. Do not wear a mask hanging from only the bottom ties or straps.
4. Pinch the metal strip at the top of the mask (if part of the mask) tightly around your nose so that it feels snug (Fig. 4-15). Fit the mask snugly around your face and below the chin.

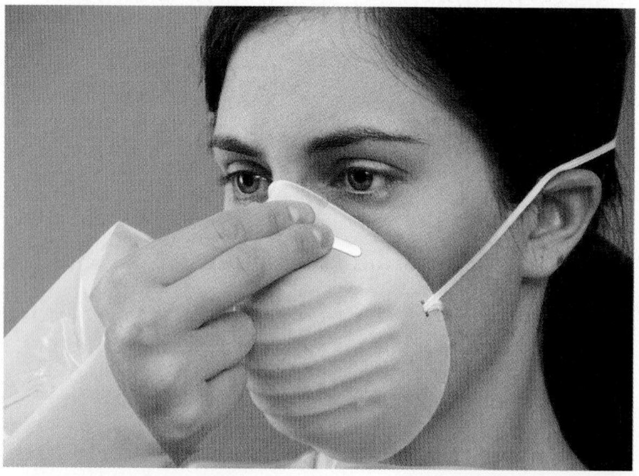

Fig. 4-15. *Adjust the metal strip until the mask fits snugly around your nose.*

5. Place the goggles over your eyes or eyeglasses. Use the headband or earpieces to secure them to your head. Make sure they are on snugly.
6. Put on gloves after putting on the mask and goggles.

Face Shields

Face shields may be worn when blood or body fluids may be splashed or sprayed into the eyes or eye area. A face shield can be substituted for a mask or goggles, or it can be worn with a mask. The face shield should cover the forehead, go below the chin, and wrap around the sides of the face. The headband can secure it to the head.

Gloves

Nonsterile gloves are used for basic care. They are available in different sizes, and may be made of nitrile, vinyl, or latex. However, due to allergy issues, some facilities have banned the use of latex gloves. In addition, in 2017 the Food and Drug Administration (FDA, fda.gov) banned the use of all powdered patient examination gloves. This is due to the powder posing numerous risks to patients and workers.

Gloves should fit the hands comfortably and should not be too loose or too tight. Facilities have specific policies and procedures on when to wear gloves. Phlebotomy technicians must learn and follow these rules. Disposable gloves can be worn only once; they cannot be washed or reused. Gloves should be changed immediately if they become wet, worn, soiled, or torn. After removing gloves, the PBT should wash or sanitize his hands before donning new gloves. Nonintact areas on the hands should be covered with bandages or gauze before putting on gloves.

Putting on (donning) gloves

1. Wash your hands.
2. If you are right-handed, slide one glove on your left hand (reverse if left-handed).
3. Using your gloved hand, slide the other hand into the second glove.
4. Interlace your fingers to smooth out folds and create a comfortable fit.

5. Carefully look for tears, holes, or discolored spots. Replace the glove if needed.
6. Adjust the gloves until they are pulled up over your wrist and fit correctly. If wearing a gown, pull the cuffs of the gloves over the sleeves of the gown (Fig. 4-16).

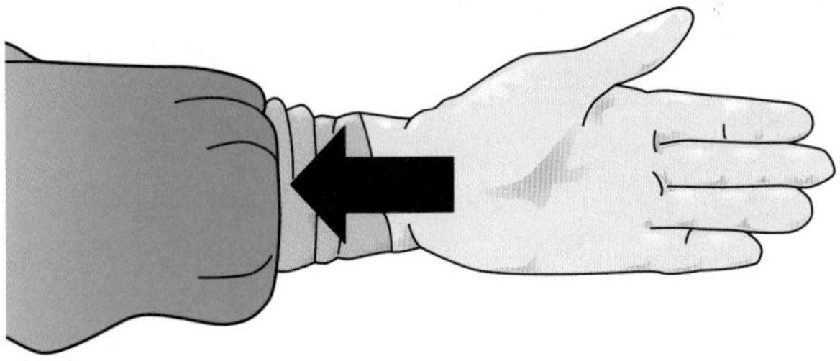

Fig. 4-16. *Adjust gloves until they are pulled up over the sleeves of the gown.*

Gloves should be removed, or doffed, promptly after use, and the PBT should wash his hands directly after removing gloves. He should be careful not to contaminate his skin or clothing when removing gloves. Gloves are worn to protect the skin from becoming contaminated. After giving care, gloves are contaminated. If the PBT opens a door with the gloved hand, the doorknob becomes contaminated. Later, anyone who opens the door with an ungloved hand will be touching a contaminated surface. Before touching surfaces or leaving the drawing station or a patient's room, the PBT must remove gloves and wash or sanitize his hands. Afterward, new gloves can be donned if necessary.

Removing (doffing) gloves

1. Touch only the outside of one glove. With one gloved hand, grasp the other glove at the palm and pull the glove off (Fig. 4-17).
2. With the fingertips of your gloved hand, hold the glove you just removed. With your ungloved hand, slip two fingers underneath the cuff of the remaining glove at the wrist. Do not touch any part of the outside of the glove (Fig. 4-18).

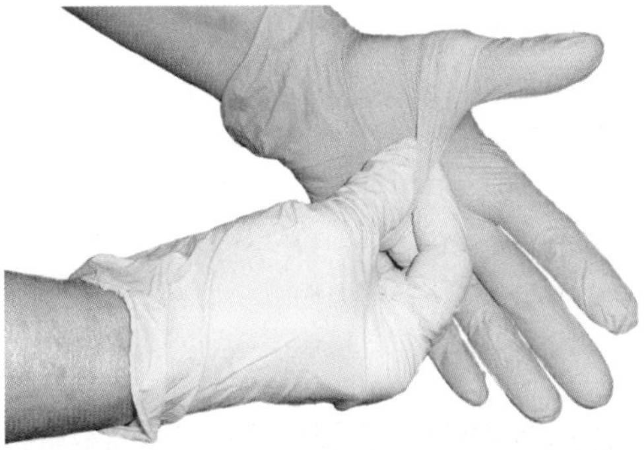

Fig. 4-17. *Grasp the glove at the palm and pull it off.*

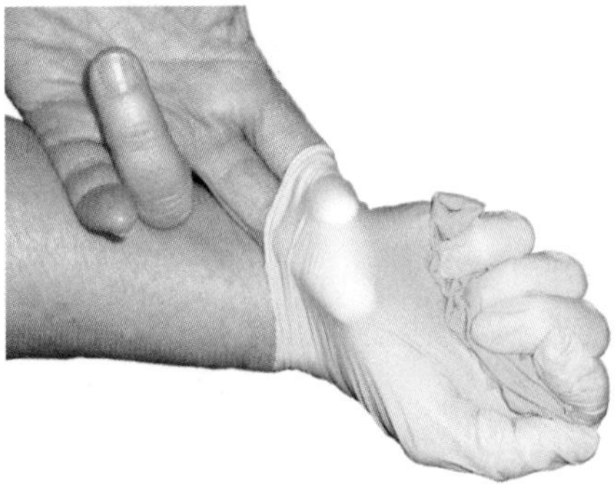

Fig. 4-18. *Reach inside the glove at the wrist, without touching any part of the outside of the glove.*

3. Pull down, turning this glove inside out and over the first glove as you remove it.
4. You should now be holding one glove from its clean inner side and the other glove should be inside it.
5. Drop both gloves into the proper container without contaminating yourself.
6. Wash your hands.

Employers provide personal protective equipment as needed. It is readily available and accessible in a variety of sizes. It is the PBT's responsibility to know where the equipment is kept and how to use it. A specific order must be followed when donning and doffing PPE.

Donning a full set of PPE

1. Wash your hands.
2. Put on the gown (Fig. 4-19).

3. Put on the mask and respirator.
4. Put on the goggles or face shield.
5. Put on gloves.

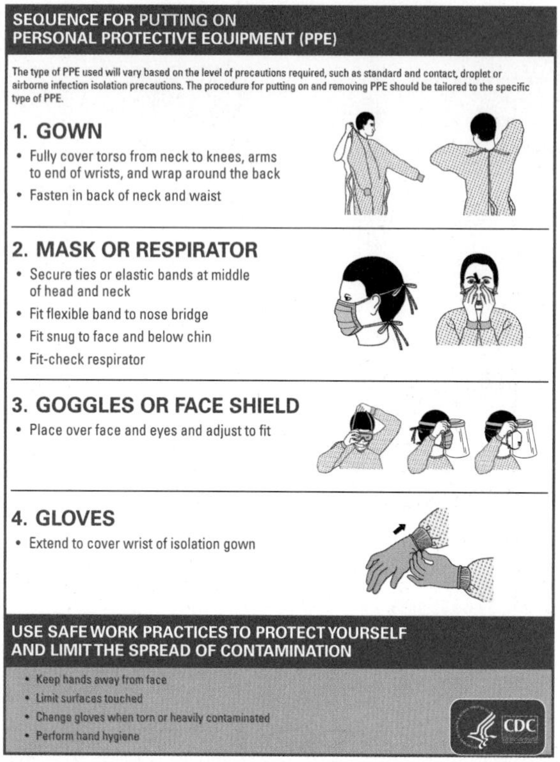

Fig. 4-19. Always follow this order when donning PPE.
(IMAGE REPRINTED FROM THE CDC'S WEBSITE, WWW.CDC.GOV/HAI/PDFS/PPE/PPE-SEQUENCE.PDF)

All personal protective equipment, except a respirator (if worn), must be removed before exiting the patient's room. A respirator is removed after leaving the room and closing the door.

Doffing a full set of PPE

1. Remove and discard gloves (Fig. 4-20).
2. Remove and discard the goggles and face shield.
3. Remove and discard the gown.
4. Remove and discard the mask.
5. Wash your hands. Washing hands is always the final step after removing and disposing of PPE.

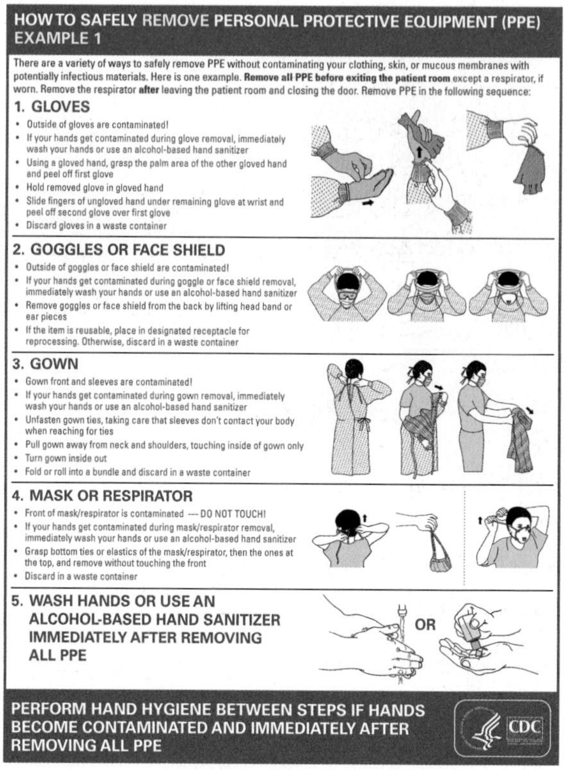

Fig. 4-20. Always follow this order when doffing PPE.
(IMAGE REPRINTED FROM THE CDC'S WEBSITE, WWW.CDC.GOV/HAI/PDFS/PPE/PPE-SEQUENCE.PDF)

Quality Counts

OSHA states that it is the employer's responsibility to instruct the staff on how to properly don PPE, how to wear PPE effectively, and how to safely doff PPE. This instruction needs to be given before the employee is in a situation requiring PPE, and as an annual review.

6. Explain Transmission-Based Precautions

The CDC set forth a second level of precautions beyond Standard Precautions. These guidelines are used for persons who are infected or may be infected with certain infectious diseases. These precautions are called **Transmission-Based Precautions**. When ordered, these precautions are used in addition to Standard Precautions. These precautions will always be listed in the patient's care plan and on the phlebotomy technician's assignment sheet. Following these precautions promotes the safety of staff members and patients.

There are three categories of Transmission-Based Precautions: Airborne Precautions, Droplet Precautions, and Contact Precautions. The category used depends on what type of pathogen or disease the person has or may have and how it spreads. These precautions may also be used in combination for diseases that have multiple routes of transmission. Conditions that require Transmission-Based Precautions in addition to Standard Precautions include the following:

- **Multidrug-resistant organisms (MDROs)** (microorganisms, mostly bacteria, that are resistant to one or more antimicrobial agents that are commonly used for treatment), such as methicillin-resistant *Staphylococcus aureus* (MRSA) and vancomycin-resistant *Enterococcus* (VRE)
- *C. diff*
- Scabies, a skin disease that causes itching
- Lice
- Influenza (during an outbreak)

Airborne Precautions

Airborne Precautions prevent the spread of pathogens that can be transmitted through the air after being expelled. The pathogens are able to remain floating in the air for some time. They are carried by moisture, air currents, and dust. Tuberculosis is an example of an airborne disease. Precautions include wearing special masks, such as N95 or HEPA respirators, to avoid being infected. The rooms of patients with airborne illnesses are likely to be specially ventilated to reduce the risk of pathogens leaving the room. This is known as an airborne infection isolation room (AIIR). When entering and exiting an AIIR, the PBT should open and close the door slowly and carefully to avoid pulling contaminated room air into the hallway.

Droplet Precautions

Droplet Precautions are used for diseases that are spread by droplets in the air. Droplets normally do not travel more than six feet. Talking, coughing, sneezing, laughing, singing, or suctioning can spread droplets. An example of a droplet disease is influenza.

Droplet Precautions include wearing a face mask when providing care and restricting visits from uninfected people. In addition, phlebotomy technicians should cover their noses and mouths with a tissue when they sneeze or cough and ask others to do the same. Used tissues should be disposed of in the nearest waste container. Used tissues should not be placed in a pocket for later use. If a tissue is not available, PBTs should cough or sneeze into their upper sleeve or elbow, not their hands. They should wash their hands immediately afterward. Patients should wear masks when being moved from room to room, and patient movement within the facility should be limited. Both the PBT and the patient should wear masks during a blood draw.

Quality Counts

The CDC has established special infection prevention measures to prevent the transmission of all respiratory infections in healthcare settings. They are a part of Standard Precautions and include the following:

1. Post visual alerts at the entrances of care facilities instructing that all patients and visitors inform staff of symptoms of respiratory infections and practice respiratory hygiene/cough etiquette.
2. All individuals with signs and symptoms of a respiratory infection must do the following:
   - Cover their noses/mouths with a tissue when coughing or sneezing.
   - Discard used tissues in the nearest no-touch waste container after use.
   - Perform hand hygiene after contact with respiratory secretions and contaminated objects.

   Healthcare facilities must make these items available to staff, patients, and visitors:
   - Tissues and no-touch receptacles for used tissue disposal
   - Conveniently located hand rub dispensers and handwashing supplies in areas where sinks are located
3. During times of increased respiratory infections, offer masks to anyone who is coughing, and

encourage coughing people to sit at least three feet away from others in waiting areas.

4. Advise healthcare personnel to observe Droplet Precautions, in addition to Standard Precautions, when examining a patient with symptoms of a respiratory infection, particularly if fever is present.

Contact Precautions

Contact Precautions are used when the patient is at risk of spreading an infection by direct contact with a person or object. The infection can be spread by touching a contaminated area on the patient's body or her blood or body fluids. It may also be spread by touching contaminated items, linen, equipment, or supplies. Conjunctivitis (pink eye) and *C. diff* infection are examples of situations that require Contact Precautions.

Contact Precautions include wearing gloves and a gown and patient isolation. To **isolate** means to keep something separate, or by itself. Contact Precautions require washing hands before and after care and not touching infected surfaces with ungloved hands or uninfected surfaces with contaminated gloves.

Staff often refer to patients who need Transmission-Based Precautions as being "in isolation." A sign should be on the door indicating *Contact Precautions* and alerting people to see the nurse before entering the room. Other guidelines for PBTs to follow include the following:

Guidelines: Isolation

G When they are indicated, Transmission-Based Precautions are always used in addition to Standard Precautions.

G Nurses will set up the isolation unit. Some facilities have a special room where isolation supplies are kept. Some facilities keep supplies within the room itself, while other facilities set up an isolation cart outside the room (Fig. 4-21). Isolation supplies consist of gloves, masks, gowns or aprons, shoe covers, and, if indicated, goggles, face shields, N95 respirators, or other forms of specialized PPE.

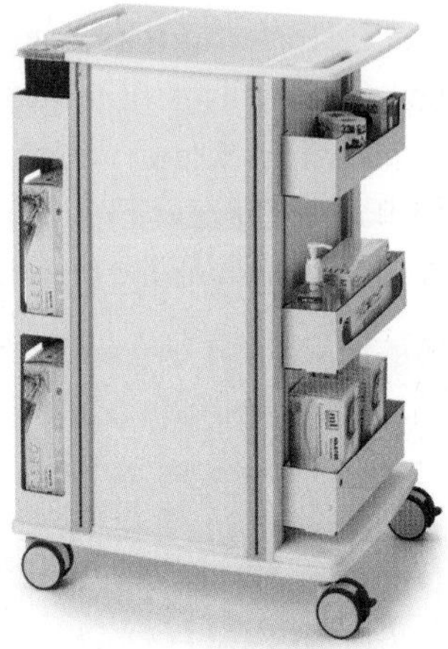

Fig. 4-21. *Isolation carts provide healthcare workers with easy access to the equipment they need to safely care for patients under Transmission-Based Precautions.*
(PHOTO COURTESY OF MARKETLAB, INC., WWW.MARKETLAB.COM)

G You will be told the proper PPE to wear for care of each patient in isolation. Make sure to put on PPE properly and remove it safely. Remove PPE and place it in the appropriate container before exiting a patient's room. PPE cannot be worn outside the patient's room. Perform hand hygiene following the removal of PPE and again after exiting the patient's room. In addition to handwashing areas inside the patient's room, there may be an alcohol-based hand rub dispenser mounted on the wall inside the room as you exit the door.

G When taking specimens from a patient in isolation, wear the proper PPE. Collect the specimen(s) and place in the appropriate container without the outside of the container coming into contact with the specimen(s). Properly remove your PPE and dispose of it in the room. Perform hand hygiene before leaving the room and transport the specimen according to facility policy.

G Do not share equipment between patients. Do not take a phlebotomy tray or caddy inside the patient's room. Use disposable supplies that can be discarded after use whenever possible. When using disposable supplies, such as tourniquets, discard them in the patient's room before leaving. Be careful not to contaminate reusable equipment by setting it on furniture or counters in the patient's room. Equipment such as blood glucose monitors and other point-of-care testing devices must be decontaminated after use if dedicated equipment (equipment that stays only with that patient) is not available.

Patients' Rights

Isolation

Basic human needs do not change while a patient is in isolation, even though physical conditions may change. The PBT should not rush through procedures with a patient in isolation or make him feel that he should be avoided. Receiving professional, empathetic, and competent care may help lessen a patient's worries or concerns about being isolated.

7. Define *bloodborne pathogens* and describe two major bloodborne diseases

Bloodborne pathogens are microorganisms found in human blood that can cause infection and disease in humans. They may also be found in body fluids, draining wounds, and mucous membranes. These pathogens are transmitted by infected blood entering the bloodstream, or if infected semen or vaginal secretions contact mucous membranes. Sharing or reusing needles is another way to spread bloodborne diseases. Infected pregnant women may transmit bloodborne diseases to their babies in the womb or at birth.

In health care, contact with infected blood or body fluids is the most common way to be infected with a bloodborne disease (Fig. 4-22). Infections can be spread through contact with contaminated blood or body fluids, needles or other sharp objects, or contaminated supplies or equipment. Following guidelines for Standard Precautions, including proper handwashing, and wearing PPE when indicated, can prevent transmission of bloodborne diseases. Employers are required by law to help prevent exposure to bloodborne pathogens (see the next learning objective for more detail).

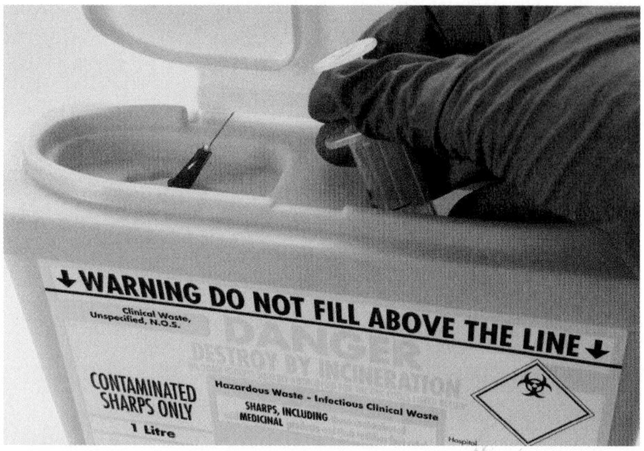

Fig. 4-22. Overfilled sharps containers increase the risk of accidental exposure to blood or body fluids.

Bloodborne diseases cannot be spread by casual contact. Phlebotomy technicians can safely touch and work with patients who have a bloodborne disease. These patients need the same thoughtful, personal attention given to all patients. PBTs need to follow Standard Precautions, but should never isolate patients emotionally because they have a bloodborne disease.

Two major bloodborne diseases in the United States are **acquired immunodeficiency syndrome** (**AIDS**) and the viral hepatitis family. *HIV* stands for **human immunodeficiency virus**, and it is the virus that can cause AIDS. Over time, HIV weakens the immune system so that the body cannot effectively fight infections. The final stage of HIV infection is AIDS. People with AIDS lose all ability to fight infection and can die from illnesses that a healthy immune system could handle. There is currently no vaccine available to prevent HIV infection.

Hepatitis is inflammation of the liver caused by certain viruses and other factors, such as alcohol abuse, some medications, and trauma. Liver function can be permanently damaged by hepatitis. Several viruses can cause hepatitis. The most common types of hepatitis are A, B, and C. Hepatitis B and C are bloodborne diseases that can cause death. Many more people have hepatitis B (HBV) than HIV. In the United States today, the risk of getting hepatitis is greater than the risk of acquiring HIV.

The virus causing hepatitis A (HAV) is a result of fecal-oral contamination, which means through food or water contaminated by stool from an infected person. HBV is a bloodborne disease. It is spread through sexual contact, by sharing infected needles, and from a mother to her baby during delivery. It can be spread through improperly sterilized needles used for tattoos and piercings and through grooming supplies, such as razors, nail clippers, and toothbrushes. It is also spread by exposure at work from accidental contact with infected needles or other sharps or from splashing blood. The hepatitis B virus can survive outside the body for at least seven days and can still cause infection in others during that time. HBV may cause few symptoms or may become a severe infection. At its most severe, HBV can cause liver damage, liver cancer, and death.

HBV is a serious threat to healthcare workers. Employers must offer phlebotomy technicians a free vaccine to protect them from hepatitis B. The hepatitis B vaccine is usually given as a series of three shots. Prevention is the best option for dealing with this disease, and employees should take the vaccine when it is offered.

Hepatitis C (HCV) is also transmitted through blood or body fluids. Hepatitis C can lead to cirrhosis and liver cancer; it can even cause death. There is no vaccine for hepatitis C and the virus can survive, and remain potentially infectious, for as long as six weeks on surfaces. Less common types of hepatitis in the United States are hepatitis D (HDV) and hepatitis E (HEV). Hepatitis D is transmitted by blood. It is found only in people who carry the hepatitis B virus. HEV is transmitted by the fecal-oral route, usually through contaminated water. Although HEV is rare in the United States, it is more common in many other parts of the world. There is no vaccine for hepatitis D or hepatitis E.

8. Explain OSHA's Bloodborne Pathogens Standard and the Needlestick Safety and Prevention Act

OSHA establishes standards for special procedures that must be followed in healthcare facilities. One of these is the **Bloodborne Pathogens Standard**. This law requires that healthcare facilities protect employees from bloodborne health hazards. By law, employers must follow these rules to reduce or eliminate the risk of exposure to infectious diseases. The standard also guides employers and employees through the steps to follow if exposed to infectious material. Significant exposures include the following:

- Exposure by injection; a needlestick
- Mucous membrane contact
- A cut from an object containing a potentially infectious body fluid (includes human bites)
- Having nonintact skin (OSHA includes acne in this category)

In 2000, the Needlestick Safety and Prevention Act was passed as an amendment to the Bloodborne Pathogens Standard. At that time, the CDC estimated that 600,000–800,000 needlestick or other sharps-related injuries occurred in healthcare settings each year. CDC research also indicated that 62–88% of these injuries could be prevented through the use of safer devices. **Engineering controls** are features incorporated in medical devices to make their use less hazardous. Retracting needles and hinged or sliding needle sheaths are engineering controls commonly used in phlebotomy (Fig. 4-23). The Needlestick Safety and Prevention Act made use of these devices mandatory.

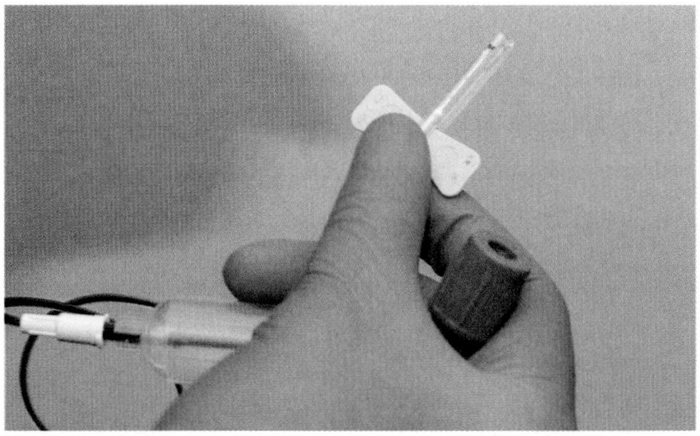

Fig. 4-23. *Engineering controls like needle sheaths can prevent accidental exposure to bloodborne pathogens.*

Guidelines employers must follow according to the Bloodborne Pathogens Standard and Needlestick Safety and Prevention Act include the following:

- Employers must have a written **exposure control plan** designed to eliminate or reduce employee exposure to infectious material. This plan identifies, step by step, what to do if an employee is exposed to infectious material (for example, if a PBT is stuck by a needle). This includes medical treatment and plans to prevent any similar exposures. It also includes specific work practices that must be followed. This plan must be accessible to all employees, and they must receive training on the plan.
- Employers must give all employees, visitors, and patients proper PPE to wear when needed at no cost. Employers must make sure PPE is available in the appropriate sizes and is readily accessible.
- Employers must make biohazard containers available for disposal of sharps and other infectious waste. These containers must be puncture-resistant, labeled or color coded, and leakproof. They must be emptied frequently to prevent overfilling.
- Employers must provide a free hepatitis B vaccine to all employees after hire.
- Warning labels must be affixed to waste containers and refrigerators and freezers that contain blood or any other potentially infectious material.
- Employers must keep a log of injuries from contaminated sharps. The information recorded must protect the confidentiality of the injured employee. Employers are also required to select safer needle devices and to involve employees in choosing these devices.
- Employers must provide in-service training on bloodborne pathogens and updates on any new safety standards at the time of hire and annually to all employees.
- When an employee is exposed to blood or other potentially infectious material, an incident report or a special exposure report form must be completed. Tests and follow-up care may be needed. The employer will take steps to prevent the employee from becoming sick. Steps will also be taken to help keep similar incidents from occurring again. Phlebotomy technicians must report any potential exposures immediately. Doing this helps protect their health and that of others. OSHA's website, osha.gov, has more information.

9. List guidelines for handling equipment and specimens

In health care, an object is called **clean** if it has not been contaminated with pathogens. An object that is **dirty** has been contaminated with pathogens. Measures such as disinfection and sterilization decrease the spread of pathogens that could cause disease.

Disinfection is a process that kills pathogens but does not destroy all pathogens. It reduces the pathogen count to a level that is considered not infectious. Disinfection is carried out with pasteurization or chemical germicides. Examples of items that are usually disinfected are countertops and other surfaces in a drawing station, collection chairs, and armrests (Fig. 4-24).

Multi-patient point-of-care testing devices such as glucose meters must also be disinfected after each use.

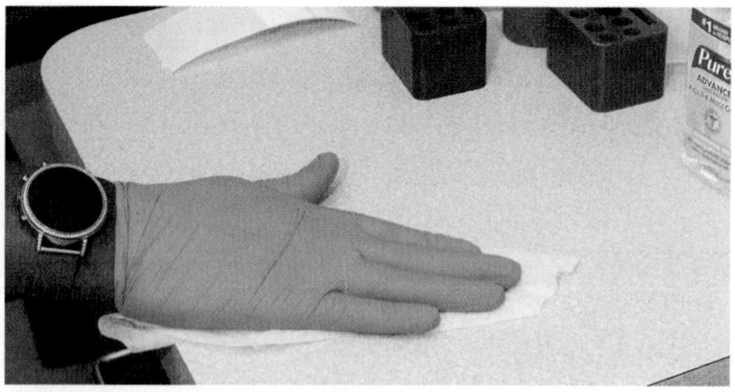

Fig. 4-24. Surfaces are disinfected after a blood draw is complete.

Sterilization is a cleaning measure that destroys all microorganisms, including pathogens. This includes those that form spores. Spore-forming microorganisms are a special group of organisms that produce a protective covering that is difficult to penetrate. Sterilization is part of surgical asepsis and is accomplished through the use of special machines and devices. An autoclave is a machine that sterilizes objects by using hot steam under pressure. Liquid or gas chemicals and dry heat are other ways to sterilize objects. Items that need to be sterilized are ones that go directly into the bloodstream or into other normally sterile areas of the body (for example, surgical instruments).

During most patient interactions, a phlebotomy technician is handling blood and needles. This creates the possibility of contact with pathogens. In following Standard Precautions, the PBT must treat every patient's blood as if it contains infectious microorganisms. This means the phlebotomy work area and patient specimens must be treated with great care.

Guidelines: Infection Prevention Measures for Handling Specimens

- G Don new gloves for every patient interaction.
- G Replace gloves any time they are wet, torn, or soiled.
- G Ensure that specimen tubes or containers are not leaking and that there is nothing on the outside of the container.
- G Place specimens in biohazard bags for transport (Fig. 4-25).
- G Follow facility policy regarding method of transport.
- G Never place needles or sharps in the transport bag or container with the specimen.
- G Follow any specific instructions/facility policy regarding specimens from patients under Transmission-Based Precautions.
- G After completing a blood draw, before calling the next patient, clean and disinfect all surfaces using a facility-approved antimicrobial agent.

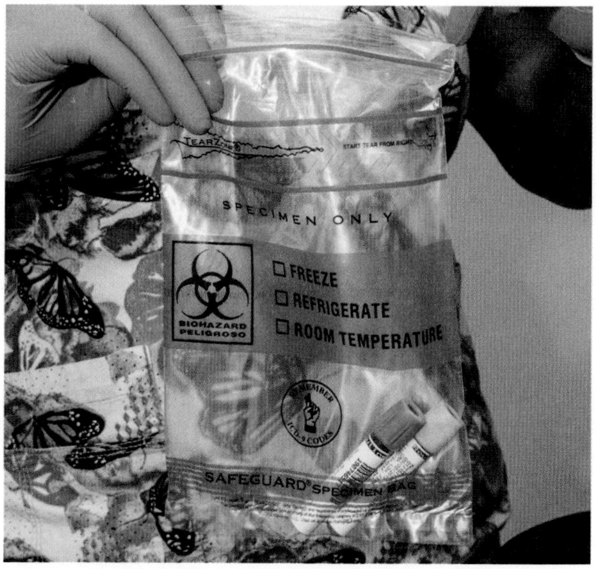

Fig. 4-25. Specimens must be transported in appropriately labeled biohazard bags or containers.

10. List employer and employee responsibilities for infection prevention

Several state and federal government agencies have guidelines and laws concerning infection prevention. OSHA requires employers to provide for the safety of their employees through rules and suggested guidelines. The CDC issues guidelines for healthcare workers to follow on the job. Some states have additional requirements. Facilities consider these rules very carefully when writing their policies and procedures. It is important that phlebotomy technicians learn these policies and procedures and follow them. They exist to protect all staff members and patients. Employers and employees both have key roles in infection prevention.

The employer's responsibilities for infection prevention include the following:

- Establish infection prevention procedures and an exposure control plan to protect workers
- Provide continuing in-service education on infection prevention, including education on bloodborne and airborne pathogens and updates on any new safety standards
- Have written procedures to follow should an exposure occur, including medical treatment and plans to prevent similar exposures
- Provide personal protective equipment for employees to use, and teach them when and how to properly use it
- Provide free hepatitis B vaccinations for all employees

The employee's responsibilities for infection prevention include the following:

- Follow Standard Precautions
- Follow all facility policies and procedures
- Follow patient care plans and assignments
- Use provided personal protective equipment as indicated or as appropriate
- Take advantage of the free hepatitis B vaccination
- Immediately report any exposure to infection, blood, or body fluids
- Participate in annual education programs covering the prevention of infection

Chapter Review

Multiple Choice

1. What is the difference between a microorganism and a microbe?
   (A) A microorganism causes disease and a microbe does not.
   (B) A microorganism is a form of bacteria and a microbe is a form of virus.
   (C) A microorganism and a microbe are the same thing.
   (D) A microorganism can be destroyed by antibacterial soap and a microbe cannot.
2. Which of the following is true of healthcare-associated infections?
   (A) They can occur anywhere in a community.
   (B) They are a concern for particular healthcare workers like doctors and nurses, but not for certified healthcare workers like PBTs and nurses' aides.
   (C) They are relatively easy to cure.
   (D) Proper hand hygiene can prevent or control their spread.
3. What is the primary route of disease transmission in a healthcare facility?
   (A) Infected needles and other sharps
   (B) Improperly sanitized equipment
   (C) The hands of healthcare workers
   (D) Infected waste from patients' rooms
4. In which of the following situations is it appropriate for a phlebotomy technician to *not* use Standard Precautions?
   (A) It is never appropriate.
   (B) When the PBT is personally familiar with the patient and knows him to be healthy
   (C) When the patient indicates she does not have any infectious diseases
   (D) When a doctor assures the PBT that the patient does not have any infectious diseases

5. OSHA's recommendation that biomedical waste be properly discarded at the point of origin means
   (A) There should be at least one appropriate container on each floor of a facility
   (B) There should be an appropriate container in every location where biomedical waste is created
   (C) If there is not an appropriate container at the site where biomedical waste is created, it should be thrown in a regular trash can
   (D) Phlebotomy technicians should tell patients they will need to return another day if there is no appropriate container available nearby

6. How long should a PBT rub hands together when washing hands with soap and water?
   (A) 10 seconds
   (B) 15 seconds
   (C) 20 seconds
   (D) 30 seconds

7. When should a phlebotomist change gloves and perform hand hygiene between patient interaction?
   (A) Always
   (B) Between patients with documented bloodborne illnesses
   (C) Between patients with any documented infectious illnesses
   (D) Between patients with any documented or suspected infectious illnesses

8. What is a precaution used to prevent the spread of influenza?
   (A) Placing a patient with known influenza in a specially sealed room
   (B) Wearing a face mask when caring for a patient with influenza
   (C) Wearing a respirator and goggles when caring for a patient with influenza
   (D) Asking the patient to wash hands before care is provided

9. What is the maximum distance usually traveled by droplets that carry viruses?
   (A) 1 foot
   (B) 2 feet
   (C) 6 feet
   (D) 10 feet

10. How is a healthcare worker most likely to be exposed to a bloodborne disease?
    (A) By contact with infected blood or body fluids
    (B) By touching or hugging an infected patient
    (C) By working in a closely confined environment with an infected patient and breathing the same air
    (D) By failing to wear a respirator and face mask when caring for an infected patient

11. One of the differences between hepatitis B and HIV is that
    (A) HIV can be deadly and hepatitis B cannot
    (B) Hepatitis B is a risk to healthcare workers and HIV is not
    (C) It is possible to tell from looking at a patient whether HIV infection is present, but this is not true of hepatitis B
    (D) There is a vaccine that protects against hepatitis B, but no vaccine to protect against HIV

12. Which of the following is an example of an engineering control?
    (A) A needle available in several different sizes
    (B) A needle that retracts (pulls back) at the push of a button
    (C) A puncture-resistant, leakproof container for sharps disposal
    (D) A cap that must be manually replaced on a needle after use

13. Blood specimens should be transported
    (A) In a lab coat pocket
    (B) In a bare hand
    (C) In sharps containers
    (D) In an appropriately labeled bag or container

14. Which of these is an employer responsibility for infection prevention?
    (A) Training employees in the use of PPE
    (B) Providing free vaccinations for all illnesses employees might be exposed to
    (C) Allowing employees to take time off when influenza or other illnesses are widespread
    (D) Providing in-service education about infection prevention if it is requested by employees

5 Safety Measures for Care Team Members and Patients

1. Discuss the importance of laboratory safety and identify OSHA's categories of common hazards

Workplace hazards may vary, but all healthcare settings can pose dangers to workers and patients alike. All staff members, including phlebotomy technicians, are responsible for safety in a facility. Recognizing and working to reduce risks will result in fewer accidents and a safer environment for everyone. OSHA identifies the following four categories of hazards in a laboratory environment:

- **Chemical.** Chemicals used in some areas of a diagnostic laboratory may create dangerous fumes. They may also be caustic (damaging to the skin or other tissues) or **flammable** (able to catch fire easily).
- **Biological.** Bloodborne pathogens are one significant biological hazard PBTs may encounter. Disease-causing bacteria, viruses, and fungi spread through the air, by droplets, or through direct contact are also biological hazards.
- **Physical.** **Ergonomics** is the science of designing equipment, areas, and work tasks to make them safer and to suit workers' abilities. Physical hazards include poor ergonomic practices. They also include exposure to radiation or to excessive noise.
- **Safety.** General safety hazards include electrical hazards, fire, burns from hot equipment, and tripping, slipping, or falling. Disaster situations can also create safety hazards.

PBTs encounter all of these types of hazards on the job. Working with sharps and blood is the central daily task of a PBT, which means exposure to biological hazards is a constant concern. Though most blood collection tubes are now made of plastic rather than glass, if tubes break or spill, there is a risk of exposure to potentially contaminated blood. PBTs may also work with equipment that could pose a risk of burns or electrical shock. They may work with harmful chemicals, including products used to disinfect surfaces or clean up spills (Fig. 5-1).

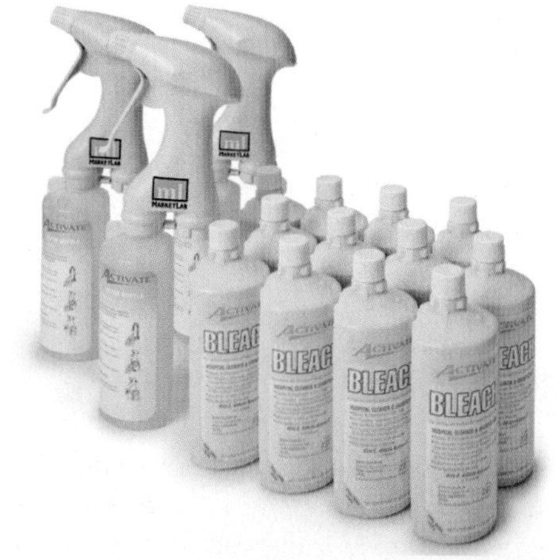

Fig. 5-1. *Cleaning products often contain potentially hazardous chemicals and should be used exactly as directed to avoid any possible harm.* (PHOTO COURTESY OF MARKETLAB, INC., WWW.MARKETLAB.COM)

Every workplace will also have its own ergonomic challenges. Factors like the height and adjustability of drawing chairs, the location of sharps containers and supply storage, and the amount of space available at a drawing station can all affect safety. Fires are a concern in any healthcare setting, but laboratories that use flammable chemicals are particularly at risk.

Patients entering a healthcare facility must be protected from harm as much as possible. PBTs should always be aware of physical dangers, such as uneven walkways or accidental exposure to heat, and dangers from electrical, biological, or chemical hazards. Emergencies such as natural disasters or active shooter situations also pose danger. Workers must know how best to protect their patients and themselves from these risks.

OSHA emphasizes the importance of preparedness in dealing with safety hazards. All healthcare facilities have policies and procedures in place for responding to hazards, and provide training on this topic at least once a year. Planning alone, however, is not enough. Training drills for fire evacuation and disaster response should be conducted regularly. Healthcare workers should review and practice safety responses so that they become automatic. Detailed guidelines for responding to common hazards are in Learning Objective 3.

Quality Counts

Regulatory and accrediting organizations emphasize the importance of continuous quality improvement in the area of workplace safety, for both patients and healthcare workers. The Joint Commission encourages healthcare facilities to adopt what it calls the qualities of a *learning organization*. It recommends that facilities create an atmosphere in which employees "report to learn." This means encouraging employees to speak up about risks and dangers so that processes can be improved. Reporting problems or potential problems should be welcomed, and blame and punishment for errors minimized. Facilities are less safe if employees fear they will be punished for reporting mistakes. Knowing about mistakes helps supervisors see where procedures might be improved.

2. Describe regulations related to safety practices in the laboratory and explain the Safety Data Sheet

The Occupational Safety and Health Act (OSH Act) of 1970 established the requirement for employers to provide a safe, hazard-free workplace. In healthcare settings, certain potential hazards are unavoidable, but employers are required to mange these hazards as effectively as possible. This may be achieved in a variety of ways:

- **Engineering controls**. These controls prevent workers from coming into contact with hazards. Retractable needles and automated lancets are examples.
- **Administrative controls**. These are policies and procedures set by employers that limit possible dangers. Developing standard operating procedures for handling blood and body fluids is an example.
- **Work practices**. These are changes to how work is done that limit exposure to hazards. Using the least caustic antimicrobial agent available for cleaning laboratory surfaces, as long as it is still effective, is an example.
- **PPE**. Personal protective equipment is essential when contact with hazards is likely. Wearing gloves when a worker might touch something contaminated with blood or body fluids is an example.

To supplement the general protections outlined in the OSH Act, OSHA developed specific regulations related to work in particular fields. Regulations that are particularly important for phlebotomists include the Bloodborne Pathogens Standard and its amendment, the Needlestick Safety and Prevention Act, the Personal Protective Equipment (PPE) Standard, and the Hazard Communication Standard.

Chapter 4 describes the Bloodborne Pathogens Standard and the Needlestick Safety and Prevention Act in detail. The **Hazard Communication**

Standard, sometimes referred to as *HazCom*, addresses the identification of potential hazards in the workplace. A series of pictograms must be used to identify hazards (Fig. 5-2), and further information must be available regarding chemical products in use. These chemicals must be clearly labeled, and all possible hazards must be clearly communicated in a document called the **Safety Data Sheet (SDS)** (formerly called *Material Safety Data Sheet*, or *MSDS*). Employers must train healthcare workers about the possible dangers of these chemicals and about measures they can take to protect themselves from harm.

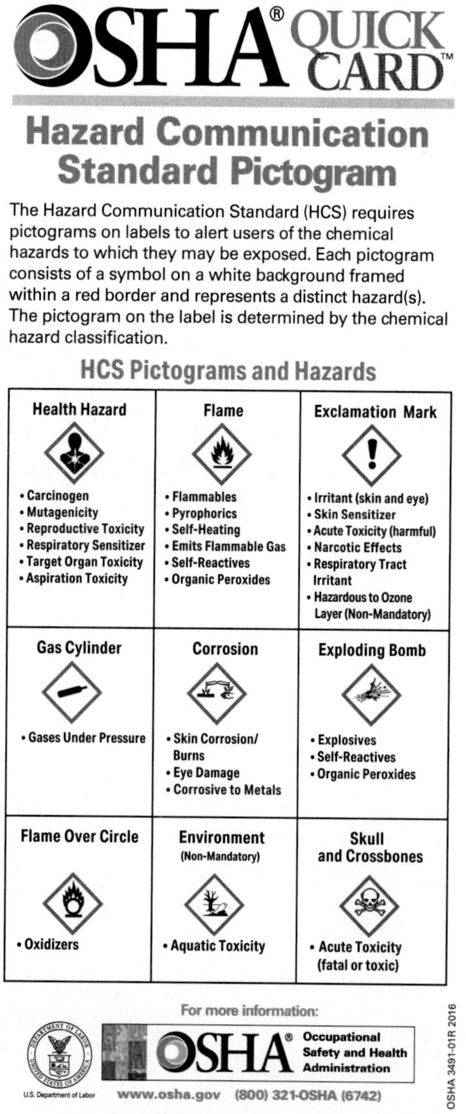
OSHA® QUICK CARD™

Hazard Communication Standard Pictogram

The Hazard Communication Standard (HCS) requires pictograms on labels to alert users of the chemical hazards to which they may be exposed. Each pictogram consists of a symbol on a white background framed within a red border and represents a distinct hazard(s). The pictogram on the label is determined by the chemical hazard classification.

HCS Pictograms and Hazards

Health Hazard	Flame	Exclamation Mark
• Carcinogen • Mutagenicity • Reproductive Toxicity • Respiratory Sensitizer • Target Organ Toxicity • Aspiration Toxicity	• Flammables • Pyrophorics • Self-Heating • Emits Flammable Gas • Self-Reactives • Organic Peroxides	• Irritant (skin and eye) • Skin Sensitizer • Acute Toxicity (harmful) • Narcotic Effects • Respiratory Tract Irritant • Hazardous to Ozone Layer (Non-Mandatory)
Gas Cylinder	**Corrosion**	**Exploding Bomb**
• Gases Under Pressure	• Skin Corrosion/ Burns • Eye Damage • Corrosive to Metals	• Explosives • Self-Reactives • Organic Peroxides
Flame Over Circle	**Environment (Non-Mandatory)**	**Skull and Crossbones**
• Oxidizers	• Aquatic Toxicity	• Acute Toxicity (fatal or toxic)

For more information:

U.S. Department of Labor OSHA® Occupational Safety and Health Administration

www.osha.gov (800) 321-OSHA (6742)

OSHA 3491-01R 2016

Fig. 5-2. These pictograms alert healthcare workers, patients, and visitors to potential hazards in a facility. (IMAGES COURTESY OF THE OCCUPATIONAL SAFETY AND HEALTH ADMINISTRATION.)

The Safety Data Sheet details the chemical ingredients, chemical dangers, and safe handling, storage, and disposal procedures for a product. Information about emergency response actions to be taken is also included. Some facilities use a toll-free number to access SDS information. These sheets must be accessible in work areas for all employees. Important information about the SDS includes the following:

- Employers must have an SDS for every chemical used.
- Employers must provide easy access to the SDS.
- Staff members must know where these sheets are kept and how to read them. They should ask for help if they do not know how to do this.

Emergency Eyewash Stations

OSHA requires that emergency eyewash stations be placed in all hazardous areas in case an eye injury occurs (Fig. 5-3). Employees must know where the closest eyewash station is and how to get there with restricted vision.

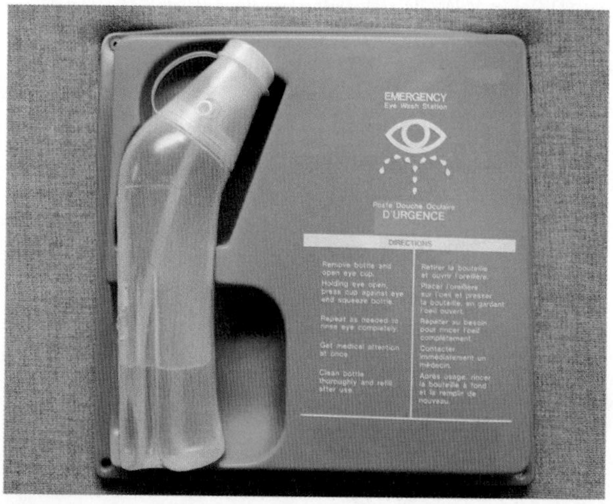

Fig. 5-3. This is one type of eyewash station.

3. List safety guidelines for common hazards in laboratory settings

The best way to avoid dangerous situations in the workplace is to develop what the CDC calls a *culture of safety*. This means the healthcare facility's policies emphasize safety and identify and address potential hazards. Healthcare workers are encouraged to speak up about possible hazards and share their ideas for avoiding them. When hazardous situations do occur, it is important for PBTs to know how best to respond.

Chemical exposure may result in harm to the skin, eyes, or mucous membranes (linings of body cavities that open to the outside of the body, such as the linings of the mouth, nose, and eyes). It can also cause breathing difficulties and a wide variety of other symptoms, depending upon the specific chemical involved. Phlebotomists work with antiseptics, which are used to reduce the number of pathogens on the body, and with disinfectants, which are used to reduce the number of pathogens on environmental surfaces. Some disinfectants can be quite damaging if spilled or used improperly. This is why it is essential that PBTs understand how and where to access Safety Data Sheets.

Guidelines: Chemical Hazards

- **G** Do not use any chemical agents you are not trained or permitted to use.
- **G** Wear appropriate gloves when using disinfectants, per facility policy, and change gloves if you are in contact with disinfectants for longer than 30 minutes. These chemicals can damage gloves over time.
- **G** Do not store food or drink in an area where hazardous chemicals are used or stored.
- **G** Do not drink or eat anything in the workplace if you are not certain of its origin. (Food and drink should be limited to break areas and never consumed in the laboratory or at drawing stations.)
- **G** Do not place pens or pencils in your mouth, apply makeup, or touch your face or eyes while working.
- **G** Always know how to access SDS information, whether in physical form or by telephone.
- **G** Know where eyewash stations, sinks, showers, and any other safety facilities are located and the quickest route to reach them.
- **G** In the case of exposure, flush with running water or wash the exposed area immediately. The length of time required for washing depends on how corrosive the chemical is. It ranges from five minutes for mildly irritating chemicals to an hour for highly corrosive chemicals. The SDS provides guidance on this topic.
- **G** Report any known or suspected exposure to hazardous chemicals to your supervisor.
- **G** Seek medical attention if needed, as directed by your supervisor.

Chapter 4 includes information about biological hazards and infection prevention. In addition to exposure to such hazards through accidental needlesticks or contact with an infected patient, PBTs may also be exposed to biological hazards through spills, leaking or broken specimen containers, or through the air during cleaning. This can happen when small particles of liquid or dried blood or body fluids are **aerosolized**, or dispersed though the air in such a way that they might be inhaled.

Guidelines: Biological Hazards

- **G** Seal tubes and other specimen containers properly to prevent leaks or spills. No part of the specimen should be on the outside of the container.
- **G** Place specimens to be carried to another area of the facility in a rigid, latching container made of a material capable of containing spills (Fig. 5-4).
- **G** In the event of broken specimen containers and/or spills, follow facility policy for cleaning. Notify your supervisor or the appropriate

person or department. Don gloves before cleaning. Special heavy-duty gloves may be required. Do not pick up any pieces of broken glass, no matter how large, with your hands. Use a dustpan and broom or other tools. Absorb the spill with whatever product is used by the facility. Apply the proper disinfectant and follow instructions regarding the amount of time it must stand before cleaning. Nonsharp waste (tissues, gauze, cloths, etc.) containing blood or body fluids should be properly bagged in a special biohazard waste bag. Anything that could pierce a biohazard bag (such as broken glass) must be placed in a puncture-proof sharps container. Follow facility policy.

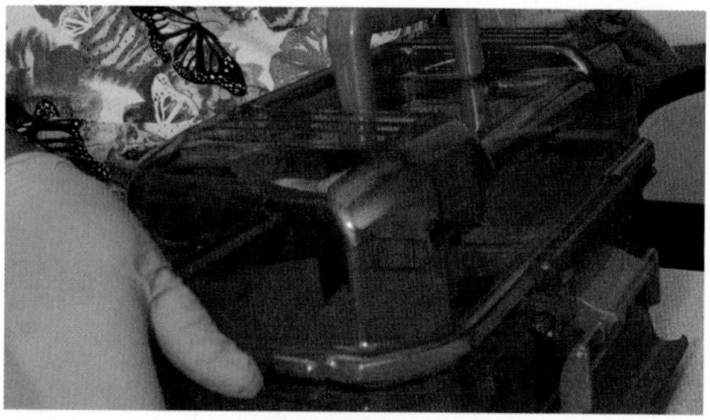

Fig. 5-4. *Tightly latch containers for transporting specimens.*

G Never scrape dried blood or other body fluids off of any surface or floor. The dried material can become aerosolized and then inhaled. Follow facility policy for cleaning dried blood and body fluids, soaking the dried materials in an antimicrobial cleaner for the required length of time.

G A **centrifuge** is a machine commonly used to separate substances in blood and other specimens through rapid spinning (Fig. 5-5). Improper use of a centrifuge can result in broken collection tubes and exposure to biological hazards. Never use equipment you have not been specifically trained to use, and always follow procedures exactly. The majority of accidental exposures to biological hazards involving a centrifuge are due to user error.

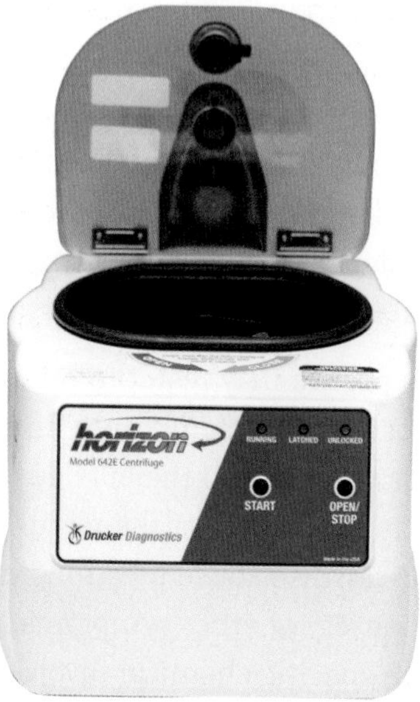

Fig. 5-5. *A centrifuge spins specimen tubes at a very high rate of speed. If the machine is not used properly, healthcare workers may be exposed to potential biological hazards.*

G Discard and reprint a paper requisition form or other paper document if it becomes wet, soiled, or potentially contaminated with blood or body fluids.

G In the case of exposure to blood or body fluids (e.g., accidental needlestick), wash or flush the area immediately with soap and water for fifteen minutes, report the exposure, and get immediate medical attention.

PBTs may also encounter physical hazards in their work spaces. Poor ergonomic practices can cause injury. Exposure to X-rays or radioactive chemicals used in some medical tests or treatments is a potential hazard. Specimens from patients who have received certain treatments or tests may have low levels of radioactivity. Noise from machinery can also be a danger if it is above a certain level.

Guidelines: Physical Hazards

G Pay attention to ergonomics. There should be room at workstations to do your job without bumping into equipment or other workers. The sharps container should be within arm's reach. You should be able to access the patient's arm (or other collection site) without stooping or bending. Supplies should be easy to reach. If this is not the case, talk to a supervisor about possible changes.

- G Standard Precautions are adequate to protect against exposure to the low-level radiation that might be present in patient samples. Wear gloves when handling any specimen containers.
- G Pay attention to signs, lights, or other warnings about X-ray and other radiation exposure. Do not enter an area in which X-rays or radioactive substances are used without following the required precautions (Fig. 5-6).
- G Follow facility policies about tracking radiation exposure. If you frequently work in areas where radiation is common, you will need to wear a *dosimeter*. This is a small clip-on badge capable of measuring radiation exposure. It must be turned in after a certain amount of time to make sure exposure levels are acceptable.
- G Use ear protection when working with noisy machines or entering rooms in which loud machines are operating, following facility policy.

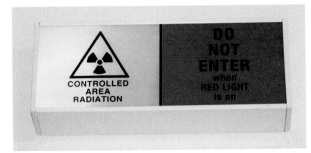

Fig. 5-6. *Lights and/or warning signs are used to indicate areas where radiation is used.*

Safety hazards can range from a loose floor mat to a fire or explosion. Natural disasters also pose safety hazards of their own, as do human-made disasters like acts of terrorism or active shooter situations. The following are general guidelines for a variety of potential safety hazards.

Guidelines: Preventing Falls and Related Injuries

- G Make sure walkways are dry and free of clutter, cords, and other tripping hazards. Floor mats should have nonslip backing and should not be uneven or have loose edges.
- G Wear nonskid, closed-toe shoes and keep shoelaces tied.
- G Uneven flooring or stairs should be marked with tape of a contrasting color to indicate a hazard.
- G Always close drawers and cabinets immediately after use.

Many phlebotomists work near electrical equipment, some of which can produce dangerous levels of heat. Damaged or improperly used electrical equipment can cause injuries or fires. Phlebotomists should never use equipment they have not been trained and assigned to use.

Guidelines: Avoiding Electrical and Burn Hazards

- G Immediately report frayed electrical cords or electrical equipment that looks unsafe. Do not use this equipment. Report it to a supervisor.
- G Do not put combustible (able to burn) material near any appliance or machine that generates heat.
- G Do not touch the surface of any appliance or machine in operation if it might be hot (e.g., an autoclave) (Fig. 5-7).
- G Do not overload electrical sockets. Report overloaded sockets if you see them.
- G Do not use extension cords or two-prong electrical plugs. Two-prong plugs do not protect against electrical surges.
- G Report damaged or malfunctioning equipment to a supervisor or the appropriate personnel right away.

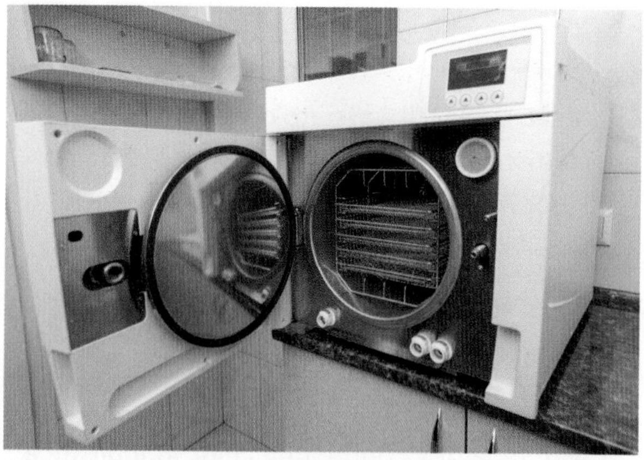

Fig. 5-7. *Autoclaves are used to sterilize equipment. The outer surfaces of some models, especially older machines, may become hot during operation.*

Fires are a risk at any healthcare facility. Laboratories can be especially dangerous in a fire because chemicals and heat-generating equipment are often present. All facilities have a fire safety plan, and all workers need to know this plan. Guidelines regarding fires and evacuations are explained to all employees. Evacuation routes are posted in facilities. Phlebotomists should read and review them often and should attend fire and disaster response trainings when they are offered.

Guidelines: Responding to Fires

- Fire alarms and exit doors should not be blocked. If they are, report this to a supervisor.
- Know the facility's fire evacuation plan.
- Stay calm. Do not panic.
- Every facility will have multiple fire extinguishers (Fig. 5-8). Learn where they are located. The PASS acronym will help you understand how to use an extinguisher:
    - **P**ull the pin.
    - **A**im at the base of the fire when spraying.
    - **S**queeze the handle.
    - **S**weep back and forth at the base of the fire.

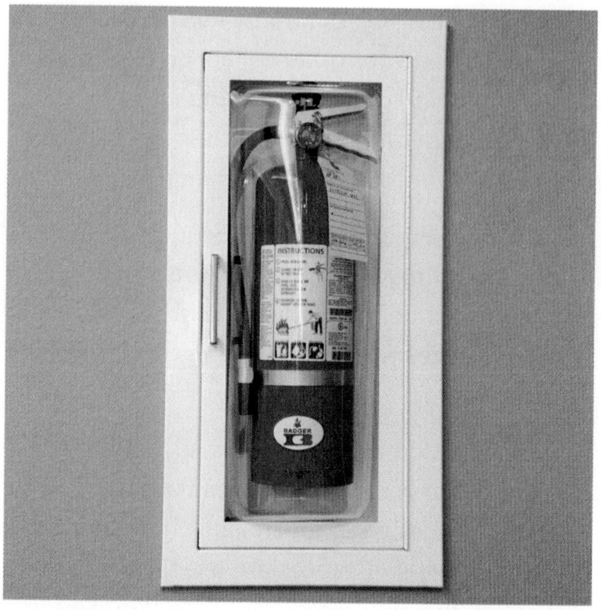

Fig. 5-8. *Know the locations of your facility's fire extinguishers and how to use them.*

In case of fire, the RACE acronym is a good rule to follow:

- **R**emove anyone in danger if you are not in danger.
- **A**ctivate alarm or call 911.
- **C**ontain the fire if possible by closing all doors and windows.
- **E**xtinguish the fire, or the fire department will extinguish it. Evacuate the area if instructed to do so.

- Follow the directions of the fire department.
- Do not get into an elevator during a fire. In certain situations, when a building has appropriate elevator equipment, firefighters may direct evacuation by elevator. This is the *only* exception to the guideline. If firefighters do not direct you to enter an elevator, always use the stairs.
- Stay low in a room to escape a fire.
- If the door of the room you are in is closed, check for heat coming from it before opening it. If the door or doorknob feels hot, stay in the room if there is no safe exit. Plug the doorway (use wet towels or clothing) to pre-

vent smoke from entering. Stay in the room until help arrives.

- Use the *stop, drop, and roll* fire safety technique to extinguish a fire on clothing or hair. Stop running or stay still. Drop to the ground, lying down if possible. Roll on the ground to try to extinguish the flames.
- Use a damp covering over the mouth and nose to reduce smoke inhalation.
- After leaving the building, move away from it.

Disasters can include fire, flood, earthquake, hurricane, tornado, or other severe weather. Human-created dangers, such as acts of terrorism, bomb threats, and active shooter situations, can pose threats to the safety of healthcare workers, patients, and visitors in a facility. Phlebotomy technicians must participate in any training or drills regarding disaster response. Emergency medical personnel, fire departments, and police may attend these drills. Taking an active role in drills can help PBTs understand the appropriate action to take if disasters occur. Preparing and practicing for emergencies is the best way to respond appropriately if one occurs. In the case of a disaster, PBTs should follow their facility's response plan and the instructions of any first responders on-site. The following guidelines apply to many disaster situations:

Guidelines: Responding to Disasters

- Remain calm.
- Know the locations of all exits and stairways.
- Know where the fire alarms and extinguishers are located.
- Know the appropriate action to take in various situations based on facility training.
- Use the internet to stay informed, or keep the radio or television tuned to a local station to get the latest information.

PBTs should also be aware of specific emergency guidelines for the geographic area in which they work. For example, a technician working where hurricanes may occur needs to know the guidelines for hurricane preparedness. The following guidelines are listed by the type of disaster:

Tornadoes

- Seek shelter inside, ideally in a steel-framed or concrete building.
- Stay away from windows.
- Stay in a hallway or basement, or take cover under heavy furniture.
- Crouch on the ground, head down. Cover your head and neck with your arms.

Power Outages

- Keep calm and take prompt action to provide light.
- Use a backup pack for electrical medical equipment, as needed.
- Backup packs do not last more than 24 hours, so contact emergency services when instructed.

Hurricanes

- Know the hurricane's category and track its expected path.
- Evacuate if advised to do so.

Earthquakes

- Drop to the ground.
- Get under a sturdy piece of furniture, such as a heavy table, if possible. Hold on until the shaking stops.
- If no table or desk is available, stay crouched down in the inside corner of a building.
- Cover your face and head with your arms.
- Stay away from windows, outside walls, and anything that might fall over or fall down.
- Do not exit a building during the shaking.

- Do not use elevators.
- If trapped under debris after an earthquake, do not light a match or ignite a lighter. Avoid kicking up dust. Breathe through a handkerchief or clothing. Make tapping noises or use a whistle, if available, to get rescuers' attention. Do not shout. Shouting could cause you to inhale dangerous amounts of dust.

Active Shooter

- Follow the facility's emergency notification procedures.
- If the area cannot be safely evacuated, stay where you are.
- Turn off the lights, secure the door, and stay hidden from outside view.
- Turn off all cell phone ringers.
- If safe to do so, call 911 and notify the operator of your exact location in the building.
- Provide information on the number and description of shooter(s), the number of victims and nature of their injuries, and their locations if known.
- Move heavy furniture to barricade the door and cover any openings or windows in the door.
- When police arrive on the scene, do not move toward any police vehicle until directed to do so by the officers. Move with hands on top of your head and follow all directions given by police.
- Remain in the area until released by police.

4. Discuss measures necessary to protect patients and keep them safe

Many of the same safety precautions described in this chapter apply to both patients and healthcare workers. Following the guidelines listed in the previous learning objective will protect patients, visitors, and members of the healthcare team. In addition, phlebotomists must always be aware of specific patient needs. PBTs can work to anticipate and prevent possible problems that could pose dangers to patients.

Listening to patients is an important step in keeping them safe. If a patient reports feeling lightheaded or faint, for instance, the PBT should respond immediately. Details for responding to fainting during a blood draw are found in Chapter 9, but if a patient reports these sensations before she is seated, she should be assisted to sit down immediately. Fainting from a standing position poses a greater risk of injury, and sitting down might relieve the sensation. In many cases, acting quickly to address patient concerns can prevent dangerous outcomes.

Pediatric and elderly patients are especially vulnerable to physical harm in healthcare facilities. When children are in a phlebotomy drawing station, the PBT should take these precautions to protect their physical safety:

Guidelines: Safety for Pediatric Patients

- Introduce yourself. Lower yourself to address the patient at eye level. Make sure he understands that he can talk to you if he is anxious or scared. This may create an atmosphere of trust, and the child may be more likely to speak up if he is hurt.
- Make sure potentially dangerous supplies are out of the child's reach.
- Make sure the sharps receptacle is within arm's reach for the phlebotomist but not within easy reach of the child.
- Do not leave a child at a drawing station unattended, even for a very short time.
- If equipment in the drawing station is not made for pediatric patients, make sure the patient is in a parent's/guardian's lap or is safely and comfortably positioned. Make sure

that you can easily access the site where you will perform the blood draw.

G If the patient is an infant, ensure that she cannot fall or roll off of facility equipment. (Details about blood draw procedures are found in Chapters 9 and 10.)

Patients' Rights

Pediatric patients matter

Pediatric patients are not small adults. Many employers do not provide much training in dealing with young patients, but their safety and well-being is just as important as every other patient's. Children might not always be able or willing to speak up if they are concerned about something they see. Part of keeping pediatric patients safe is communicating to them that their voices are valued and heard. Speaking directly to children, not lying to them, and seeking their input will help protect their rights and promote their safety.

Elderly patients require special precautions as well. They may have reduced senses of vision or hearing, or may be less steady on their feet. Canes or walkers may make maneuvering in small areas more challenging. Elderly patients have more fragile bones, more delicate skin, and may be injured more easily than younger patients.

Guidelines: Safety for Geriatric Patients

G Be sure the patient has a clear path to the drawing station.

G Take care to point out any uneven walkways or steps/stairs along the patient's path.

G If the patient uses an aid such as a cane or walker, ensure that she can reach the chair without difficulty, assisting as needed (Fig. 5-9). Store the cane or walker in a location that will not interfere with your access to the patient.

G Follow the communication guidelines in Chapter 3 to ensure proper and clear communication.

G Take care in handling elderly patients' limbs and be gentle with their skin (see Chapters 9 and 10 for procedure-specific details).

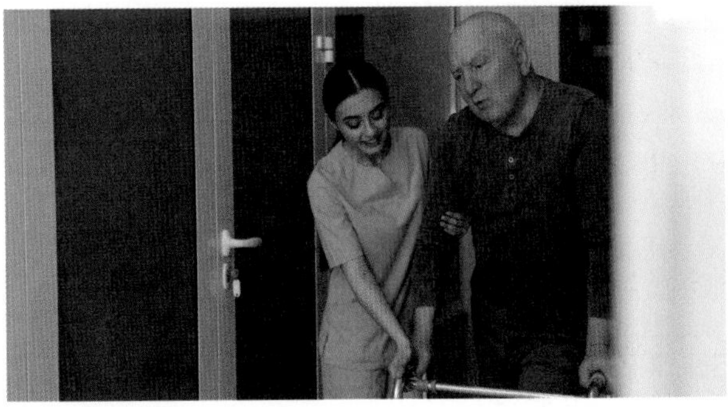

Fig. 5-9. *Walkers provide extra stability but can sometimes be difficult to maneuver in tight spaces.*

Chapter Review

Multiple Choice

1. What are the four categories of hazards OSHA has identified in laboratory settings?
   (A) Immediate, delayed, prolonged, and brief
   (B) Chemical, biological, physical, and safety
   (C) Chemical, biological, tactical, and long-range
   (D) Physical, safety, human-made, and natural

2. Which of the following is an example of a biological hazard?
   (A) Exposure to radiation
   (B) Exposure to a chemical solvent
   (C) Exposure to faulty electrical wiring
   (D) Exposure to bloodborne pathogens

3. Which of the following is a *policy control* to reduce a workplace risk?
   (A) Pressure is placed on a venipuncture site immediately after the needle is withdrawn.
   (B) Needles have sliding sheaths to cover the point after use.
   (C) Gloves protect a healthcare worker's hands from becoming contaminated.
   (D) Healthcare workers are not allowed to have food or drinks in patient care areas.

4. The Safety Data Sheet must include this information about a chemical:
   (A) Brand names of all products containing the chemical
   (B) Directions for manufacturing the chemical
   (C) Emergency response actions for exposure to the chemical
   (D) A direct line to a scientist who can provide specific advice about the chemical

5. What does the Hazard Communication Standard address?
   (A) The identification of potential hazards in the workplace
   (B) The treatment of biological hazards in the workplace
   (C) The precautions required when working with bloodborne pathogens
   (D) The responsibility of employers to train employees in a variety of safety drills

6. Why should healthcare workers avoid actions that might aerosolize dried blood or other body fluids?
   (A) Because they might stain clothing
   (B) Because they might be inhaled
   (C) Because doing so makes it more difficult to clean them
   (D) Because they must then be rehydrated for testing

7. Which of the following explains why fires are of particular concern in a laboratory?
   (A) Laboratories are often stocked with flammable substances.
   (B) Laboratories do not usually have fire exits.
   (C) Fire extinguishers cannot be used in laboratories because they will destroy specimens.
   (D) Laboratory technicians are often so engaged in their work that they might not notice a fire.

8. Fall risks
   (A) Are not relevant for phlebotomists
   (B) Are only dangerous for elderly patients
   (C) Are always created by carelessness
   (D) May be caused by a building's physical structure

9. A PBT is collecting supplies for a blood draw on a 4-year-old child. She normally gathers supplies on a tray right beside the patient's chair. Which of these actions is most important to protect the child's safety?
   (A) The PBT should show the patient each item and describe what it is as she places it on the tray, noting which items are dangerous.
   (B) The PBT should make sure the tray is not within the child's reach.
   (C) The PBT should ask the child to hold the tray for her as she places the supplies on it, but to not touch the supplies.
   (D) The PBT should not gather supplies in advance to avoid frightening the child.

10. An elderly patient with a walker is having difficulty getting to a PBT's drawing station. There is enough room, but the patient is having difficulty maneuvering. What is the best and safest response from the PBT?
   (A) "Just take the walker back out and leave it in the waiting room."
   (B) "If you give it a good push, I know it can fit through."
   (C) "Let me help you with that."
   (D) "You can just leave it there and walk around to the chair."

6
Overview of the Human Body

Note: The circulatory system is covered in depth in the following chapter, so it is not included here.

1. Describe body systems and define key anatomical terms

Bodies are organized into body systems. Each system in the body has a condition under which it works best. **Homeostasis** is the name for the condition in which all of the body's systems are balanced and are working together to maintain internal stability. To be in homeostasis, the body's **metabolism**, or physical and chemical processes, must be working at a steady level. When disease or injury occurs, the body's metabolism is disturbed, and homeostasis is lost.

Changes in metabolic processes are called *signs* (objective information) and *symptoms* (subjective information). For instance, changes in the amounts of certain substances in the blood might be signs of liver damage in a patient. Fatigue, or feeling tired even when rested, might be a symptom of a condition like heart disease. A blood test conducted as part of a routine examination may be the first indication that the body's homeostasis is disturbed. Testing may also help a doctor whose patient is experiencing symptoms to determine what changes are taking place in the body's systems. This information can aid diagnosis and treatment. Blood tests can also be helpful in measuring progress back toward homeostasis and improved health. The phlebotomist makes this process possible by drawing high-quality specimens.

Each system in the body has its own unique structure and function. The body's systems can be organized in different ways. In this book, the human body is divided into ten systems:

1. Integumentary (skin)
2. Musculoskeletal
3. Nervous
4. Circulatory (covered in the next chapter)
5. Respiratory
6. Urinary
7. Gastrointestinal
8. Endocrine
9. Reproductive
10. Immune and Lymphatic

Body systems are made up of **organs**. An organ has a specific function. Organs are made up of **tissues**. Tissues are made up of groups of cells that perform a similar task. For example, in the gastrointestinal system, the stomach is one of the organs. It is made up of tissues and cells. **Cells** are the building blocks of the body. Living cells divide, grow, and die, renewing the tissues and organs of the body.

Anatomical terms of location are descriptive terms to help identify positions or directions of the body. Here are some anatomical terms used to describe location in the human body (Fig. 6-1):

- Anterior or ventral: the front of the body or body part
- Posterior or dorsal: the back of the body or body part
- Superior: toward the head
- Inferior: away from the head
- Medial: toward the midline of the body
- Lateral: to the side, away from the midline of the body
- Proximal: closer to the torso
- Distal: farther away from the torso

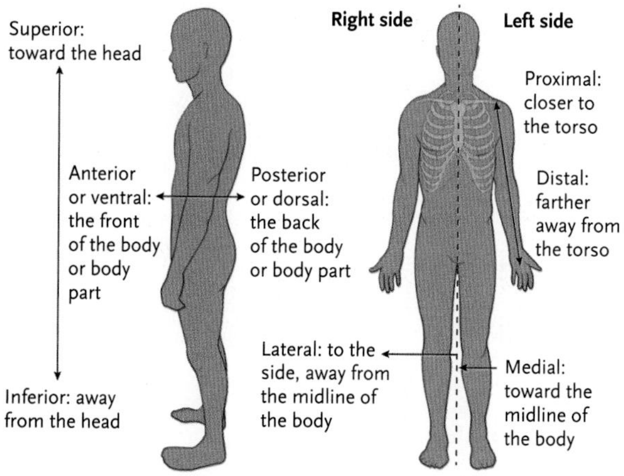

Fig. 6-1. Phlebotomists should understand the terms used to indicate location or direction on the human body.

2. Describe the integumentary system

The largest organ and system in the body is the skin, a natural protective covering, or **integument**. Skin prevents injury to internal organs, and it protects the body against entry of bacteria. Skin also prevents the loss of too much water, which is essential to life. Skin is made up of layers of tissues. Within these layers are sweat glands, which secrete sweat to help cool the body when needed, and sebaceous glands, which secrete oil (sebum) to keep the skin lubricated. There are also hair follicles, many tiny blood vessels (capillaries), and tiny nerve endings (Fig. 6-2).

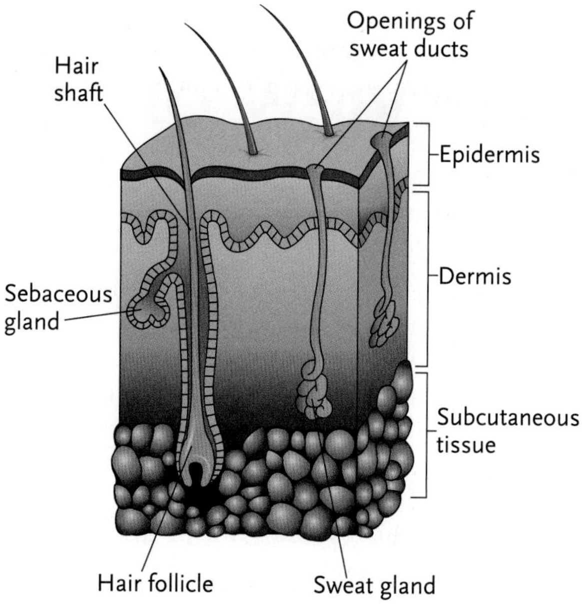

Fig. 6-2. Cross-section showing details of the integumentary system.

The skin is also a sense organ that feels heat, cold, pain, touch, and pressure. It then tells the brain what it is feeling. Body temperature is regulated in the skin. Blood vessels **dilate**, or widen, when the outside temperature is too high. This brings more blood to the body's surface to cool it off. The same blood vessels **constrict**, or narrow, when the outside temperature is too cold. By restricting the amount of blood reaching the skin, the blood vessels help the body retain heat.

Capillaries, the smallest blood vessels in the body, are located in the dermis, which is the inner layer of skin. (Because of this, the specimen collection procedure called *capillary puncture* is also known as *dermal puncture*.) The dermis also contains nerves, sweat glands, sebaceous (oil) glands, and hair roots. Sweat glands help control body temperature by secreting sweat. Sweat is made up of mostly water, but it also contains salt and a small amount of waste products. Sweat comes to the body's surface through pores, or tiny openings in the skin. It cools the body as it evaporates. Sebaceous glands in the dermis secrete sebum (oil). Sebum comes to the skin surface through hair follicles, or roots. Sebum keeps the skin and hair lubricated.

No blood vessels and only a few nerve endings are located in the epidermis, which is the outer layer of skin. Thinner than the dermis, the epidermis contains both dead and living cells. The dead cells begin deeper in the epidermis. They are pushed to the surface as other cells divide and are eventually worn off. The epidermis also contains pigment cells that give skin its color.

Hair grows from roots located in the dermis. It grows through hair follicles that extend through the epidermis to the outside of the body. Hair protects the body from heat and cold. Hair inside the nose and ears keeps out particles and bacteria trying to enter the body.

The functions of the integumentary system are to protect internal organs from injury, protect the body against bacteria, and prevent the loss of too much water. It also responds to heat, cold, pain, touch, and pressure, and it regulates body temperature.

PBT Connection

Allergies occur due to an overactive response by the immune system, but they often produce symptoms in the integumentary system. Hives and rashes might indicate an allergic response. Blood testing can help determine whether allergy plays a role in integumentary system problems. Blood tests for IgE, a type of **antibody** (protein made by the body to protect against foreign substances), may be ordered. IgE is produced as part of an allergic reaction. A *complete blood count* (*CBC*) may also be ordered, as allergies can increase the number of a particular type of white blood cell in a person's blood.

3. Describe the musculoskeletal system

Muscles, bones, ligaments, tendons, and cartilage give the body shape and structure. They work together to move the body. The skeleton, or framework, of the human body has 206 bones (Fig. 6-3). In addition to allowing the body to move, bones also protect organs. For example, the skull protects the brain and the vertebrae protect the spinal cord. Bones are hard and rigid, but are made up of living cells. Blood vessels supply oxygen and nutrients to the bones, as well as to other tissues of the body.

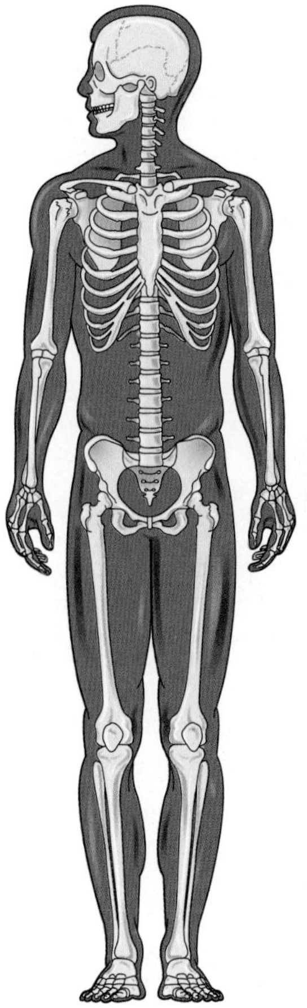

Fig. 6-3. *The skeleton is composed of 206 bones that aid movement and protect organs.*

Two bones meet at a **joint**. Some joints, such as the ball-and-socket joint, make movement possible in all directions. This joint is a type of synovial joint. In this joint, the round end of one bone fits into the hollow end of the other bone, which allows it to move in all directions. The hip and shoulder joints are examples.

Other joints permit movement in one direction only. The hinge joint is another example of a synovial joint. Like the hinge of a door, a hinge joint permits movement in one direction only. The elbow and knee are hinge joints. They bend in one direction only (Fig. 6-4).

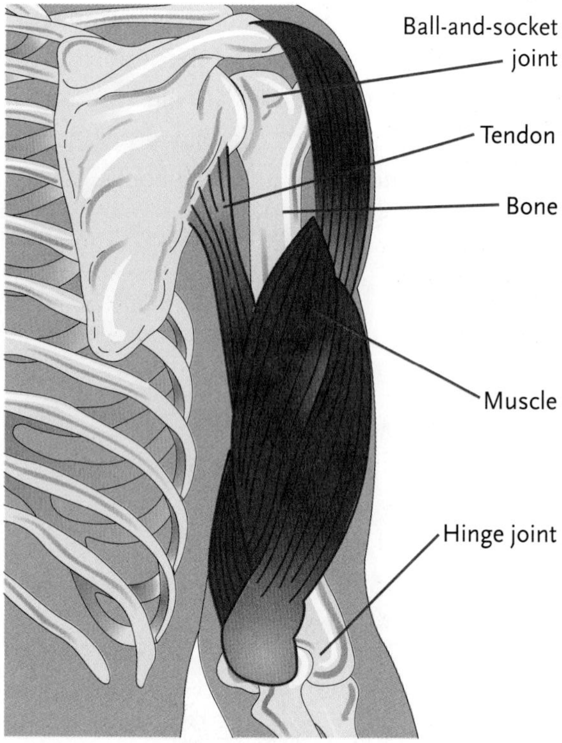

Fig. 6-4. *Muscles are connected to bones by tendons. Bones meet at different types of joints. The ball-and-socket joint and the hinge joint are shown here.*

Muscles provide movement of body parts to maintain posture and to produce heat. Muscles can be voluntary or involuntary. Voluntary muscles are also called skeletal muscles. They are attached to bones and can be moved when a person wants them to move. Examples of voluntary muscles are the arm and leg muscles, which are consciously controlled. Involuntary muscles cannot be consciously controlled. They automatically regulate the movement of organs and blood vessels. An example of an involuntary muscle is the heart.

The functions of the musculoskeletal system are to give the body shape and structure, to allow the body to move, to protect body organs, to maintain posture, and to produce heat.

PBT Connection

There are several different blood tests associated with the musculoskeletal system. One test, the *erythrocyte sedimentation rate* (*ESR*), measures the rate at which red blood cells settle to the bottom of a test tube. When the cells settle quickly, this can indicate inflammation, though the test does not reveal the cause. Tests for certain antibodies may help diagnose arthritis. Levels of muscle enzymes may be measured to determine if muscle tissue is being damaged or destroyed by a disease process. These same tests can also help monitor progress in the treatment of musculoskeletal disorders.

4. Describe the nervous system

The nervous system is the control and message center of the body. It controls and coordinates all body functions. The nervous system also senses and interprets information from outside the human body.

The neuron, or nerve cell, is the basic unit of the nervous system. Neurons send messages or sensations from the receptors in different parts of the body, through the spinal cord, to the brain.

The nervous system has two main parts: the **central nervous system** (**CNS**) and the **peripheral nervous system** (**PNS**). The central nervous system is composed of the brain and spinal cord. The peripheral nervous system deals with the periphery, or outer part, of the body via the nerves that extend throughout the body (Fig. 6-5).

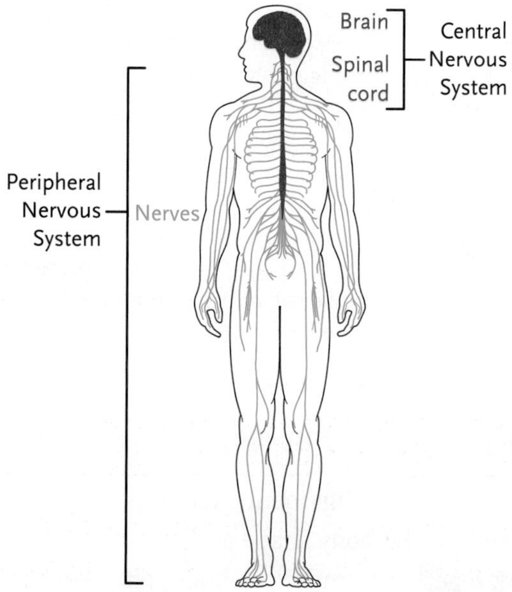

Fig. 6-5. *The nervous system includes the brain, spinal cord, and nerves throughout the body.*

The Central Nervous System

The brain is housed within the skull. The spinal cord is housed within the spinal column. The spinal column extends from the brain into the trunk of the body. Both the brain and the spinal cord are covered by a protective membrane made up of three layers. Between two of these layers is the cerebrospinal fluid. This fluid circulates around the brain and spinal cord. It provides a cushion against injuries.

The brain has three main sections: the cerebrum, the cerebellum, and the brainstem (Fig. 6-6). The largest section of the human brain is the cerebrum. The outside layer of the cerebrum is the cerebral cortex. The cerebral cortex is the part of the brain in which thinking, analysis, association of ideas, judgment, emotions, and memory occur. The cerebral cortex also

- Directs speech and emotions
- Interprets messages from the eyes, ears, nose, tongue, and skin
- Controls voluntary muscle movement

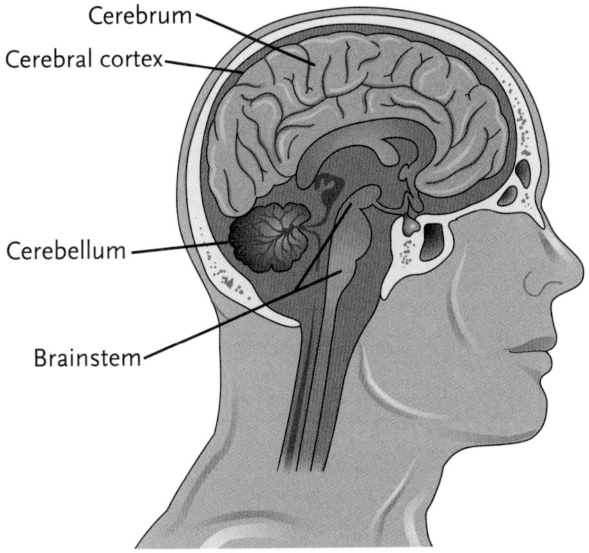

Fig. 6-6. *The three main sections of the brain are the cerebrum, cerebellum, and brainstem.*

The cerebrum is divided into right and left hemispheres. The right hemisphere controls movement and function in the left side of the body. The left hemisphere controls movement and function in the right side of the body (Fig. 6-7). Any illness in or injury to the right hemisphere affects functions on the left side of the body. Illness in or injury to the left hemisphere disrupts function on the right side.

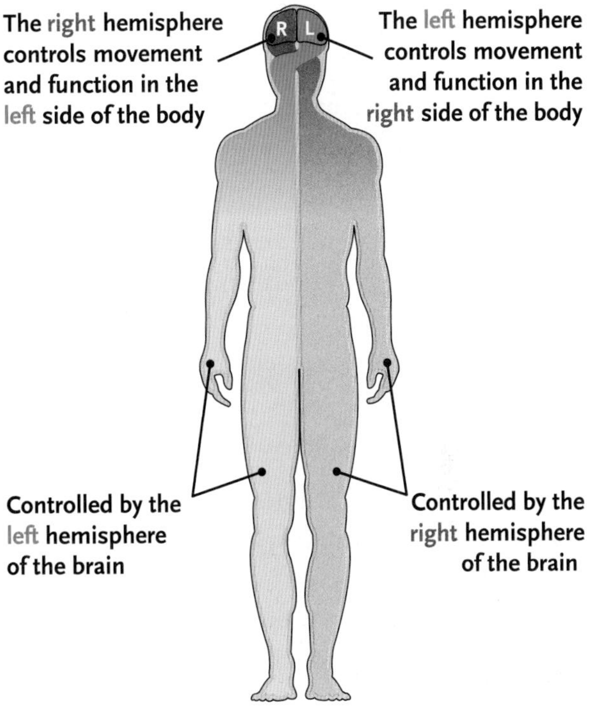

Fig. 6-7. *The right hemisphere controls movement and function in the left side of the body. The left hemisphere controls movement and function in the right side of the body.*

The cerebellum controls balance and regulates the body's voluntary muscles. It produces and coordinates smooth movements. Someone who has a problem in the cerebellum will be uncoordinated and have jerky movements and muscle weakness.

The cerebrum and cerebellum are connected to the spinal cord by the brainstem. The brainstem contains a kind of regulatory center called the *medulla oblongata*. It controls heart rate, breathing, swallowing, coughing, vomiting, and closing/opening of blood vessels.

The spinal cord is connected to the brain. It is protected by the bones of the spinal column. Nerve pathways run through the spinal cord. They conduct messages between the brain and the body. Cranial nerves attach to the brain and brainstem. Some of these nerves bring information from the sense organs to the brain. Some control muscles, and others are connected to glands or organs, such as the lungs. There are 12 pairs of cranial nerves. Nerves that are attached to the spinal cord and connect the spinal cord to other parts of the body are called *spinal nerves*. The brain communicates with most of the body through the spinal nerves. There are 31 pairs of spinal nerves.

The functions of the nervous system are to control and coordinate all body functions and to sense, interpret, and respond to changes occurring both inside and outside the human body.

The Nervous System: Sense Organs

The eyes, ears, nose, tongue, and skin are the body's major sense organs. They are considered part of the central nervous system because they contain receptors that receive impulses from the environment. They relay these impulses to the nerves.

The eye, which is about an inch in diameter, is located in a bony socket in the skull (Fig. 6-8). The bony socket protects the eye, which is surrounded by muscles that control its movements.

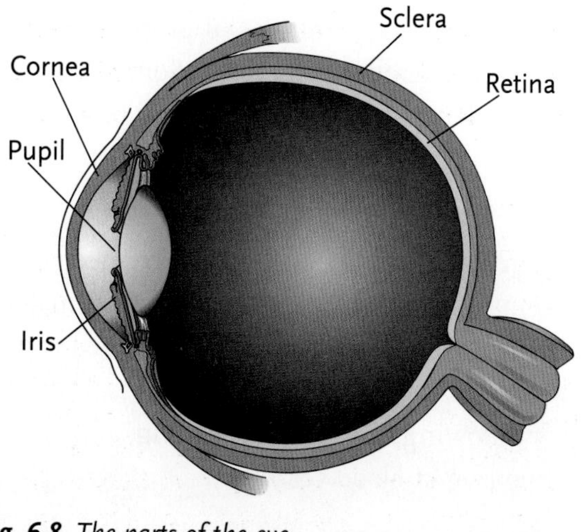

***Fig. 6-8.** The parts of the eye.*

The outer part of the eye is called the sclera. The sclera appears white, except in front, where it is called the cornea. The cornea is actually clear, but it appears colored because it lies over the iris, or the colored part of the eye. The pupil, or black circle in the center of the iris, widens or narrows to adjust the amount of light that enters the eye. Inside the back of the eye is the retina. The retina contains cells that respond to light and send a message to the brain, where the picture is interpreted so a person can see.

The ear is a sense organ that provides balance and hearing. It is divided into three parts: the outer, middle, and inner ear (Fig. 6-9). The outer ear is the funnel-shaped outer part, sometimes called the auricle or pinna. It guides sound waves into the auditory canal. This canal is about one inch long and contains many glands that secrete earwax. Earwax and hair in the ear protect the ear from foreign objects. The eardrum, or tympanic membrane, separates the outer ear from the middle ear.

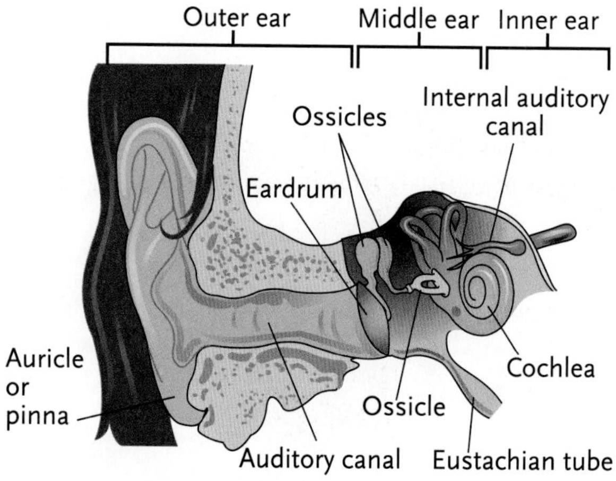

***Fig. 6-9.** The outer ear, middle ear, and inner ear are the three main divisions of the ear.*

The middle ear consists of the eustachian tube and three ossicles, small bones that amplify sound. The ossicles transmit sound to the inner ear. The eustachian tube connects the middle ear to the throat. It functions to allow air into the middle ear to equalize pressure on the tympanic membrane. The inner ear contains fluid that carries sound waves from the middle ear to the auditory nerve. The auditory nerve then transmits the impulse to the brain. The inner ear also contains structures that help in maintaining balance.

PBT Connection

Cerebrovascular accident, or stroke, is one of the most common disorders of the nervous system. It occurs when the blood supply to a part of the brain is blocked, or when a blood vessel leaks or ruptures within the brain. There is no blood test that can detect or confirm a stroke, but when stroke is suspected, blood tests will be ordered to rule out other possible causes of the patient's symptoms. Blood tests might also provide clues to possible causes of stroke, such as indications of abnormal blood clotting. Nervous system disorders like Parkinson's disease and multiple sclerosis cannot be diagnosed by blood test, but blood tests are likely to be ordered for patients in whom these illnesses are suspected. They can help the doctor determine if other problems might be causing the patient's symptoms. Researchers are working to develop blood tests that can diagnose these and other nervous system illnesses. Most of this research centers on testing the patient's blood for biological markers associated with certain diseases.

5. Describe the respiratory system

Respiration, or the body taking in oxygen and removing carbon dioxide, involves breathing in, inspiration, and breathing out, expiration. The lungs accomplish this process (Fig. 6-10).

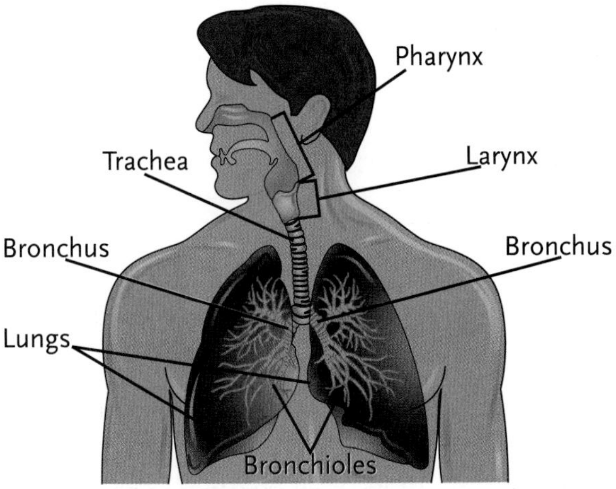

Fig. 6-10. *The respiratory process begins with inspiration through the nose or mouth. The air travels through the trachea and into the lungs via the bronchi, which then branch into bronchioles.*

As the lungs inhale, the air is pulled in through the nose and into the pharynx, a tubular passageway for both food and air. From the pharynx, air passes into the larynx, or voice box. The larynx is located at the beginning of the trachea, or windpipe. The trachea divides into two branches at its lower portion, the right and left bronchus, or bronchi. Each bronchus leads into a lung and then subdivides into bronchioles. These smaller airways subdivide further. They end in alveoli: tiny, one-cell sacs that appear in grape-like clusters. Blood is supplied to the alveoli by capillaries. Oxygen and carbon dioxide are exchanged between the alveoli and capillaries.

Oxygen-saturated blood then circulates through the capillaries and venules (small veins) of the lungs into the pulmonary vein and left side of the heart. The carbon dioxide is exhaled through the alveoli into the bronchioles and bronchi of the lungs, through the trachea, through the larynx and the pharynx, and out the nose and mouth.

Each lung is covered by the pleura, a membrane with two layers. One is attached to the chest wall. The other is attached to the surface of the lung. The space between the layers is filled with a thin fluid that lubricates the layers, preventing them from rubbing together during breathing.

The functions of the respiratory system are to bring oxygen into the body and to eliminate carbon dioxide produced as the body uses oxygen.

PBT Connection

Blood gas testing is commonly used to evaluate the function of the respiratory system. Blood is usually drawn from an artery (*arterial blood gas test*), but in some cases may be drawn from a vein or from the capillaries (especially in infants). The pH (acid/base balance), oxygen level, and carbon dioxide level of the blood is tested, showing medical professionals how well the lungs are working. Phlebotomists do not generally collect arterial blood specimens, but they may draw other specimens for blood gas testing. Blood tests are also important in the diagnosis of cystic fibrosis, a genetic disorder (passed down through families) that, among other symptoms, causes recurring respiratory illnesses. Newborn infants are screened, through blood tests, for a number of illnesses, including cystic fibrosis.

6. Describe the urinary system

The urinary system is composed of two kidneys, two ureters, one urinary bladder, a single urethra, and a meatus (Figs. 6-11 and 6-12).

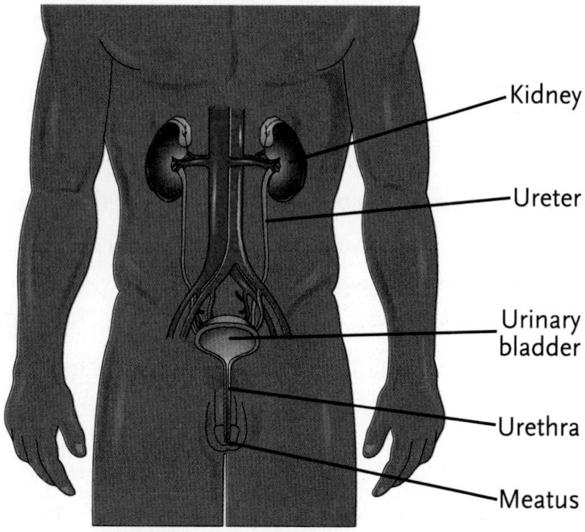

***Fig. 6-11.** The urinary system consists of two kidneys and two ureters, the bladder, the urethra, and the meatus. This is an illustration of the male urinary system.*

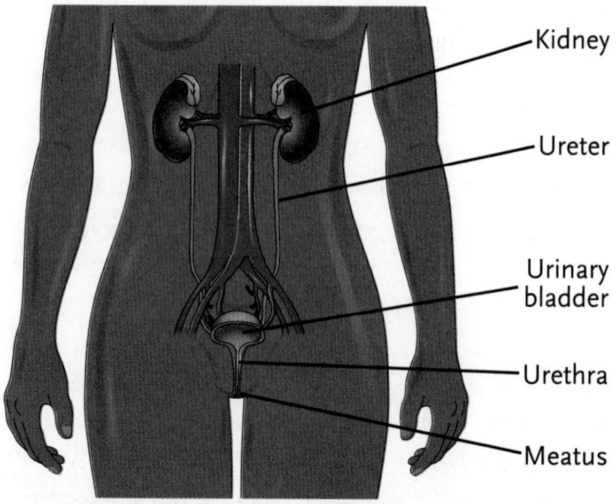

***Fig. 6-12.** The female urethra is shorter than the male urethra. This is one reason why the female bladder is more likely to become infected by bacteria.*

The kidneys are located in the upper part of the abdominal cavity on each side of the spine. These two bean-shaped organs are protected by the muscles of the back and the lower part of the rib cage. When blood flows through the kidneys, waste products and excess water are filtered out. Necessary water and substances are reabsorbed into the bloodstream. Waste and the remaining fluid form urine. The body must maintain a proper balance between water absorbed in the body and waste fluids that are released from the body.

Each kidney has a ureter, which is attached to the bladder. Urine flows through the ureters to the bladder, a muscular sac in the lower part of the abdomen. Urine flows from the bladder through the urethra. It then passes out of the body through the meatus, the opening at the end of the urethra. In the female, the meatus is located in the genital area just in front of the opening of the vagina. In the male, the meatus is located at the end of the penis.

The urinary system has two important functions. Through urine, the urinary system eliminates waste products created by the cells. The urinary system also maintains the water balance in the body.

PBT Connection

Urinary tract infections are among the most common disorders of the urinary system. They are usually detected through urinalysis, or the examination of a patient's urine. Many phlebotomy technicians are trained to collect urine specimens. Urinalysis and blood tests are both used in the diagnosis of kidney disorders. When a doctor is assessing a patient for possible kidney disease, she will test the patient's blood for the presence of certain waste products. The presence of these wastes indicates that the kidneys are not filtering the blood as effectively as they should be. The series of tests ordered to evaluate kidney health is known as a *renal panel.*

7. Describe the gastrointestinal system

The gastrointestinal (GI) system, also called the *digestive system,* is made up of the gastrointestinal tract and the accessory digestive organs (Fig. 6-13). The gastrointestinal tract is a long passageway extending from the mouth to the anus, the opening of the rectum. Food passes from the mouth through the pharynx, esophagus, stomach, small intestine, and large intestine, then out of the body as solid waste (*feces* or *stool*). The teeth, tongue, salivary glands, liver, gallbladder, and pancreas are the accessory organs to digestion. They help prepare the food so that it can be absorbed.

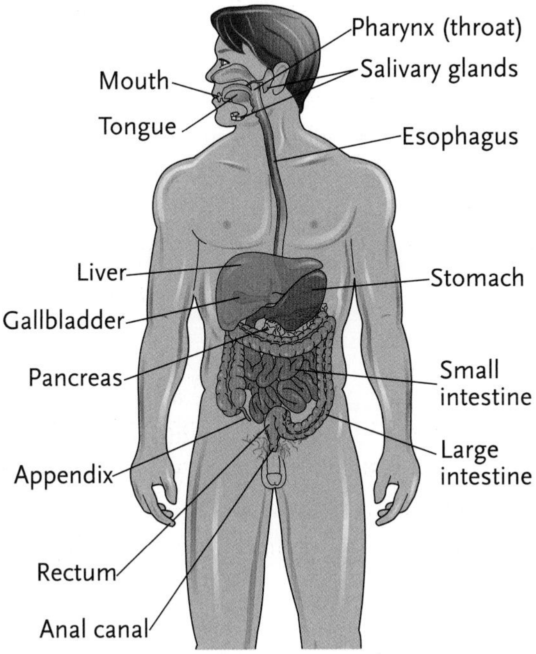

Fig. 6-13. *The GI system consists of all the organs needed to digest food and process waste.*

Food is first placed in the mouth. The teeth chew it by cutting it, then chopping and grinding it into smaller pieces that can be swallowed. Saliva moistens the food and begins chemical digestion. The tongue helps with chewing and swallowing by pushing the food around between the teeth and then into the pharynx. The pharynx is a muscular structure located at the back of the mouth. It extends into the throat. It contracts with swallowing and pushes food into the esophagus. The muscles of the esophagus then move food into the stomach through involuntary contractions called *peristalsis*.

The stomach is a muscular pouch located in the upper left part of the abdominal cavity. It provides physical digestion by stirring and churning the food to break it down into smaller particles. The glands in the stomach lining aid in digestion. They secrete gastric juices that chemically break down food. This process turns food into a semiliquid substance called *chyme*. Peristalsis continues in the stomach, pushing the chyme into the small intestine.

The small intestine is about 20 feet long. Here enzymes secreted by the liver and the pancreas finish digesting the chyme. Bile, a green liquid produced by the liver, is stored in the gallbladder and released into the small intestine. Bile helps break down dietary fat. The liver converts fats and sugars into glucose, a sugar that can be carried to cells by the blood. The liver also stores glucose. The pancreas produces insulin, a hormone that works to move **glucose**, or natural sugar, from the blood and into the cells for energy for the body.

The chyme is moved by peristalsis through the small intestine. There villi, tiny projections lining the small intestine, absorb the digested food into the capillaries.

Peristalsis moves the chyme that has not already been digested through the large intestine. In the large intestine, most of the water in the chyme is absorbed. What remains is feces, a semisolid material of water, solid waste material, bacteria, and mucus. Feces passes by peristalsis through the rectum, the lower end of the colon. It moves out of the body through the anus, the rectal opening.

The gastrointestinal system has the following functions: digestion, absorption, and elimination. *Digestion* is the process of preparing food physically and chemically so that it can be absorbed into the cells. *Absorption* is the transfer of nutrients from the intestines to the cells. *Elimination* is the process of expelling wastes (made up of the waste products of food and fluids) that are not absorbed into the cells.

PBT Connection

Common blood tests associated with gastrointestinal diseases and disorders include tests for antibodies often present in patients with digestive illnesses such as Crohn's disease or ulcerative colitis. There are also many blood tests related to the health of the liver. These tests, known as a *hepatic function panel*, check the levels of certain substances and enzymes in the blood. The results can help a doctor determine if a patient's liver is functioning properly. Phlebotomists may also assist in collecting stool samples or in conducting CLIA waived tests such as checking stool for the presence of hidden (occult) blood, which can be an indicator of colon or rectal cancer.

8. Describe the endocrine system

The endocrine system is made up of glands in different areas of the body (Fig. 6-14). *Glands* are organs that produce and secrete chemicals called hormones. **Hormones** are chemical substances created by the body that control numerous body functions. Hormones are carried in the blood to various organs.

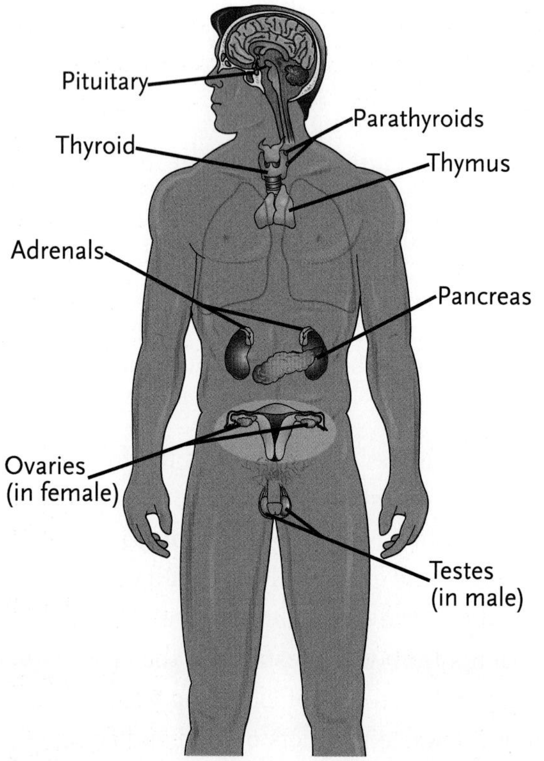

Fig. 6-14. *The endocrine system includes organs that produce hormones that regulate essential body processes.*

The pituitary gland, called the *master gland,* is located behind the eyes at the base of the brain. It secretes key hormones that cause other glands to produce other hormones. The following are some hormones secreted by the pituitary gland:

- Growth hormone, which regulates growth and development
- Antidiuretic hormone (ADH), which controls the balance of fluids in the body
- Oxytocin, which causes the uterus to contract during and after childbirth

The pituitary gland also produces hormones that regulate the thyroid gland and the adrenal glands. The thyroid gland is located in the neck in front of the larynx. It produces thyroid hormone, which regulates metabolism, the burning of food for heat and energy.

The parathyroid glands secrete a hormone that regulates the body's use of calcium. Nerves and muscles require calcium to function smoothly. A deficiency of this hormone can cause severe muscle contractions and spasms. It can be fatal if untreated.

The pancreas, a gland located in the upper midsection of the abdomen, secretes insulin. Insulin is a hormone that works to move glucose (natural sugar) from the blood and into the cells for energy for the body.

Two adrenal glands are located at the tops of the kidneys. They produce hormones that are essential to life. These hormones are important because they help the body regulate carbohydrate metabolism. They also control the body's reaction to stress and regulate salt and water absorption in the kidneys. Adrenal glands also produce the hormone adrenaline, which regulates muscle power, heart rate, blood pressure, and energy levels during stressful situations or emergencies.

Gonads, or sex glands, produce hormones that regulate the body's ability to reproduce. The testes in the male secrete testosterone. The ovaries in the female secrete estrogen and progesterone.

The functions of the endocrine system are to maintain homeostasis through hormone secretion, influence growth and development, maintain blood sugar levels, and regulate levels of calcium and phosphate in the body. The endocrine system also regulates the body's ability to reproduce and determines how fast cells burn food for energy.

PBT Connection

Many blood tests are associated with diseases and disorders of the endocrine system. **Diabetes** is an illness in which the pancreas does not produce enough insulin or does not produce any insulin. Blood tests to determine how much glucose is present in the blood aid in the diagnosis and management of diabetes. Patients with diagnosed diabetes may test their own blood regularly, and phlebotomists may also be trained to perform CLIA waived tests for blood glucose levels. Phlebotomists may also assist in performing glucose challenge or glucose tolerance tests, in which a patient drinks a very sweet liquid and then has her blood drawn for testing at certain intervals. These tests are commonly performed during pregnancy to check for **gestational diabetes**, a form of diabetes associated with pregnancy. Blood tests are also commonly used to diagnose and monitor treatment for other endocrine system disorders such as hyperthyroidism and hypothyroidism. In these disorders the levels of thyroid hormone, which controls many body processes, are either too high (*hyper*) or too low (*hypo*).

9. Describe the reproductive system

The reproductive system is made up of the reproductive organs, which are different in men and women. The reproductive system allows human beings to reproduce, or create new human life. Reproduction begins when a male's and female's sex cells (sperm and ovum) join. These sex cells are formed in the male and female sex glands. These sex glands are called the gonads.

In the male, the sex glands or gonads are the testes or testicles. The two oval glands are located outside the body in the scrotum. The scrotum is a sac made of skin and muscle that is suspended between the thighs. The testes produce the male sex cells, called sperm, and testosterone (Fig. 6-15). Testosterone is the hormone needed for the male reproductive organs to function properly. Testosterone also promotes development of male secondary sex characteristics such as growth of facial and body hair and deepening of the voice.

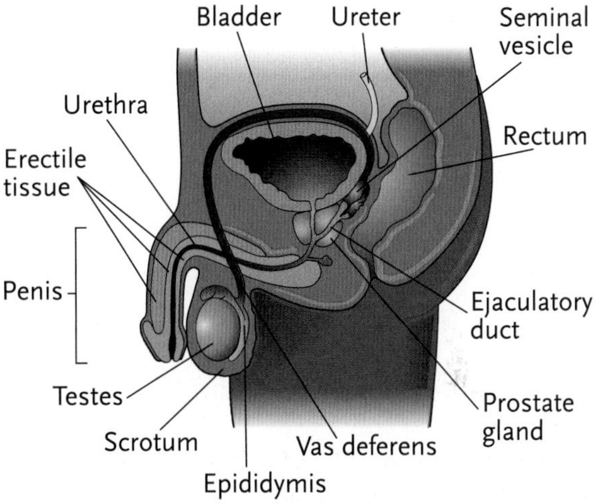

Fig. 6-15. *The male reproductive system.*

In the female, the gonads are two oval glands called the ovaries. There is one ovary on each side of the uterus (Fig. 6-16). The ovaries make the female sex cells or eggs (ova). They release the hormones estrogen and progesterone. Each month, from puberty to menopause, an egg is released from an ovary. This cycle is maintained by estrogen and progesterone. These hormones control development of female secondary sex characteristics, such as increased breast size and growth of pubic and underarm hair.

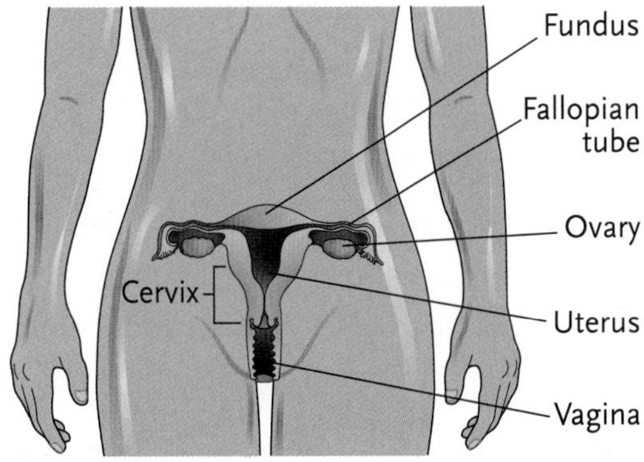

Fig. 6-16. *The female reproductive system.*

For males, the function of the reproductive system is to manufacture sperm and the hormone testosterone. For females, the reproductive system manufactures ova (eggs) and the hormones estrogen and progesterone. It also provides an environment for the development of a fetus and produces milk for the nourishment of a baby after birth.

PBT Connection

Blood tests are used to confirm pregnancy by measuring the level of hCG, a pregnancy-related hormone, in a patient's blood. Throughout a woman's pregnancy, blood tests are ordered at various times to screen for potential problems or defects in the fetus. They may also be used in various ways during the course of infertility treatment.

10. Describe the immune and lymphatic systems

The immune system protects the body from disease-causing bacteria, viruses, and microorganisms in two ways. **Nonspecific immunity** protects the body from disease in general. **Specific immunity** protects against a particular disease that is invading the body at a given time.

Nonspecific Immunity

To protect itself against disease in general, the body has several defenses:

- Anatomic barriers include the skin and the mucous membranes. They provide a physical barrier to keep foreign materials—bacteria, viruses, or microorganisms—from invading the body. Saliva, tears, and mucous secretions also help protect the body by washing away substances.
- Physiologic barriers include body temperature and acidity of certain organs. Most organisms that cause disease cannot survive high temperatures or high acidity. When the body senses foreign organisms, it can raise its temperature (by running a fever) to kill off the invaders. The acidity of organs like the stomach keeps harmful bacteria from growing there.
- Inflammatory response refers to the body's ability to fight infection through inflammation or swelling of an infected area. When inflammation occurs, it indicates that the body has sent extra disease-fighting cells and extra blood to the infected area to fight the infection.

Specific Immunity

To protect itself against specific diseases, the body makes different types of cells that will fight a range of different invaders. Once it has successfully eliminated an invader, the immune system records the invasion in the form of antibodies. Antibodies are carried within cells. They prevent a disease from threatening the body a second time.

Acquired immunity is a kind of specific immunity. The body acquires it either by fighting an infection or by vaccination. For example, a person can acquire immunity to a disease like the measles in two ways:

1. The person gets measles. His body forms antibodies to the disease to make sure he will not get it again; or
2. The person gets a vaccine for the measles. This causes his body to produce the same antibodies to protect him from the disease.

The lymphatic system removes excess fluids and waste products from the body's tissues. It also helps the immune system fight infection. It is closely related to both the immune and the circulatory systems. The lymphatic system consists of lymph vessels and lymph capillaries in which a fluid called lymph circulates (Fig. 6-17). **Lymph** is a clear yellowish fluid that carries disease-fighting cells called lymphocytes.

When the body is fighting an infection, swelling may occur in the lymph nodes. These are oval-shaped bodies that can be as small as a pinhead or as large as an almond. Located in the neck, groin, and armpits, the lymph nodes filter out germs and waste products carried from the tissues by the lymph fluid. After lymph fluid has been filtered in the lymph nodes, it flows into the bloodstream.

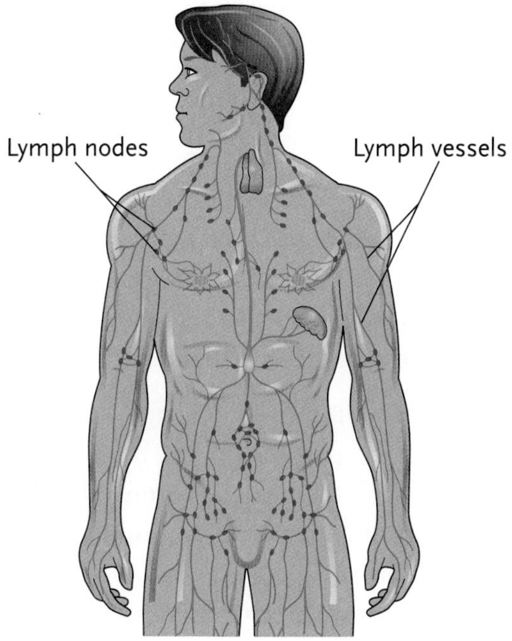

Fig. 6-17. *Lymph nodes work to fight infection and are located throughout the body.*

Unlike the circulatory system, in which the heart functions as a pump to move the blood, the lymph system has no pump. Lymph fluid is circulated by muscle activity, massage, and breathing. A sore muscle may feel better if it is rubbed. The rubbing action helps the lymph fluid circulate, carrying waste products away from the tired muscle.

The functions of the immune and lymphatic systems are to protect the body against disease-causing bacteria, viruses, and microorganisms and to remove excess fluids and waste products from the body's tissues.

PBT Connection

Immune system disorders might be caused by overactive or underactive immune responses. In some disorders, a person's immune system attacks and damages the person's own cells or tissues. This is called an *autoimmune* disorder, and different autoimmune disorders may affect different body systems. Rheumatoid arthritis and Guillain-Barré syndrome are examples. In other disorders, the immune system either does not respond or does not respond enough to true threats from pathogens. This is called *immune deficiency*. Blood tests can be used to analyze the presence or absence of particular antibodies, and can also determine the speed and efficiency of the immune system's response.

Chapter Review

Multiple Choice

1. Which of the following is an example of a *sign*?
   (A) Patient reports dizziness
   (B) Patient looks tired
   (C) Patient's heart rate is elevated and irregular
   (D) Patient reports feelings of anxiety
2. The condition in which the body's systems are working together to maintain health and stability is known as
   (A) Homeostasis
   (B) Homogeneity
   (C) Hemogenesis
   (D) Homeodynamism
3. Blood vessels and nerve endings are concentrated in the
   (A) Epidermis
   (B) Dermis
   (C) Subcutaneous tissue
   (D) Sebaceous glands
4. One of the functions of muscles is to
   (A) Supply oxygen and nutrients to the body
   (B) Provide heat
   (C) Direct and coordinate the movements of the body
   (D) Rid the body of wastes

5. How does the nervous system send messages to the brain?
   (A) Through the blood that flows to the head
   (B) Through a network of special vessels carrying neuron-filled fluid
   (C) Through neurons, from receptors throughout the body and then through the spinal cord
   (D) From the right hemisphere of the cerebrum to the left hemisphere

6. Which of the following is part of the peripheral nervous system?
   (A) The brainstem
   (B) The spinal cord
   (C) The cerebral cortex
   (D) The nerves

7. Peristalsis is the process that
   (A) Transmits information from the sense organs to the brain
   (B) Moves food through the gastrointestinal system
   (C) Causes blood to clot
   (D) Secretes hormones that regulate body processes

8. This gland is also known as the *master gland*:
   (A) The pituitary gland
   (B) The parathyroid gland
   (C) The adrenal gland
   (D) The pancreas

9. Progesterone is a hormone associated with
   (A) The male reproductive system
   (B) Regulation of calcium levels in the blood
   (C) The female reproductive system
   (D) Movement of glucose from the blood into the cells of the body

10. Which of the following describes a type of acquired immunity?
    (A) A person is exposed to influenza, but does not become ill because he had received an influenza vaccine three weeks before.
    (B) A person is exposed to influenza, but does not become ill because he is always very careful about washing hands.
    (C) An infant does not become sick with influenza, despite being too young to receive the vaccine, because everyone around him has received the vaccine.
    (D) A person is exposed to influenza, but does not become ill because he was wearing a mask at the time.

11. Lymph is a fluid that circulates
    (A) With the pumping of the heart
    (B) Through the spinal column
    (C) Through muscle activity, massage, and breathing
    (D) Only in times of strong immune system response

7
The Circulatory System in Depth

1. Describe the circulatory system and the structure and function of the heart

The circulatory, or cardiovascular, system is made up of the heart, blood vessels, and blood (Fig. 7-1). A healthy circulatory system is essential for life. Phlebotomists are responsible for drawing blood from patients, so it is important that they understand basic facts about how the circulatory system works.

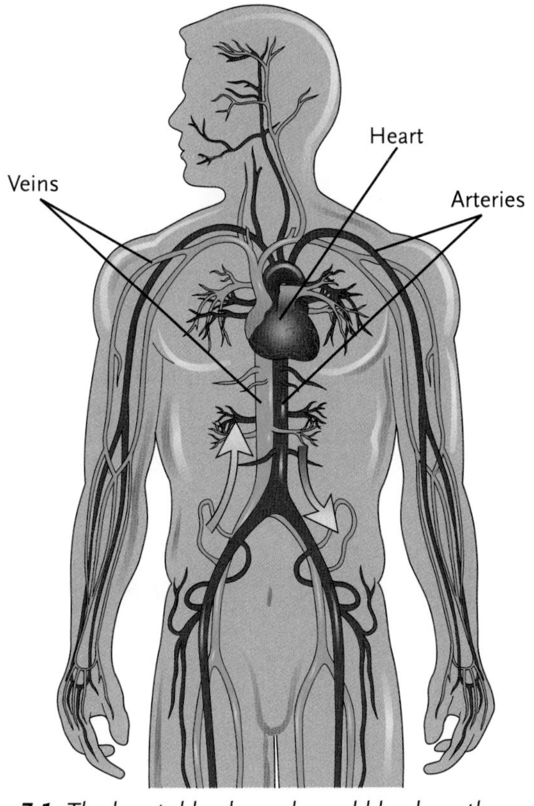

Fig. 7-1. *The heart, blood vessels, and blood are the main parts of the circulatory system.*

The heart is located between the lungs, and its center is just left of the midline of the body. The top of the heart, known as the *base,* points toward the right shoulder. The bottom of the heart, known as the *apex,* points toward the left hip. The heart can be described as a double pump, pumping deoxygenated blood into the lungs and pumping oxygenated blood to the body. The right side of the heart receives deoxygenated blood from the body through the veins and pumps it to the lungs. In the lungs, the blood receives oxygen again. The left side of the heart receives the oxygenated blood from the lungs and pumps it out to the body through the arteries.

The right and left sides of the heart are separated by a wall called a **septum**. The heart has two upper chambers called **atria** (singular: atrium) and two lower chambers called **ventricles**. The chambers contract and relax in a rhythmic pattern to produce blood flow.

The atria contract while the ventricles relax, and then the atria relax while the ventricles contract. This back-and-forth action between the upper and lower chambers allows the chambers to fill with blood before they contract to pump the blood.

Blood always flows through the heart in a distinct path. First, the right atrium receives deoxygenated blood from the body and pumps it to the right ventricle. The right ventricle pumps the deoxygenated blood to the lungs through the pulmonary arteries. The lungs oxygenate the blood, which then returns to the heart through the pulmonary veins.

The left atrium receives blood from the pulmonary veins and pumps it to the left ventricle. The left ventricle pumps oxygenated blood out of the heart via the aorta, the largest artery in the body.

A series of valves ensures that blood flows in the correct direction as it is pumped through the heart. The four major valves of the heart are the **tricuspid valve**, the **pulmonary valve**, the **bicuspid valve**, and the **aortic valve** (Fig. 7-2). During a normal heart cycle, the tricuspid and bicuspid valves will be closed, and the pulmonary and aortic valves open, when the ventricles contract.

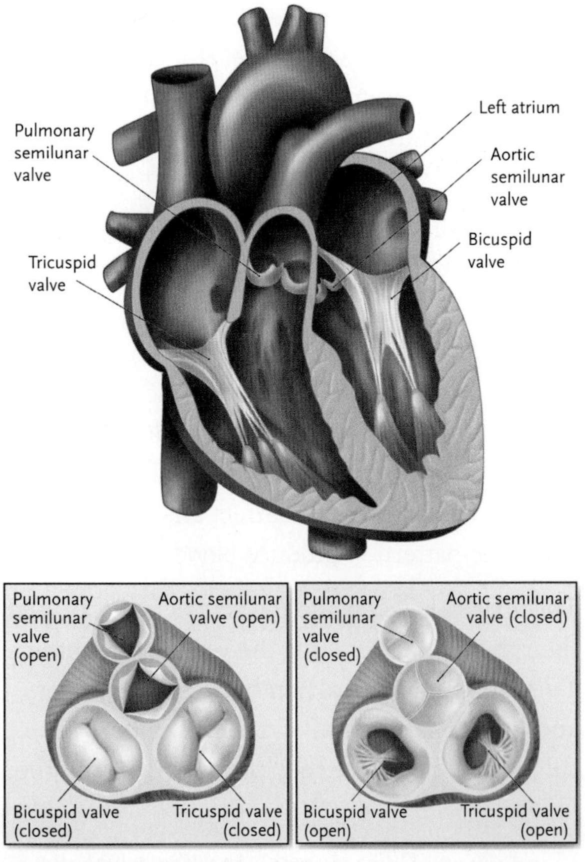

Fig. 7-2. *The valves of the heart work to ensure proper blood flow.*

2. Explain the cardiac conduction system

In order for the heart to pump blood throughout the body, the heart muscle and valves must be healthy, and there must be enough blood in an intact system of blood vessels. There is also another essential factor in proper heart function: a system of specialized cardiac tissue capable of generating electrical signals. The actions of the heart muscle are prompted by electrical signals. Specialized heart tissue begins, or *initiates*, these electrical impulses, then *conducts*, or carries, them through the heart. These impulses are the "spark" that triggers the mechanical actions of the heart muscle. This network of signal-conducting tissue is known as the **cardiac conduction system** (Fig. 7-3).

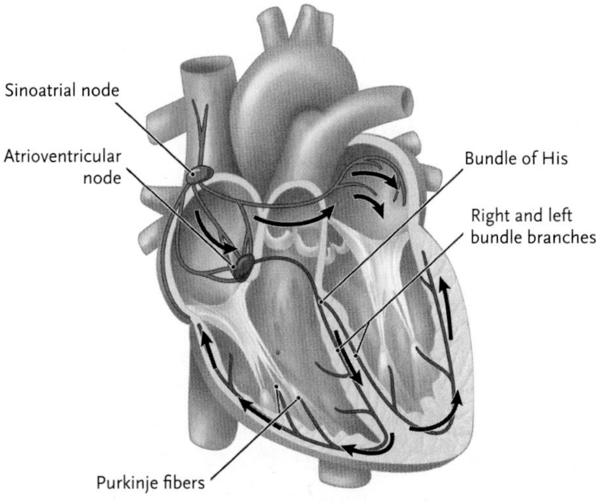

Fig. 7-3. *Electrical impulses are conducted through the heart, causing the heart muscles to contract in a regular rhythm to pump blood.*

The cardiac conduction system begins in the upper part of the right atrium and continues through the heart to the walls of the ventricles. The **sinoatrial node**, sometimes called the *SA node* or *sinus node*, is in the upper part of the right atrium and is the main pacemaker of the heart. This means it sets the timing of the heart's contractions.

From the SA node, the electrical impulse travels to the **atrioventricular node**, also called the *AV node,* at the bottom of the right atrium, behind the tricuspid valve. As the impulse enters the AV node it is slowed down slightly. Without this delay the atria and ventricles would contract at the same time. Instead, this delay allows the atria to empty of blood and the ventricles to fill before they contract.

The electrical impulse then travels through an area known as the **atrioventricular (AV) junction** to the **bundle of His**, or *AV bundle*. The bundle of His is located in the upper part of the wall between the left and right ventricles. Fibrous connective tissue surrounds the conductive tissue in the bundle of His and makes sure that the impulse travels the correct route.

The bundle of His divides into the right and left **bundle branches**. These branches carry the electrical impulse to the walls of the ventricles. The bundle branches continue to divide into smaller branches and then form the **Purkinje fibers**.

3. Describe blood vessels

There are three main types of blood vessels found in the body: arteries, capillaries, and veins. **Arteries** carry oxygenated blood away from the heart to all cells in the body (Fig. 7-4). The aorta, the largest artery in the body, receives blood from the left ventricle when the heart contracts. Arteries become smaller and connect with arterioles, or small arteries, before connecting with capillaries.

The capillaries are very small blood vessels where exchanges are made. Exchanges of oxygen and carbon dioxide, and of nutrients and waste products, take place between the blood and the cells in areas called **capillary beds** (Fig. 7-5). The capillaries connect to venules, or small veins, which then connect to larger veins. The veins carry blood containing waste products and carbon dioxide back to the heart (Fig. 7-6). The **inferior vena cava**, carrying blood from the legs and trunk, and the **superior vena cava**, carrying blood from the arms, head, and neck, empty into the right atrium of the heart.

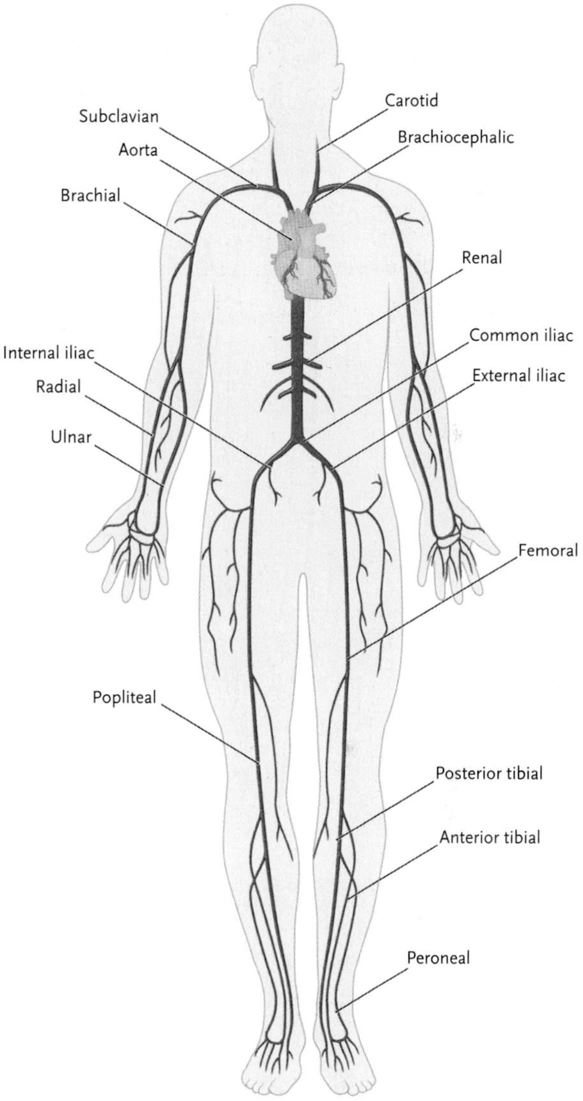

Fig. 7-4. *These are the major arteries of the body.*

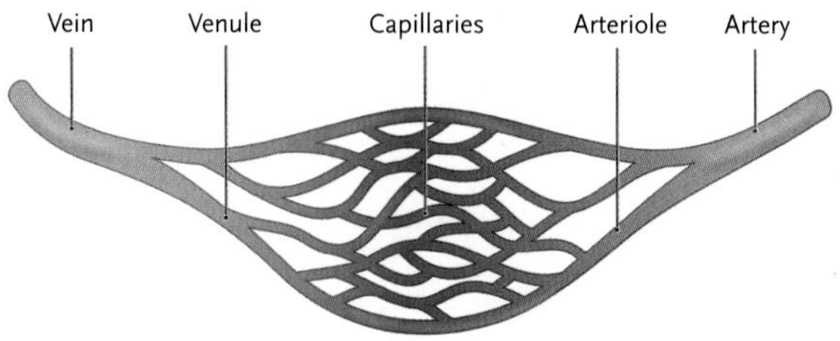

Fig. 7-5. *Networks of capillaries allow for the exchange of gases, nutrients, and wastes.*

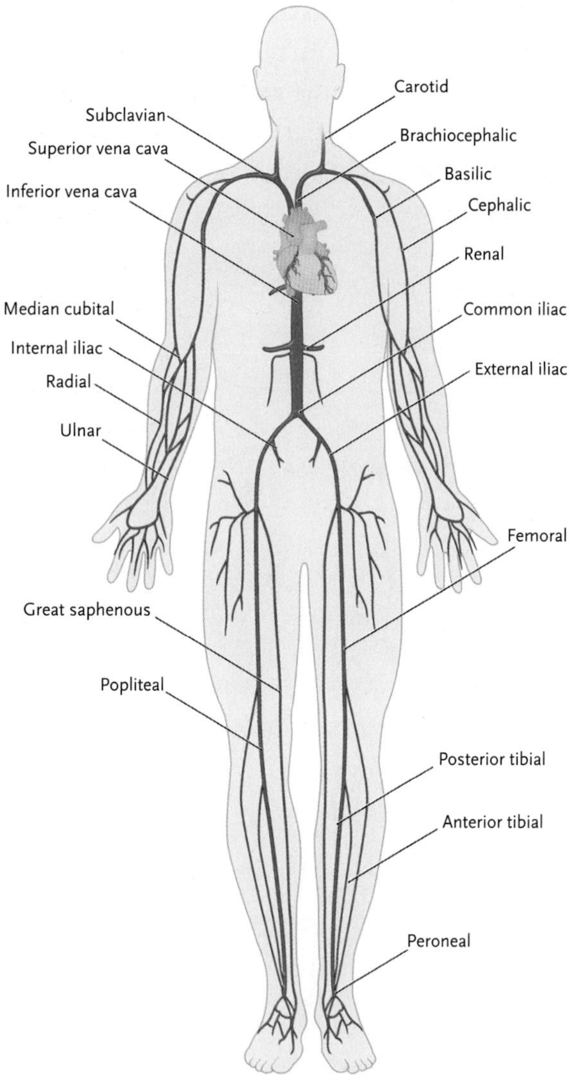

Fig. 7-6. *These are the major veins of the body.*

The structure of veins and arteries is similar. However, arteries have thicker walls to withstand the pressure of the beating heart. When felt through the skin (or **palpated**), arteries feel stiff and firm. It is also possible to feel the pulsing of blood through the arteries when the heart beats. Veins have thinner walls, and many veins also have internal valves that help to keep blood moving in the right direction, back toward the heart. When palpated, healthy veins feel more springy or bouncy than arteries, and there is no pulse present.

The walls of veins and arteries are composed of three layers: an outer layer, called the **tunica adventitia**; a middle layer, called the **tunica media**; and an inner layer, called the **tunica intima** (Fig. 7-7). The middle layer, which is composed of muscle tissue and elastic fibers, is considerably thinner in veins than it is in arteries. The thinner walls of the veins increase their capacity to hold blood. At any given time about 70% of the body's blood is found in the veins.

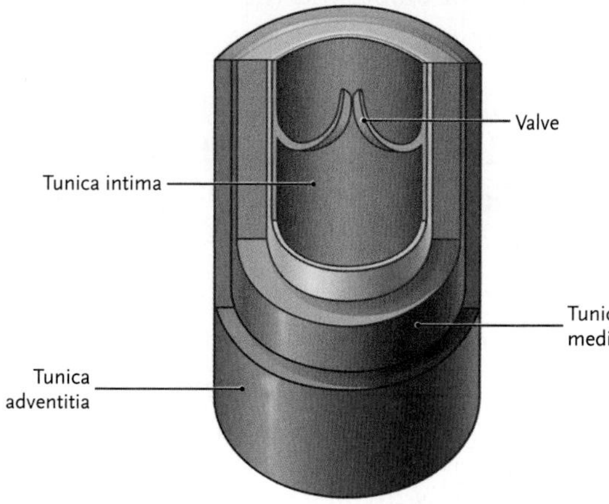

Fig. 7-7. *Vein walls are made up of three layers. Valves may be present to help direct the flow of blood.*

The blood vessels of the body circulate blood between the heart and the lungs (called the **pulmonary circuit**) and between the heart and the rest of the body (called the **systemic circuit**). After the venae cavae (plural for *vena cava*) deliver deoxygenated blood to the right atrium, the blood flows to the right ventricle. There it is pumped to the lungs through the pulmonary arteries (the only arteries in the body that carry deoxygenated blood). At the end of the respiratory tract are tiny, elastic sacs called *alveoli* that are surrounded by capillaries. Oxygen and carbon dioxide are exchanged between the alveoli and capillaries. Oxygenated blood goes from the pulmonary capillaries to venules. Then it travels to the pulmonary veins (the only veins in the body that carry oxygenated blood) before arriving at the left atrium (Fig. 7-8).

The systemic circuit is the constant, closed circuit that delivers substances needed by the cells and removes waste products at exchange sites throughout the body. It begins when the left ventricle pumps blood to the aorta. That blood is eventually returned to the right atrium through the superior and inferior venae cavae.

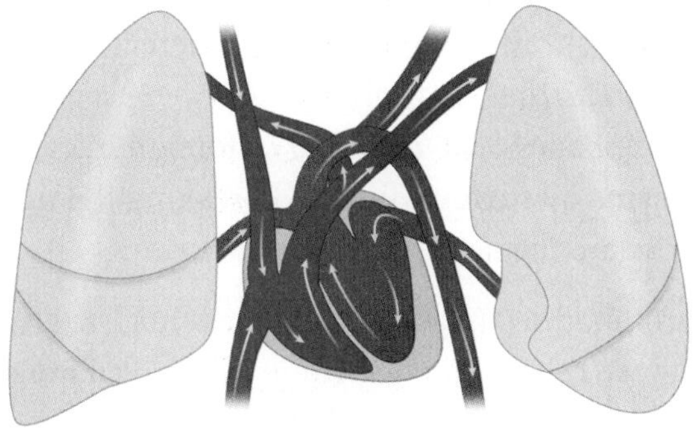

Fig. 7-8. The pulmonary circuit is the path deoxygenated blood follows from the heart to the lungs and back to the heart.

4. Describe the components of blood

The average healthy adult has five to six liters of blood, consisting of a liquid component called **plasma** and solid components called **formed elements** (Fig. 7-9). Blood transports gases, nutrients, wastes, and hormones throughout the body. It also protects against infections, forms clots to stop blood loss in the case of injury, regulates body temperature, and helps the body maintain homeostasis.

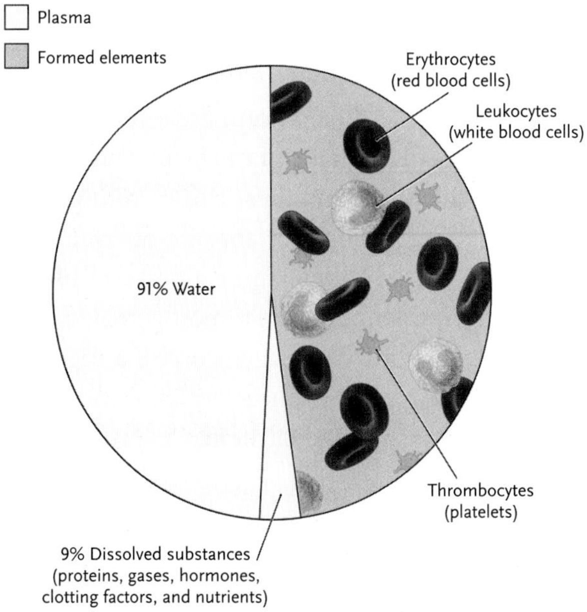

Fig. 7-9. Blood is made up of liquid and solid components.

About 55% of the total blood volume is made up of plasma, which is a clear, straw-colored fluid. Plasma is about 91% water and 9% dissolved substances, including proteins, gases, hormones, and nutrients. Some of the proteins in the plasma are important for proper blood clotting.

Formed elements make up about 45% of the blood volume and include red blood cells (RBCs), also called **erythrocytes**, several types of white blood cells (WBCs), also called **leukocytes**, and platelets, also called **thrombocytes** (Fig. 7-10). Erythrocytes contain hemoglobin, a protein that transports oxygen and carbon dioxide. Leukocytes protect the body against foreign substances such as bacteria and viruses. Thrombocytes play a role in blood clotting (see Learning Objective 7).

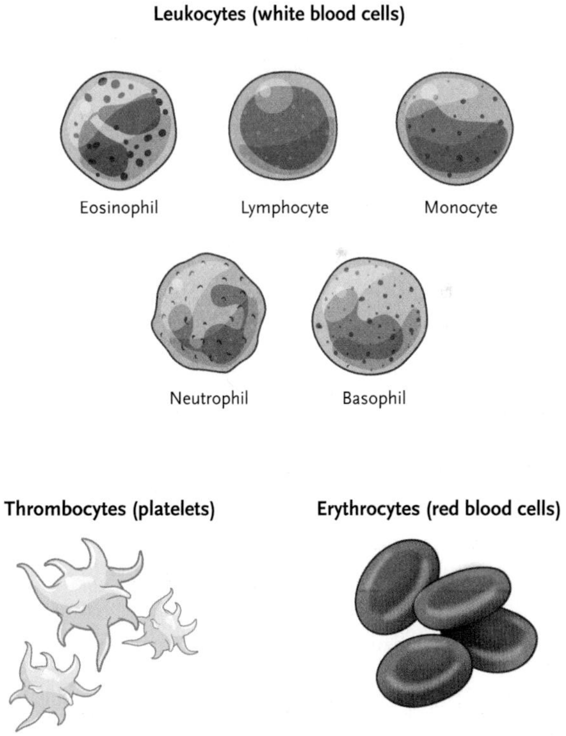

Fig. 7-10. Each solid component of blood has its own unique form and appearance.

Erythrocytes are the most common of the blood cells. They make up about 40% of total blood volume. They are generated from **stem cells**, or cells that can become any type of cell, in the bone marrow. They mature over the course of about seven days and live for approximately 120 days. They are disc-like with a center indented on both sides. Their shape allows them to bend to fit into blood vessels of all sizes. Some capillaries are so small that erythrocytes must go through them one by one or even distort themselves in order to fit.

Leukocytes are much fewer in number, accounting for around 1% of total blood volume. There are several different types of leukocytes. The most common is the **neutrophil**. Neutrophils make up approximately 1/2 to 2/3 the total number of white blood cells. Neutrophils are also generated from stem cells in the bone marrow, and they are the body's first defense against illness. Related to the neutrophils, but less numerous, are the **eosinophils** and **basophils**. Together these three types of white blood cells are known as **granulocytes**. Granulocytes are very short-lived. Any given cell lasts less than a full day, so they must be generated constantly.

Approximately 20–30% of the white blood cells are **lymphocytes**. They play a number of roles in boosting the body's immune system. These cells also originate in the bone marrow. Some remain in the marrow and mature into a type of lymphocyte known as **B cells**. Some move to the thymus, an organ in the lymphatic system, and become **T cells**. Some types of T cells give chemical signals to the body to regulate immune response and some fight infected cells directly. B cells, with the help of signals from the T cells, produce antibodies. Antibodies bind to **antigens**, or proteins that mark foreign substances and cause immune response. Lymphocytes circulate in the blood but are also present in high concentrations in the lymph nodes, tonsils, and spleen. Most lymphocytes live only a few weeks, but some can live for years. This provides the body's immune system with a "memory" of antigens it has encountered in the past. It allows for a more rapid response when the body is exposed to them again.

Up to 10% of the white blood cells in the human body are **monocytes**. After entering the bloodstream from the bone marrow, monocytes move to tissues throughout the body. There they mature further into cells called *macrophages*. Macrophages "eat" invading or foreign microorganisms by surrounding and breaking them up. These are the largest of the leukocytes.

Thrombocytes (platelets) are not actually cells; they are cell fragments. Large cells called **megakaryocytes** are produced in the bone marrow, and these cells fragment into platelets. Platelets are important in the beginning stages of blood clotting (see Learning Objective 7).

PBT Connection

The **complete blood count** (**CBC**) is a common test used to check the composition of a patient's blood. It allows a doctor to determine how many red blood cells, white blood cells, and platelets are in a patient's blood. In some variations the test may further measure how many of each type of white blood cell is present. This is called a complete blood count *with differential*. **Anemia** is a condition in which a person has either too few red blood cells or too little hemoglobin in the blood. A CBC may be used to diagnose anemia.

5. Explain the ABO blood group system and the Rh factor

The surfaces of red blood cells have certain antigens (substances that can cause an immune response) attached, and these differ from person to person. The presence or absence of specific antigens is tested to determine a person's **blood type**. The antigens most commonly present on RBCs are known as A antigens and B antigens. People may have one of these antigens, both of these antigens, or none of them.

People with blood type A have A antigens. Because the body of a person with type A blood recognizes A antigens as part of itself, it does not create antibodies to attack them. It does, however, create antibodies to attack B antigens (called *anti-B antibodies*). People with blood type B have B antigens and anti-A antibodies. People with both A and B antigens are said to have type AB blood. Because their bodies recognize both A and B antigens as "self," they do not possess anti-A or anti-B antibodies. Individuals with neither A nor B antigens have type O blood, and have both anti-A and anti-B antibodies (Fig. 7-11). This system of classifying blood types is called the **ABO blood group system**.

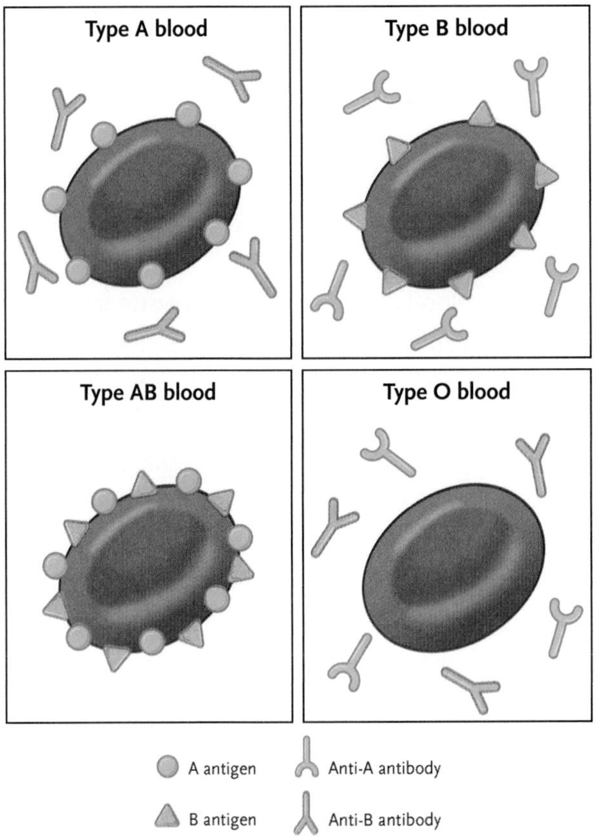

Fig. 7-11. *Blood type is determined based on the type of antigens present on a person's red blood cells.*

Another variation in red blood cells involves the presence or absence of a protein called **Rh factor**. Individuals who have Rh factor on their red blood cells are said to be **Rh positive**. Those who do not have the protein are considered **Rh negative**. *Negative* or *positive* is usually attached to the description of a person's blood type to indicate absence or presence of Rh factor. For example, a person with *O positive* blood has type O blood with Rh factor present.

Rh factor and blood type are genetically determined, meaning a person's blood type results from the combination of genes passed down from both parents. While people with A antigens naturally possess anti-B antibodies and vice versa, people who are Rh negative do not naturally possess anti-Rh antibodies. They only develop these antibodies when their blood is exposed to Rh-positive blood.

This can happen in the case of a **transfusion** (a transfer of blood from one person to the bloodstream of another) from an Rh-positive donor, or in certain situations when an Rh-negative woman is pregnant with an Rh-positive fetus. The first time an Rh-negative person's blood encounters Rh-positive blood, the resulting reaction is generally mild. The antibodies have not yet developed in great number. The second time, however, dangerous or even fatal complications can occur. In the case of a mother and fetus or infant, a second Rh-positive child is at greater risk than the first. Because of this, women are tested for blood type and Rh factor early in pregnancy. Medicine can be given to the mother to suppress her body's response to Rh factor, and the fetus can be monitored for signs of red blood cell destruction.

Before a patient receives a blood transfusion or an organ transplant, her blood is tested for blood type and for the presence of Rh factor. Because of the antibodies that are present with certain blood types or that may develop in Rh-negative recipients, not all blood can be transfused into all people. For example, a person with type A blood possesses anti-B antibodies and so cannot receive type B or type AB blood. Further, if the recipient is Rh negative, the donor blood must also be Rh negative. Table 7-1 summarizes the donor and recipient restrictions for each blood type.

Because AB blood type, Rh-positive individuals can receive blood from any ABO and Rh type, they are known as *universal recipients*. And

BLOOD TYPE (ABO AND RH)	APPROXIMATE PERCENTAGE OF PEOPLE WITH THIS TYPE	CAN DONATE TO	CAN RECEIVE FROM
A, Rh positive (A+)	36%	A+, AB+	A+, A-, O+, O-
A, Rh negative (A-)	6%	A+, A-, AB+, AB-	A-, O-
B, Rh positive (B+)	9%	B+, AB+	B+, B-, O+, O-
B, Rh negative (B-)	2%	B+, B-, AB+, AB-	B-, O-
AB, Rh positive (AB+)	3%	AB+	All ABO and Rh types/ everyone
AB, Rh negative (AB-)	Less than 1%	AB+, AB-	A-, B-, AB-, O-
O, Rh positive (O+)	37%	A+, B+, AB+, O+	O+, O-
O, Rh negative (O-)	7%	All ABO and Rh types/ everyone	O-

Table 7-1. *Blood type determines the type(s) of blood people can receive and to whom they can donate.*

because O blood type, Rh-negative individuals can donate blood to any ABO and Rh type, they are called *universal donors.*

Quality Counts

Patients must always be identified before providing care. In the case of blood typing and blood transfusions, the risks associated with failure to identify patients and/or label specimens clearly and accurately can be deadly. Even a small amount of the wrong type of blood transfused into a patient can cause a series of effects that can lead to serious damage or death. PBTs must always remember that following policies about patient identification and specimen labeling can be a life-or-death issue.

6. Describe the qualities of arterial, venous, and capillary blood

Although all blood in the body has the same basic composition of plasma and formed elements, blood found in different types of blood vessels will have different qualities.

Blood in the arteries, or **arterial blood**, has been pumped out from the heart to be carried throughout the body. With the exception of blood in the pulmonary arteries, arterial blood is oxygenated. Oxygen is transported by the protein hemoglobin, which is present in red blood cells. Hemoglobin contains iron and gives blood its red color. Oxygenated arterial blood is bright red. Arterial wounds can bleed forcefully, possibly spurting or spraying due to the pressure created by the beating heart.

Although blood in the veins, or **venous blood**, is usually depicted as blue in illustrations and may appear blue under the skin, it is not blue at all. Veins return blood to the heart, and in all cases other than the pulmonary veins, they carry deoxygenated blood. The color of this blood is a darker, deeper red. The blue color of veins under the skin is a trick of light, and when venous blood flows into a collection tube its deep, nearly maroon color is visible (Fig. 7-12).

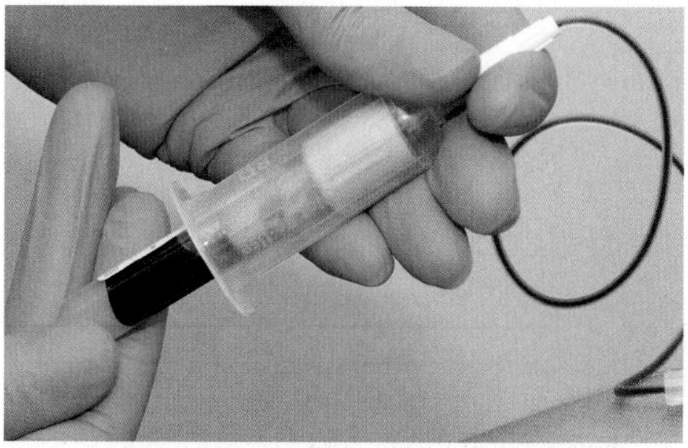

Fig. 7-12. *Venous blood is very dark red in color.*

Venous blood does not flow with the same amount of pressure as arterial blood. It does not spurt or pulse when a vein is breached. In fact, taking venous blood from a patient requires some amount of force to pull, or draw, the blood from the veins. Venous blood is usually collected either in a tube emptied of air to create a vacuum that draws in the blood, or through the use of a **syringe**, a tubular device with a plunger that draws blood from the veins when pulled.

The capillaries are the smallest blood vessels in the body. They are the exchange sites between veins and arteries. **Capillary blood** contains a mixture of arterial and venous blood. Nutrients and wastes are also exchanged in capillary beds, so capillary blood will also contain these substances. Its color is somewhere between the bright red of arterial blood and the deep red of venous blood.

7. Discuss hemostasis and coagulation and related conditions

An anticoagulant is a substance that prevents blood from clotting. The innermost lining of blood vessels releases natural anticoagulants to keep blood moving within the body and to prevent **thrombosis**, or the formation of a clot within the blood vessel. When this lining is disturbed by an injury, the body is able to repair the injury while maintaining the flow of blood in the rest of the circulatory system. This is called **hemostasis**.

When tissue outside the inner lining of the blood vessels is exposed to blood, this triggers a series of reactions. First, the muscular tissue in the tunica media constricts, or narrows, at the site of the injury. This **vasoconstriction** limits the amount of blood flowing to the area around the injury (Fig. 7-13). Second, nearby platelets are activated, or made to stick to the site of the injury and to each other. **Enzymes** are substances in the body that speed up specific reactions. An enzyme in the plasma called **thrombin** controls the platelet response. Thrombin activates only the platelets in the area immediately around the wound (Fig. 7-14). The formation of this platelet plug is known as **primary hemostasis**.

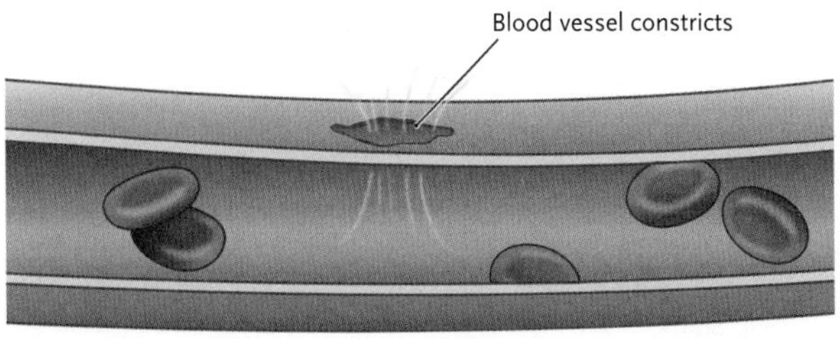

Fig. 7-13. *After an injury to a blood vessel, such as one caused by a needle during a blood draw, the blood vessel constricts to reduce the flow of blood.*

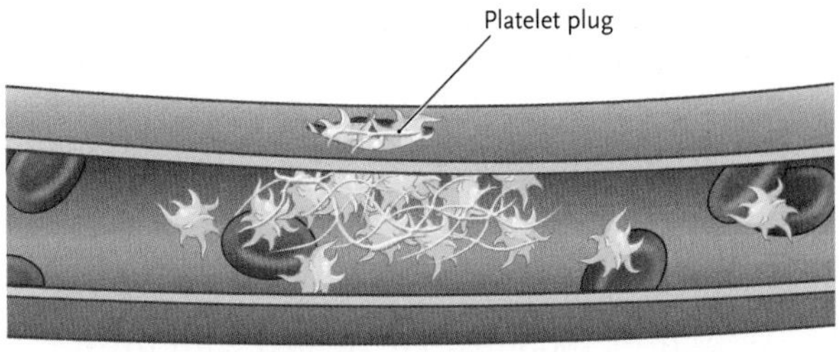

Fig. 7-14. *Platelets are quickly activated to start plugging the wound.*

Thrombin is also key in changing a protein called **fibrinogen**, which is present in the plasma, to **fibrin**, a protein that cannot be dissolved. Together, fibrin and the activated platelets form a mesh at the injury site to create a **hemostatic plug**, stopping blood loss (Fig. 7-15). This phase is known as **secondary hemostasis**. When an injury heals, a process called **fibrinolysis** breaks down the clot. An enzyme called **plasmin** is key to breaking apart the fibrin in the clot. Fibrinolysis is a complementary process to hemostasis, preserving the balance between blood flow and clotting.

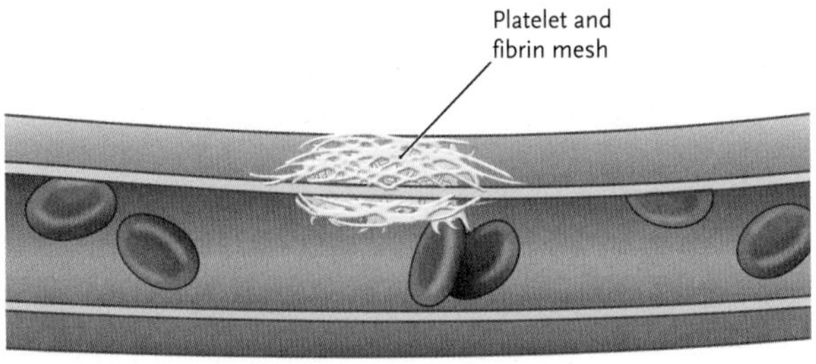

Fig. 7-15. *The hemostatic plug is made up of platelets and fibrin.*

Hemostasis and blood clotting are very complicated processes, involving a large number of blood proteins (known as **clotting factors**) and enzymes. The term **coagulation cascade** describes this series of changes that prevent blood loss while also avoiding unnecessary and dangerous excessive clotting. Certain disorders can cause either excessive clotting or excessive bleeding. **Hemophilia** is a disorder that can cause excessive bleeding. **Thrombophilia** is a disorder that can cause excessive clotting. A clot formed inside a blood vessel is called a **thrombus**. This is especially dangerous when it occurs in deep veins; these clots can come loose, move, and cause **pulmonary embolism**, a potentially deadly disorder involving blood clots in the lungs.

People with hemophilia are treated with infusions of the clotting factors they lack. People with thrombophilia may be treated with anticoagulant medications. These medications are also used in certain other situations. Some types of abnormal heart rhythms or the presence of artificial heart valves might increase a patient's risk for abnormal blood clotting and require the use of anticoagulant therapy. Blood testing may be required to monitor these conditions.

Quality Counts

When a PBT performs venipuncture or capillary puncture, the process of hemostasis repairs the wound. Applying pressure to the puncture site aids in vasoconstriction and speeds the process along. Bleeding from a capillary puncture site is likely to stop more quickly than bleeding from a venipuncture site. It is important for the PBT to ensure bleeding has stopped before allowing a patient to leave. In patients taking anticoagulant medications this process can take a bit longer.

Blood does not just clot in or on the body. Blood specimens that are not treated with an anticoagulant will clot after a certain amount of time (usually 30–60 minutes). When processing blood specimens, some tests require that the blood be allowed to clot in the collection tube. Some require that the blood remain uncoagulated. Collection tubes contain a variety of **additives**, or chemical agents that affect how the blood can be processed and tested. The tubes are color coded to indicate the type of additive contained (more detail about the tubes and the color coding system is found in Chapter 8).

After a specimen is collected, it may need to be processed for testing. Often this involves allowing the tube(s) to sit for a specific amount of time and then spinning them in a centrifuge, which separates the liquid and solid components. Blood specimens spun in a centrifuge after coagulation are different from blood specimens collected in a tube with an anticoagulant additive (Fig. 7-16).

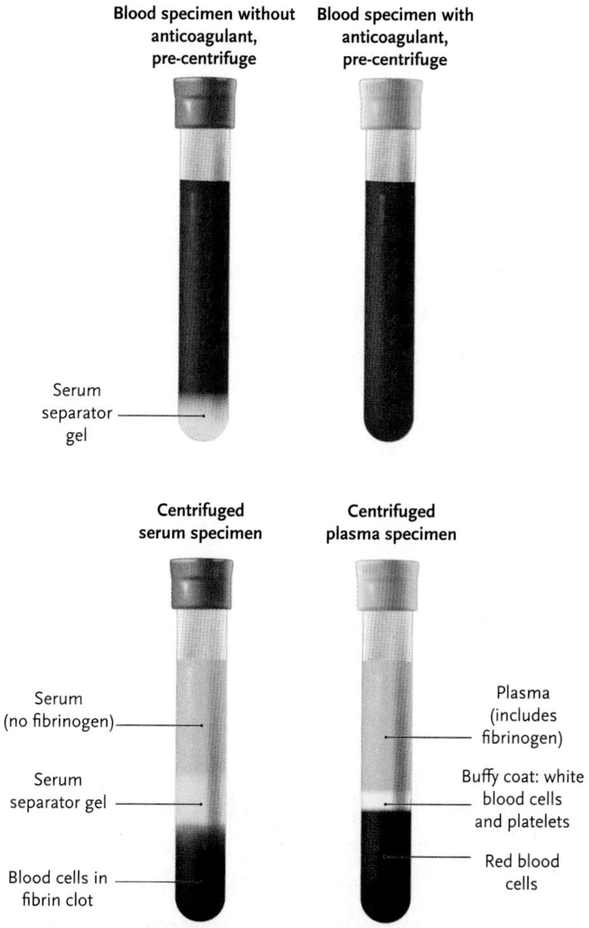

Fig. 7-16. *Blood specimens that have been allowed to coagulate are different from blood specimens collected in tubes with an anticoagulant additive.*

After centrifuging, a coagulated specimen contains blood cells in a fibrin clot at the bottom. At the top, the specimen contains a liquid portion known as **serum**. Serum is distinct from plasma. Serum lacks fibrinogen, which is present in plasma. Some collection tubes for serum samples will contain a gel that separates the serum from the solid blood components.

Before an anticoagulated specimen is spun, it is known as a **whole blood specimen**. Because the anticoagulant prevents clotting, the tube contains all components of the blood, more or less as they exist in the body. When an anticoagulated specimen is spun, it divides into three layers. The bottom layer includes red blood cells. The thin middle layer contains white blood cells and platelets, and is known as the **buffy coat**. The top layer contains plasma, including fibrinogen.

Some diagnostic tests, such as tests related to immunology, require serum specimens. Some, such as tests related to hematology, require anticoagulated specimens. These specimens may be either in whole blood form or centrifuged into solid and liquid components. It is important for phlebotomists to know the difference between the composition of these specimens.

Chapter Review

Multiple Choice

1. The circulatory system is also known as the
   (A) Cardiovascular system
   (B) Vein system
   (C) Oxygen exchange system
   (D) Arterial system
2. The heart pumps deoxygenated blood to the ____________ and oxygenated blood to the ____________.
   (A) entire body, lungs
   (B) limbs, brain
   (C) extremities, heart muscle
   (D) lungs, entire body
3. The valves of the heart function to
   (A) Keep blood flowing in the correct direction through the heart
   (B) Protect the arteries from extreme pressure
   (C) Send electrical signals that cause the heart to contract
   (D) Measure the amount of blood flowing through the heart
4. Which of the following is the main pacemaker of the heart?
   (A) The aorta
   (B) The semilunar valve
   (C) The sinoatrial node
   (D) The atrioventricular node
5. The smallest blood vessels are called
   (A) Capillaries
   (B) Venules
   (C) Arterioles
   (D) Erythrocytes
6. These blood vessels almost always carry oxygenated blood:
   (A) Veins
   (B) Arteries
   (C) Pulmonary arteries
   (D) Venules
7. The layer in blood vessels made up mostly of muscle tissue and elastic fibers is known as the
   (A) Tunica intima
   (B) Tunica media
   (C) Tunica adventitia
   (D) Tunica variegata
8. Which type of blood vessel typically holds about 70% of the body's blood?
   (A) The veins
   (B) The arteries
   (C) The chambers of the heart
   (D) The capillaries

9. Which of these sets of words best describes how a healthy vein feels when palpated?
   (A) Firm, rope-like
   (B) Dense, tight
   (C) Soft, spongy
   (D) Springy, bouncy

10. The formed elements make up
    (A) About 1/3 of blood volume
    (B) A bit less than 1/2 of blood volume
    (C) A bit more than 1/2 of blood volume
    (D) About 2/3 of blood volume

11. The liquid portion of blood is
    (A) Entirely made of water
    (B) Entirely made of oxygen in oxygenated blood and carbon dioxide in deoxygenated blood
    (C) What gives blood its red color
    (D) A combination of water and dissolved substances

12. Which type of blood cell contains hemoglobin?
    (A) Granulocytes
    (B) Erythrocytes
    (C) Lymphocytes
    (D) Monocytes

13. Which of the following parts of the body is associated with the creation of blood cells?
    (A) The heart
    (B) The kidneys
    (C) The tendons
    (D) The bone marrow

14. What can be said about a person with blood type A negative?
    (A) She has type A antigens, anti-B antibodies, and no Rh factor.
    (B) She has type B antigens, anti-A antibodies, and no Rh factor.
    (C) She has type A antigens, anti-B antibodies, and Rh factor.
    (D) She will naturally possess anti-Rh antibodies.

15. Who could safely donate blood for a patient with the blood type AB negative?
    (A) Someone with AB positive blood
    (B) Someone with O negative blood
    (C) Someone with A positive blood
    (D) Someone with B positive blood

16. Venous blood is
    (A) Deep, dark red
    (B) Blue
    (C) Bright red
    (D) Bluish purple

17. _______________ is a term describing the process that keeps blood flowing normally through the rest of the body while clotting at the site of an injury.
    (A) Homeostasis
    (B) Hematology
    (C) Coagulation
    (D) Hemostasis

18. This is the body's first line of defense when a blood vessel is injured:
    (A) The heart rate slows to reduce blood loss.
    (B) Platelets and fibrin form a plug at the site of the injury.
    (C) The blood vessel constricts to reduce blood loss.
    (D) The blood vessel expands to allow clotting materials to flow out.

19. Which of these terms describes the complex series of events within the body related to blood clotting?
    (A) The coagulation cascade
    (B) The anticoagulative factor
    (C) The clotting stream
    (D) The antibody response

20. What does blood plasma contain that blood serum does not?
    (A) Red blood cells
    (B) Water
    (C) White blood cells
    (D) Fibrinogen

21. A specimen containing an anticoagulant additive and not spun in a centrifuge is called a(n) ____________________ specimen.
    (A) Whole blood
    (B) Representative
    (C) Undifferentiated
    (D) Routine

22. The buffy coat in a centrifuged specimen contains
    (A) Red and white blood cells
    (B) White blood cells and platelets
    (C) Fibrinogen and platelets
    (D) White blood cells and fibrinogen

8

Preparing for Specimen Collection

1. Discuss venipuncture and capillary puncture and identify different types of specimens collected by phlebotomy technicians

The primary job of a phlebotomist is to collect blood specimens for analysis. Most specimens are collected by venipuncture, or the puncture of a vein. Some tests require specimens collected by capillary (dermal) puncture (Fig. 8-1). In adults and in children over 1 year old, capillary puncture is performed on the fingertip. For infants, capillary puncture is performed at the heel.

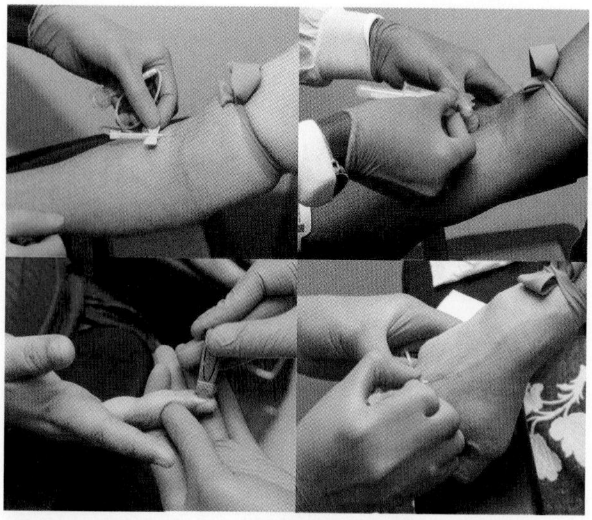

Fig. 8-1. *Blood specimens are collected by puncturing a vein or by puncturing the skin to access the capillaries below.*

Blood specimens are usually collected in tubes. The tubes can vary in size and shape, and many contain chemical additives that act to prepare the blood for testing. Tubes used to collect venipuncture specimens are larger than those used to collect capillary specimens. Pediatric tubes are smaller than tubes used for adults. Some tests do not require that blood be collected in a tube at all. One example is point-of-care blood tests, which generally require that blood from a capillary puncture be placed directly onto a test strip that is inserted into a machine for analysis. Another example is a test commonly performed on newborns that requires capillary blood to be dripped onto filter paper.

Some blood tests, such as a **blood culture**—which involves testing blood for the presence of bacteria—require the use of special equipment. Blood culture testing involves collecting samples in bottles that allow any bacteria in the blood to multiply. A preparation called a **peripheral blood smear** requires the phlebotomist to smear a drop of capillary blood or blood from a venous collection tube onto a microscope slide. More details about these types of collections and preparations are found in Chapters 9 and 10.

2. Describe the importance of avoiding errors before and during specimen collection

Although phlebotomists do not diagnose illnesses or plan treatment, their work is essential to patient health and well-being. When blood is drawn for testing, actions taken or not taken by the phlebotomist have a significant impact on the quality of the sample and the results. If a specimen is not collected properly, the results may not be accurate, and the patient may not receive the right treatment. If a specimen is not handled, processed, or transported correctly, test results can be affected. The patient's doctor will make decisions based on inaccurate information. If a patient or specimen is misidentified, the resulting errors can be deadly. PBTs must understand the value of their work and perform procedures accurately.

Errors that occur prior to testing a specimen are called **preanalytical errors**. Careful PBTs can avoid these errors most of the time. Misidentification of a patient or specimen is one of the most common errors in phlebotomy. It is also one of the most dangerous. Before a specimen is drawn, the PBT must identify the patient by two unique identifiers. Most commonly this means asking the patient to state and spell her first and last names and state her date of birth. This information must be checked against the patient's wristband (at facilities where they are used) and against the requisition form and specimen labels (Fig. 8-2). Learning Objective 7 has more detailed instructions for patient identification.

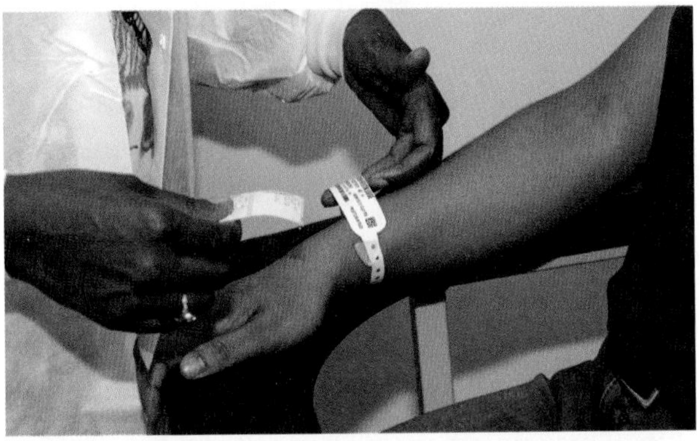

Fig. 8-2. *A patient's stated name and date of birth must be checked against the wristband, requisition form, and specimen labels.*

Errors can also occur when a requisition form is not filled out legibly or when the tests ordered are not clearly marked. Before performing a blood draw the phlebotomist must examine the form closely. The patient's name on the requisition must match the patient, and the form itself should not contain obvious errors. Every requisition must list the ordering provider. If duplicate tests are ordered or if anything is unclear, the PBT should contact the ordering provider or his supervisor before proceeding.

The requisition indicates any special requirements related to timing or to patient preparation. The PBT is responsible for confirming that the patient has followed any instructions—such as **fasting**, or not eating or drinking anything except water for 8–12 hours prior to the test—before completing the blood draw. Common requirements include the following:

- Fasting for a specified amount of time
- Achieving a **basal state**, or a rested state in which food and beverage (except water) have not been consumed in the last 12 hours and no strenuous exercise has been performed. **Note:** For most patients this will mean an early morning blood draw is necessary. For patients who have unusual schedules, basal state may be achieved at another time of day.
- Taking the proper dose of a medication within a certain window of time prior to the blood draw

Preanalytical errors can occur at every stage of blood collection. The following are errors the PBT must avoid, followed by the learning objective (LO) or chapter in which more detailed information is found:

- Use of needles or collection equipment not well suited to the test or the patient (LO 3)
- Use of incorrect tubes for the tests ordered (LO 4)
- Improper mixing of the specimen with the tube additive (LO 4)
- Failure to follow correct **order of draw**, the standard sequence in which tubes must be filled (LO 5)

- Failure to fill tubes to full capacity (LO 5)
- Lack of careful technique during the blood draw (Chapters 9 and 10)
- Improper handling, processing, or transportation of specimens (Chapters 9, 10, and 11)

Phlebotomy technicians do a very important job. They must understand how significant the consequences can be when they do not work carefully and precisely.

3. Discuss common blood specimen collection systems and identify equipment used for venipuncture and capillary puncture

Venipuncture requires the use of a hollow needle to access the patient's vein. In most cases, the needle is used along with a system that allows a single puncture to collect as much blood as necessary for the tests ordered. A double-sided needle allows the PBT to insert, fill, and remove multiple collection tubes. One side of the needle enters the patient's vein, and the other side screws into a rigid plastic holder and punctures the stoppers of collection tubes. The tubes are emptied of air during the manufacturing process and designed to draw in the exact amount of blood needed to complete the specimen. The double-sided needle, holder, and vacuum tube together are called an **evacuated tube system** (Fig. 8-3).

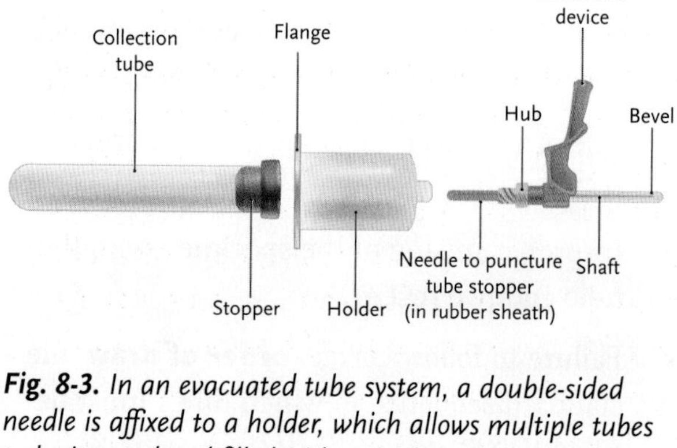

Fig. 8-3. In an evacuated tube system, a double-sided needle is affixed to a holder, which allows multiple tubes to be inserted and filled with a single venipuncture.

Manufacturers produce a number of different needle and holder styles, all of which are fitted with safety devices to reduce chances of accidental needlesticks. Some needles have protective shields that slide or swing into place after use. Others have blunting mechanisms that eliminate the sharp point of the needle before it is even removed from the patient's vein. The basic concept is the same for all of these systems. A double-sided hollow needle, called a **multisample needle**, is either premounted or screwed into a tube holder using a threaded **hub** (Fig. 8-4). After use the entire assembly is immediately placed in a sharps disposal container.

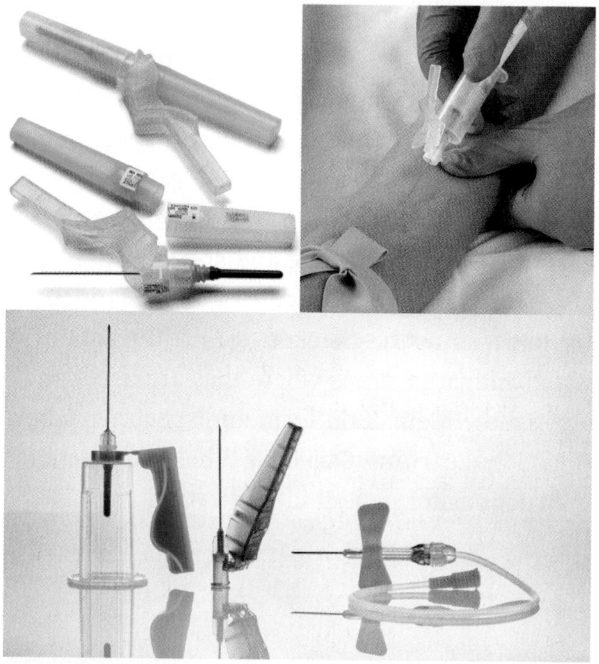

Fig. 8-4. Multisample needles and holders come in a variety of styles and with different safety mechanisms. (TOP IMAGES COURTESY AND © BECTON, DICKINSON AND COMPANY. BOTTOM PHOTO COURTESY OF GREINER BIO-ONE, WWW.GBO.COM)

The opening of a venipuncture needle is slanted so that there is a sharp point for piercing the skin. This angled opening is called a **bevel** (Fig. 8-5). Needles are available in a variety of sizes. Multisample needles are usually 1"–1.5" long, and are also categorized by diameter (the width of the needle), or **gauge**. The hollow space inside the needle is called the **lumen**. A lower gauge number indicates a wider needle and a lumen with a larger diameter. A higher number indicates a thinner needle and a lumen with a smaller diameter. The needles used most commonly in venipuncture for adults are 21-gauge. However, 22- or 23-gauge needles may sometimes be used in patients with smaller or fragile veins or in pediatric draws (which may even require a 25-gauge needle). Blood donation requires the collection of a large amount of blood and so a larger needle is used, usually 16-gauge. Manufacturers color-code the hubs of needles according to gauge and PBTs should be familiar with the coding system used at their facilities.

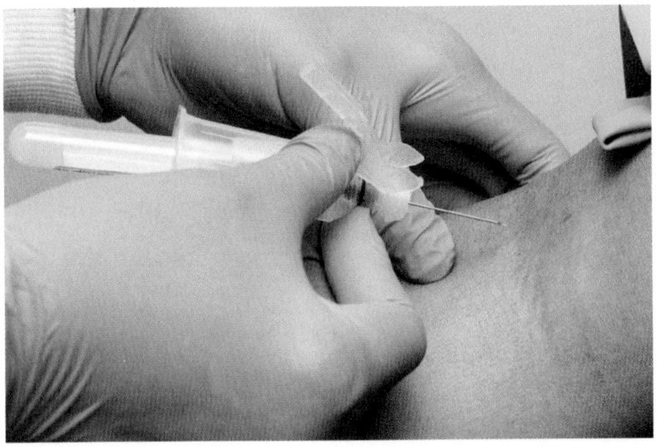

Fig. 8-5. *The needle's bevel is the angled opening that allows it to puncture the skin and allows the patient's blood to flow to the collection tube.*

In addition to straight multisample needles, phlebotomy technicians also use a type of needle called a **winged collection set**, commonly known as a *butterfly needle* (Fig. 8-6). This needle is generally shorter than a straight needle (3/4"–1"). At the base of the needle there is a pair of flaps ("wings") that allow the phlebotomist to guide the needle as it is inserted in the patient's skin and vein. Rather than connecting directly to a tube holder, the winged collection set includes a thin, flexible tube through which blood flows. This tube connects to the wider, rigid tube holder. This allows the PBT to change tubes without any risk of moving the needle or placing added pressure on the patient's vein. Skilled phlebotomists can change tubes in a straight needle system with little or no needle movement, but the flexible tubing in the butterfly system makes this easier.

Like straight needles, butterfly needles come in a variety of gauges. The most common are 21- and 23-gauge needles, but 25-gauge winged needles are also available. This type of needle is often used when drawing blood from patients with small or fragile veins. It is also used when blood is drawn from the back of the hand. Some collections, such as blood cultures, are routinely performed using a butterfly assembly (see Chapter 9). Butterfly needles are also usually used when drawing a specimen with a syringe.

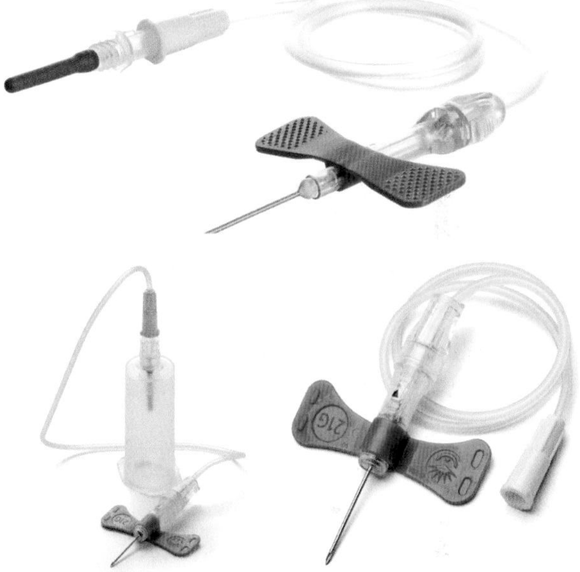

Fig. 8-6. *Winged collection, or butterfly, systems are often used for patients who are elderly, very young, or medically fragile (seriously ill patients who may be undergoing complicated or difficult treatments).* (TOP PHOTO COURTESY OF GREINER BIO-ONE, WWW.GBO.COM; BOTTOM PHOTOS COURTESY AND © BECTON, DICKINSON AND COMPANY)

Collection tubes also come in a variety of sizes (Fig. 8-7). Larger tubes create a stronger pull on the patient's vein. Because of this, and because lower volumes of blood should be drawn from children, pediatric collection tubes are smaller (1–2 mL) than tubes used for adults (3–5 mL). Children's veins are smaller and more likely to collapse when exposed to the greater pressure created by a large tube. Smaller tubes may also be necessary for patients who are elderly or ill (such as those undergoing chemotherapy), or for hospitalized patients whose blood is being drawn frequently.

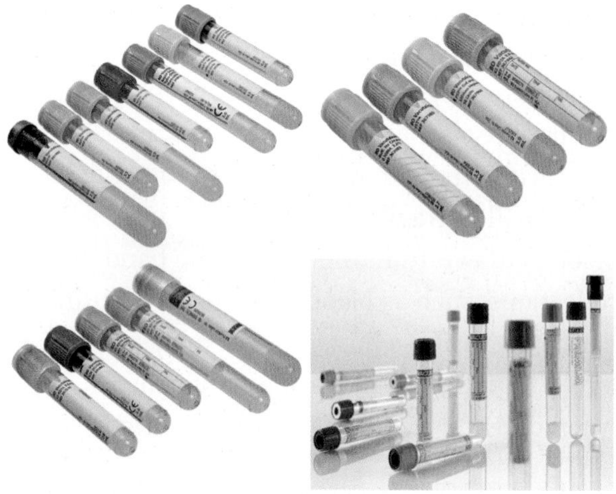

Fig. 8-7. Venipuncture collection tubes range widely in size. (TOP AND BOTTOM LEFT PHOTOS COURTESY AND © BECTON, DICKINSON AND COMPANY; BOTTOM RIGHT PHOTO COURTESY OF GREINER BIO-ONE, WWW.GBO.COM)

Because of the pressure created by evacuated tube systems, these systems are not appropriate for all patients. Thin or fragile veins may not be able to withstand the pull without collapsing, causing the blood flow to stop and possibly compromising the specimen. In these situations, the PBT will need to use a syringe and a **syringe transfer device** to collect the specimen (Fig. 8-8). A syringe is a barrel-shaped device with a plunger that is pulled to draw in blood. The needle (either a standard multisample needle or a winged collection set) is affixed to the syringe. The PBT collects the blood by gently pulling back on the plunger. Blood is then transferred to evacuated tubes (procedure in Chapter 9).

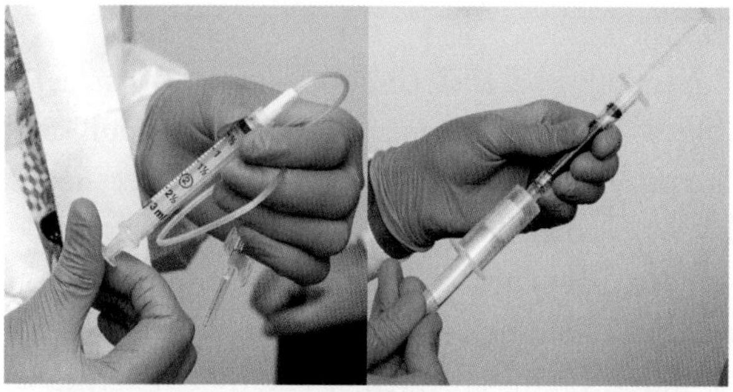

Fig. 8-8. A syringe and syringe transfer device may be necessary for patients with fragile veins.

With most blood collection systems, the phlebotomy technician must choose either to use a multisample needle and tube holder or to use a syringe and transfer the specimen to an evacuated tube. At least one collection system involves tubes with plungers incorporated in the tube design. These can either be used as a syringe or can be pulled out to an indicated mark prior to a blood draw and then broken off. This creates a vacuum as in an evacuated tube system. Facilities using this type of tube will provide training in its use.

In addition to the devices required for puncturing the vein and collecting the blood, phlebotomists also need the following supplies for each draw:

- **Gloves**. New gloves must be used for each patient. Some patients may be sensitive or even highly allergic to latex. Facilities will have nonlatex gloves available, or may exclusively use nonlatex gloves. Although an allergy to latex should be noted on the requisition form, it is a good idea to ask the patient. Gloves should always be inspected for holes and discarded if defective. PBTs should never tear off glove fingertips to palpate veins. Gloves should not interfere with the ability to feel the patient's veins.
- **Antiseptic solution**. The venipuncture site must be cleaned before the procedure is performed. In most cases a 70% **isopropyl alcohol** pad is used to do this. Sometimes other antiseptics may be used. **Chlorhexidine gluconate** (ChloraPrep is a common brand name) is often used for blood culture preparation. **Povidone-iodine**, **benzalkonium chloride**, or **iodine tincture** may also be used. Iodine solutions, however, can cause allergic reactions in patients with shellfish allergies.
- **Tourniquet**. A tourniquet is a band that temporarily restricts the return of venous blood below the area where is it applied (Fig. 8-9). This allows for easier identification of and access to the patient's veins. Most facilities use disposable, nonlatex tourniquets, as reuse of tourniquets can pose a contamination risk.

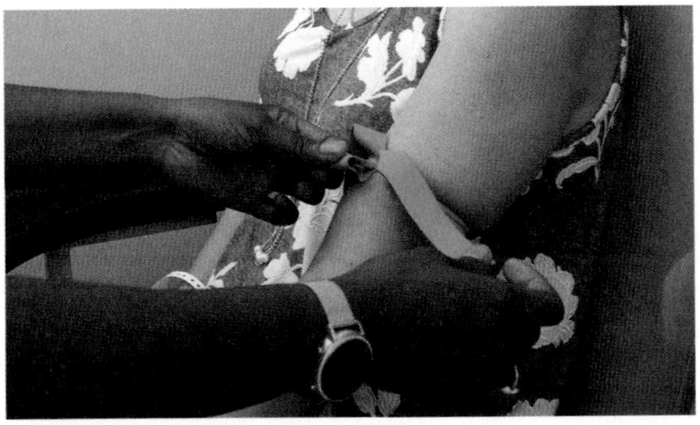

Fig. 8-9. Tourniquets are applied above the venipuncture site. They restrict venous blood return, causing the veins below to fill and expand. This makes it easier to locate and puncture a vein.

- **Gauze**. Gauze is applied to the puncture site immediately following venipuncture. Applying pressure on the gauze will help stop the flow of blood.
- **Bandage**. Either a standard adhesive bandage or a self-adhesive wrap is placed over the gauze. This ensures that the clot at the puncture site is not dislodged (Fig. 8-10). Coban is a common brand name for wrap bandages. Adhesive bandages sometimes contain latex. PBTs should ensure only latex-free bandages are used on patients with a sensitivity to latex.

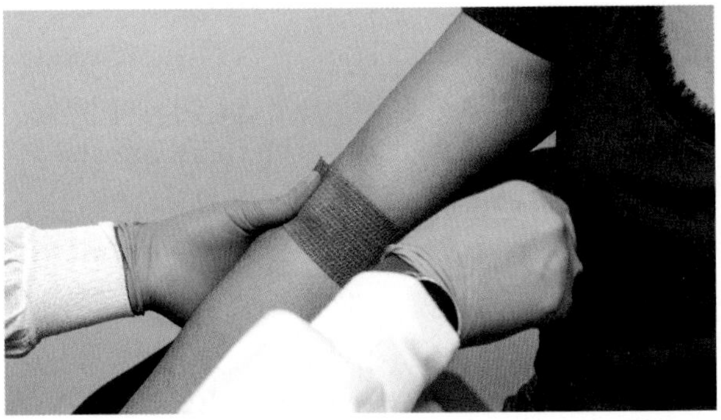

Fig. 8-10. Self-adhesive wrap bandages are often used after blood draws. They are gentle on the patient's skin and easy to remove.

In some situations, warming packs may be required to assist in accessing the patient's veins. Some facilities may have electronic devices called *venoscopes* to assist with vein location. Phlebotomists will be trained in the use of these devices if they are available. They may be helpful in caring for patients who are obese, because in these patients the veins may be more difficult to locate by palpation.

Much of the same equipment used for venipuncture is also used for capillary puncture. Gloves, antiseptic pads, gauze, and bandages are all necessary. Collection tubes may be used as well, although the tubes are not evacuated tubes and are designed to contain a much smaller volume of blood (Fig. 8-11). In general, collection tubes for capillary puncture have a volume ranging from 125 to 600 microliters (µL). One microliter is one thousandth (1/1000) of a milliliter. They may be referred to as **microcollection tubes**.

Some microcollection tubes have a straw-like attachment allowing blood to be easily channeled from the puncture site into the tube. Others have spout-like openings under their caps to facilitate blood collection. Sometimes capillary blood is not collected in tubes with lids but in very thin, straw-like tubes that hold a very small amount of blood (often 75 µL) and are sealed with clay or another substance. These tubes may be referred to as **capillary tubes**. Some are treated with the anticoagulant heparin. Color indicates which tubes are heparinized and which are not. Heparinized capillary tubes are usually marked with a red or green line, while tubes without heparin are marked with a blue line.

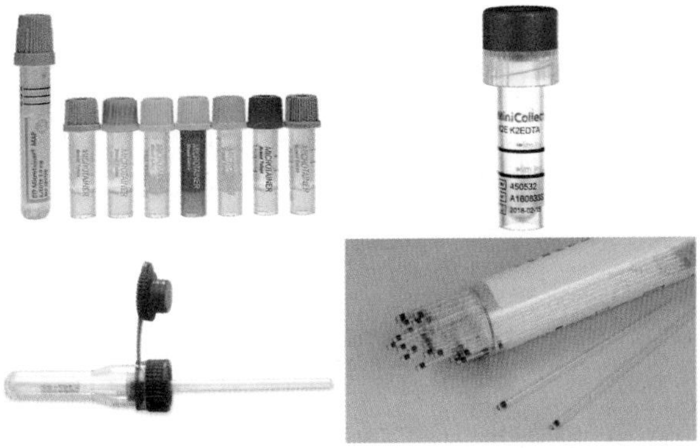

Fig. 8-11. Capillary collection tubes are much smaller than venipuncture tubes. They might have straw-like lids to make collection easier. Capillary blood may also be collected in tiny straw-like tubes. (FIRST PHOTO COURTESY AND © BECTON, DICKINSON AND COMPANY; SECOND PHOTO COURTESY OF GREINER BIO-ONE, WWW.GBO.COM; THIRD PHOTO COURTESY OF MARKETLAB, INC., WWW.MARKETLAB.COM; FOURTH PHOTO COURTESY OF GLOBE SCIENTIFIC, INC., WWW.GLOBESCIENTIFIC.COM)

Establishing blood flow for capillary specimens requires a lancet. A lancet is a device containing a small, sharp retractable blade or needle (Fig. 8-12). Depending on the design, the PBT either presses a button or presses the device against the patient's skin to activate the blade or needle, which punctures the skin and then retracts. All lancets are disposable, single-use items and are discarded in a sharps container after use. Lancets come in a variety of shapes and sizes, and are set to puncture the skin at different depths, ranging from 0.85 millimeters (mm) for premature infants to 2.4 mm. The range of 1.8 mm–2.2 mm is recommended for adults, while 2 mm is the maximum puncture depth for small children. (More information regarding lancet selection is in Chapter 10).

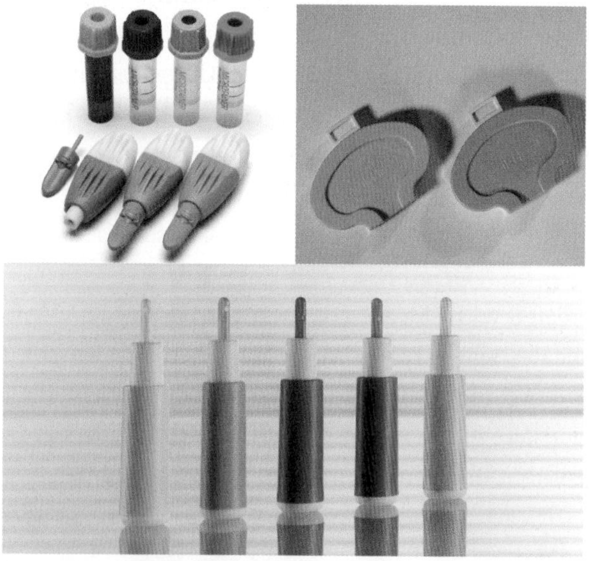

Fig. 8-12. *Lancets for finger sticks and infant heel sticks come in a variety of styles. Some are adjustable and others puncture at a preset depth.* (TOP IMAGES COURTESY AND © BECTON, DICKINSON AND COMPANY; BOTTOM IMAGE COURTESY OF GREINER BIO-ONE, WWW.GBO.COM)

To improve blood flow, warming packs may be used for infant heel sticks or for finger sticks in patients of any age. Other necessary equipment may include filter paper for certain blood tests (e.g., PKU, a required screening for newborns) or test strips for glucose monitoring and PT/INR testing (a test to assess blood clotting time, often used to monitor the effectiveness of certain anticoagulant medications). Adhesive bandages are generally used after capillary puncture, but never on infants and toddlers, as the bandages can loosen and become choking hazards.

4. Identify additives to blood specimens and describe the color coding of collection tubes

Even as blood is being collected, additives in the collection tubes are preparing it for testing. The substances studied in diagnostic tests are called **analytes**. Using a tube with the correct additive ensures that the analytes for each test are preserved properly and accurately reflect the blood in the patient's bloodstream. Complete blood counts, for instance, require whole blood. Specimens for complete blood counts are collected in tubes with an anticoagulant additive because a clotted specimen will not allow for an accurate count. Many tests are performed on blood serum. Specimens used for serum testing must be allowed to clot before tests can be performed. Most requisition forms indicate the type of tube needed for each test, and most electronic systems print specimen labels that indicate the type of tube required.

Tube stoppers are color coded to indicate the type of additive inside. The colors of some tubes may vary between manufacturers, but in most cases the colors are similar. The tubes are also labeled with the name of any additives, as well as an expiration date (Fig. 8-13). They may have a fill line or arrow to indicate the capacity of the tube. Phlebotomists should check all of this information prior to using a collection tube.

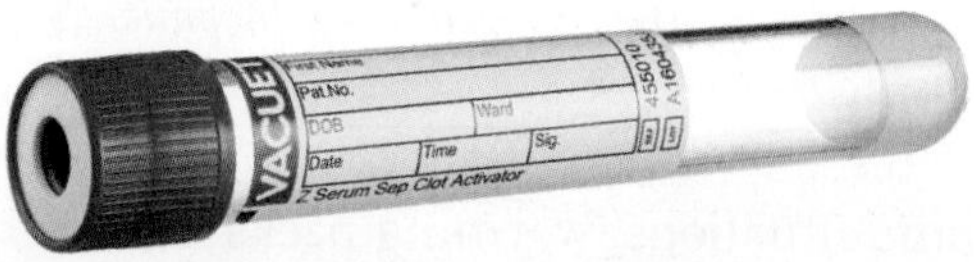

Fig. 8-13. *It is important to check the tube label as well as the stopper. Not all manufacturers use the same shades or colors for each additive. Some stopper colors are associated with more than one type of additive.* (PHOTO COURTESY OF GREINER BIO-ONE, WWW.GBO.COM)

There are two different categories of tubes: those containing anticoagulants and those without anticoagulants. Some tubes without anticoagulants include clot activators to speed the coagulation process. Different anticoagulants act in different ways. Some bind calcium in the blood, making it unavailable. Because calcium is one of the key substances in blood clotting, this has an anticoagulant effect. Others stop the action of thrombin, the enzyme that causes fibrin to form. These different means of preventing coagulation make each additive suited to particular blood tests.

Because centrifuged specimens containing anticoagulants divide into plasma and cellular components, anticoagulant tubes are sometimes called *plasma tubes. Serum tubes* allow the blood to clot, yielding serum and clotted cells after centrifugation. In addition to chemical additives that act on the blood, tubes may contain a gel that, when the specimen is centrifuged, forms a barrier between the liquid and solid components. The separator gel generally forms this barrier without affecting analytes in the blood, but certain tests (e.g., tests for the level of particular drugs in the body) may be affected, so PBTs should check tube requirements carefully.

It is important to follow manufacturer instructions for mixing blood specimens with tube additives. Immediately after collection, a specimen with an additive must be gently turned upside down and then brought upright several times. More information about this process is in Chapter 9. Descriptions of color coding of plasma and serum tubes are listed in Tables 8-1 and 8-2.

Other tubes may be used in addition to the common tubes listed in these tables. Tan-topped tubes contain the same additive as lavender tubes (see table), but are certified to be essentially lead-free. They are often used to test lead levels. Phlebotomists should always follow facility policy regarding which collection tubes to use, and should ask a supervisor if there is any doubt.

SERUM TUBES	
Red. Tubes with red stoppers either contain a clot activator (plastic tubes) or no additive (glass tubes). The inside of the tube is coated with silicone to prevent the blood cells from sticking to the tube. Serum tubes are used for certain chemistry, **serology**, and immunology tests. *Serology* is the study of blood serum.	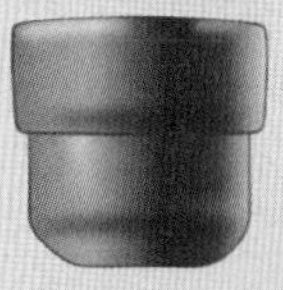
Gold or mottled red and gray (tiger top). Tubes with either gold or mixed red and gray stoppers contain both a clot activator and a separator gel. They are commonly called **serum separator tubes** (**SSTs**). Like other serum tubes, SSTs are used for chemistry, serology, and immunology testing. They should not be used when testing for therapeutic drug levels.	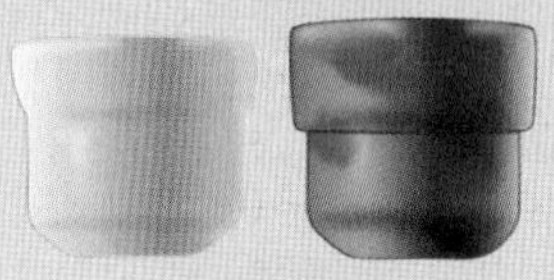
Orange. Tubes with an orange stopper are **stat serum tubes** and contain a fast-acting clot activator. These tubes are used for testing that must be conducted very quickly, and they are available with or without separator gel.	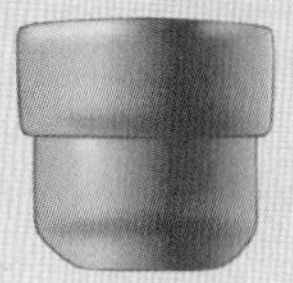

Table 8-1. *Serum tubes may or may not contain clot activators and/or separator gel.*

ANTICOAGULANT (PLASMA) TUBES	
Light blue. Tubes with light or sky blue stoppers contain an anticoagulant additive called **sodium citrate**. They are often referred to as *citrate tubes* and are used for coagulation studies. Sodium citrate acts by binding calcium and its action is reversible, which means technicians in the laboratory can also perform clotting time tests on blood collected in these tubes. These tubes must be filled completely for the proper balance of blood to additive.	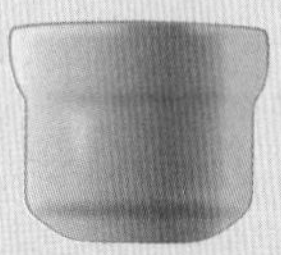
Green. Tubes with green stoppers (sometimes light, sometimes dark, and sometimes speckled green) contain the anticoagulant **heparin**. Heparin acts by preventing thrombin from acting to form fibrin. Sodium heparin and lithium heparin are two different tube additives, both with the same anticoagulant action (deactivating thrombin). Light green usually indicates that the tube contains a separator gel, and these tubes may be referred to as **plasma separator tubes** (**PSTs**). These tubes are most often used for routine chemistry tests and certain types of genetic testing. Because heparin is an anticoagulant that does *not* bind calcium, it is often used when calcium levels are tested. Green-topped tubes may also be used for stat chemistry tests, as there is no need to wait for clotting and centrifuging when green tubes are used.	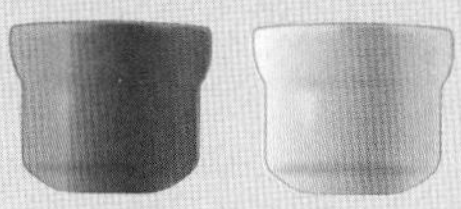
Lavender, pink, or white. Tubes with lavender (light purple), pink, or pearly white stoppers contain the additive **EDTA**. This anticoagulant acts by inhibiting the action of calcium in a patient's blood. EDTA tubes are typically used for hematology studies (e.g., complete blood count). Pink-topped tubes are used for blood bank specimens (blood type and matching for transfusion, called *type and crossmatch*).	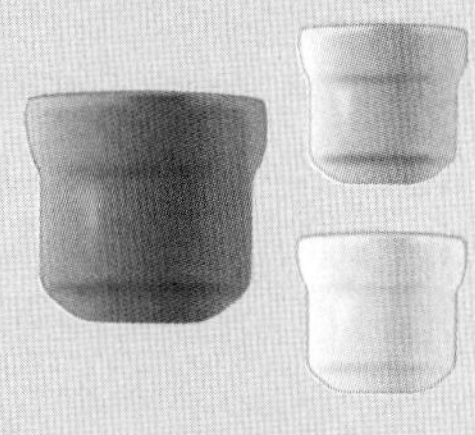
Gray. Tubes with gray stoppers usually contain two types of additive: an anticoagulant in the form of either sodium or potassium oxalate and a substance called sodium fluoride that prevents the deterioration of glucose, or blood sugar. This process of deterioration, called **glycolysis**, affects certain test results if it is not prevented. Glucose testing is generally done using specimens in gray-topped tubes (also called *oxalate tubes*). **Note:** Although oxalate/sodium fluoride is the most common additive combination in gray-topped tubes, some may contain EDTA as an anticoagulant. All gray-topped tubes contain sodium fluoride to prevent glycolysis.	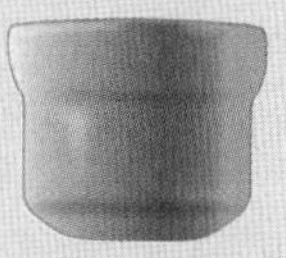
Yellow. Tubes with yellow stoppers contain either acid citrate dextrose (ACD) or sodium polyanethol sulfonate (SPS) as an anticoagulant additive. They are not as commonly used as the other anticoagulant tubes. ACD tubes are generally used to collect whole blood specimens for DNA analysis (e.g., paternity testing) or testing prior to organ transplant. SPS tubes are used for microbiology studies such as blood culture. *It is very important to check the label to verify the additive in a yellow tube.*	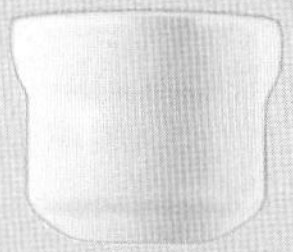
Royal blue. Tubes with royal blue stoppers usually contain EDTA, although they may also contain heparin or no additive. A colored stripe on the label shows the additive: usually lavender for EDTA, green for heparin, and red for no additive. These tubes are certified to be free of *trace elements*, or chemical elements present in tiny amounts. They are used for trace element, toxicology, and nutrition testing. *Due to the possibility of different additives, royal blue tubes should be checked closely before use.*	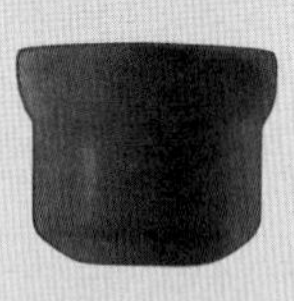

Table 8-2. *Different anticoagulant additives are used for specific diagnostic tests.*

5. List the order in which collection tubes must be filled (order of draw)

Because chemical additives may carry over from one tube to the next, there is a specific tube order required when multiple specimens are collected. This order prevents clot activators, for example, from entering a citrate tube and interfering with the action of the anticoagulant. It also reduces the risk of any kind of contamination entering a blood culture specimen. This order is known as the order of draw, and following order of draw is an essential part of a phlebotomist's job. It is one of the key steps in ensuring that the laboratory receives the best quality specimens, reducing the risk of inaccurate test results for the patient.

The CLSI standard for filling tubes for any type of venipuncture collection, regardless of the system used to collect the specimens, is as follows:

1. Blood culture (may be yellow-topped SPS tubes or special blood culture bottles)
2. Sodium citrate tubes (light blue tops)
3. Serum tubes, with or without separator gel or clot activator (mottled red/gray, gold, red, or orange tops)
4. Heparin tubes (green tops, all shades)
5. EDTA tubes (lavender, pink, or pearly white tops)
6. Oxalate tubes (gray tops)

Although it is not specifically mentioned in CLSI's order of draw, yellow-topped ACD tubes are usually drawn after oxalate tubes. For collection of tubes not listed above and for collection of gel and non-gel tubes of the same type (e.g., heparin tubes with and without separator gel), facility policy should be followed. The manufacturer of the collection tubes most commonly used in the US recommends that, within each category, gel tubes be collected before non-gel tubes.

Quality Counts

Most requisitions require only tubes listed in CLSI's order of draw. Sometimes, however, specialized tests require adjustments to this order. Royal blue-topped tubes are manufactured to be free of trace elements, and tan-topped tubes are free of lead. The stoppers of other tubes may contain enough of these substances to interfere with trace element or lead testing. Because of this, order of draw may need to be rearranged when this testing is performed along with other tests. Royal blue and tan-topped tubes should be filled first, before any other tubes. After they are filled, a **discard tube** must be filled before continuing. A discard tube is one that will not be tested, and it does not need to be filled completely. It is drawn to ensure that the additives from the royal blue or tan-topped tube will not carry over to the next tubes. In this situation, the discard tube should either be a tube with no additive at all (e.g., a red-topped glass tube) or a tube with the same additive as the next tube to be drawn. For example, if a heparin tube is the next tube needed, the discard tube should be a heparin tube or a nonadditive tube. Another option when drawing for lead or trace element testing is to draw the remaining tests from a separate venipuncture site. PBTs should know and follow facility procedures.

When collecting specimens by capillary puncture, a different order applies. The portion of the multisample needle that punctures the collection tubes is the source of possible contamination in venipuncture collections, and this is not a factor in capillary collections. This order is used, not to prevent cross-contamination, but because of the qualities of capillary blood. As blood is collected from a capillary puncture site, the composition of the blood changes. The first blood collected more closely resembles arterial blood, and as the collection continues, the blood becomes more like venous blood. Another change also occurs as time passes after a capillary puncture: platelets begin to collect at the puncture site, causing the blood to be less representative of the patient's blood overall.

This order applies to capillary collection:

1. Specimens to measure blood gases (this test is most often performed on arterial blood,

but the first capillary blood can be close to arterial blood in composition)

2. EDTA tubes (often used for complete blood count, and should be filled before platelets accumulate excessively)
3. Tubes with other additives
4. Serum tubes

For collections both from capillary puncture and venipuncture, it is also important to fill each tube to the proper level before switching tubes. If a requisition requires the use of an unfamiliar tube, the PBT should ask a supervisor for help regarding where the tube falls in the order of draw.

6. Describe considerations for timing of blood draws

Various factors determine the order in which patients are seen for blood draws. In many settings the order of patients will be determined by someone other than the phlebotomist, but it is still good practice to check requisitions and make sure there are no timing factors that have been overlooked.

A patient whose requisition is for a *stat* blood test must be drawn immediately, if possible, and no later than 10 minutes after the order is issued. The specimen is then processed according to facility policy. Often orange-topped tubes are used for stat orders, shortening the clotting time from the typical 30–60 minutes to approximately five minutes and centrifuge time from 15 minutes to as little as three minutes. Green tubes are also frequently used for stat chemistry testing.

An order requiring that a test take place **ASAP** means that it should occur *as soon as possible.* As a general guideline, orders marked *ASAP* should be drawn within half an hour. They are not as urgent as stat orders but they are still time-sensitive. **Routine** tests are less urgent but should not be delayed unnecessarily. In many cases patients with routine test orders have been fasting and should not be made to wait unless it is unavoidable. Not only can fasting be unpleasant for patients, but fasting beyond 14 hours will affect certain analytes and could make test results less accurate.

Some blood draws, especially those monitoring the effect of medications, are **timed draws**. The blood may need to be drawn at the **peak**, or highest, level of the medicine's effect, or at the **trough**, or lowest, level of the medicine's effect. Because exact timing is important to achieving the most accurate results, these orders should be completed within five minutes of the time indicated. The phlebotomist should verify the timing of the patient's last medication dose.

Quality Counts

Getting a patient's medication dose right can be complicated. Sometimes blood is drawn to check medication levels and to ensure that the patient is receiving the best therapeutic dose: not too much and not too little. Measuring a patient's medication levels at trough times ensures that the drug is still acting just before a new dose is taken. Trough levels are most accurately measured right before the next dose is scheduled. Measuring a patient's medication levels at peak times ensures that there is not a potentially harmful level of medication in the patient's system. The timing for measuring peak levels varies according to the medicine and how it is given to the patient. Medicines delivered intravenously will peak more quickly than medicines taken by mouth. A general guideline for IV medications is that peak levels occur 15–30 minutes after the dose has been given. For oral medications, peak time is usually considered to occur an hour after the medication was swallowed. PBTs should always confirm the time of the patient's last dose with the nurse, and should document the time of the last dose and the time of draw.

Another common timed draw is a **glucose tolerance test**. This test is generally performed when testing for diabetes or to test for gestational diabetes (a type of diabetes that only occurs during pregnancy). The patient has her blood drawn at the beginning of the test, then drinks a very sweet beverage and has her blood drawn at various intervals to track her body's response to the sugar in the drink. In order to ensure accuracy of results, the draws should be completed as close as possible to the timing indicated on the order.

If a PBT ever has questions about the timing of a test or the order in which patients should be seen, she should ask her supervisor or the ordering care provider. Depending on the tests ordered and the reasons for testing, timing can be an essential factor in the quality of specimens drawn.

7. Discuss the steps required to properly identify patients and specimens

Patient identification is a critical part of preparing for specimen collection. Incorrect identification of a patient can result in a variety of serious problems:

- Inconvenience and pain caused by additional blood draws if incorrect orders are applied to a patient
- Delay in diagnosis and treatment due to incorrect tests performed
- Inaccurate diagnosis or treatment due to misidentification of patient/specimen
- Prolonged hospital stay if diagnosis or treatment is handled improperly due to misidentification
- Increased costs for the patient and healthcare system due to repeated testing or care given to correct errors
- Illness or death if transfusion or medication is administered based on faulty patient identification
- Possible legal action against the phlebotomist and/or facility

There are several steps to properly identifying a patient. The first involves asking a patient to provide two uniquely identifying pieces of information about herself. The standard information used to identify a patient is full name (first and last) and date of birth. Information such as room number at a hospital or long-term care facility is not uniquely identifying and should not be used to confirm a patient's identity. CLSI recommends that patients should both speak and spell first and last names, and speak their date of birth, including month, date, and year (Fig. 8-14).

The next step in identifying the patient is checking the information provided by the patient against the requisition/specimen labels and the patient's wristband (Fig. 8-15). It is important that the patient provide the identifying information without prompting. In other words, the phlebotomist should not simply read out the name and birth date and ask for confirmation.

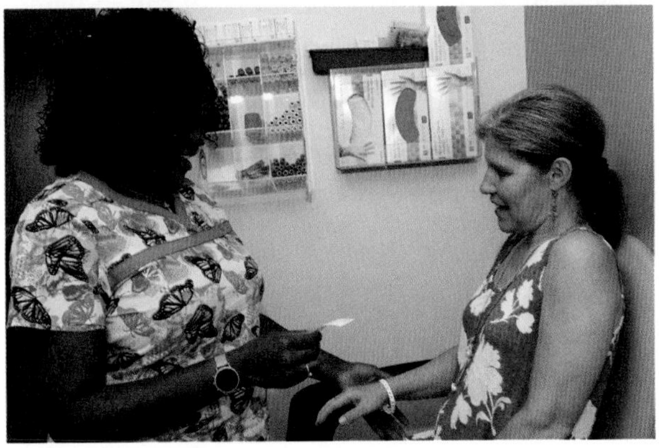

Fig. 8-14. The patient should state and spell her name and state her date of birth.

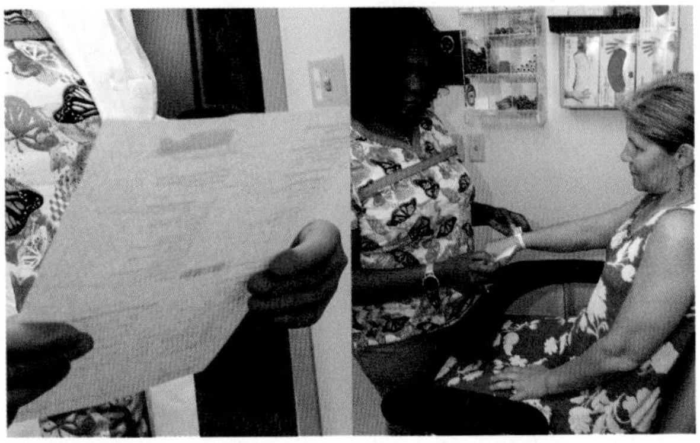

Fig. 8-15. The patient's stated name and date of birth should be checked against all materials related to the collection.

The patient's wristband must be on his body in order to be considered a valid form of identification. A wristband affixed to a hospital bed rail or sitting on a bedside table is not valid. That patient's identity must be confirmed by other means. In this situation, the PBT should check the patient's photo ID or request that a nurse responsible for the patient confirm his identity and reaffix the bracelet before completing the draw. The name of the person who confirms the patient's identity should be documented.

Nonverbal patients or patients who cannot respond due to use of a ventilator or other equipment that limits speech must be identified by matching full name and date of birth on an identification bracelet to the requisition. This identification must also be confirmed by a photo ID or through the recognition of a family member or nurse familiar with the patient. The PBT should then document the name of the individual who confirmed the patient's identity and his relationship to the patient.

If at any point there is doubt about the patient's identity, or whether the requisition contains the correct patient information, these issues must be resolved before any procedure is performed. If there is a mismatch between the patient's stated and spelled name/date of birth and the requisition, specimen labels, or wristband, the PBT should discuss the differences with a supervisor or with the ordering care provider. If an error was made on the requisition or labels, it should be corrected and the requisition or labels reprinted before any specimens are collected. All specimens collected must be labeled with the patient's identifying information and initialed by the PBT in front of the patient after the draw is completed but before the patient leaves the drawing station or before the PBT leaves the patient's bedside. The patient should confirm that the labels are accurate (Fig. 8-16).

Quality Counts

Because the consequences of incorrectly identifying a patient are grave—even potentially deadly—the PBT must properly identify each patient. When a patient has hearing loss, speaks a language other than English, or is cognitively impaired, errors are more likely to occur if identification protocol is not followed carefully. People with very common names, or names that sound similar to other names (e.g., Jan/Ann, Bob/Rob) are also at risk for misidentification. Carefully following CLSI identification standards for every patient interaction guarantees that the correct patient is linked to the correct specimens. If a PBT feels she does not have time to perform these checks, she should speak to her supervisor.

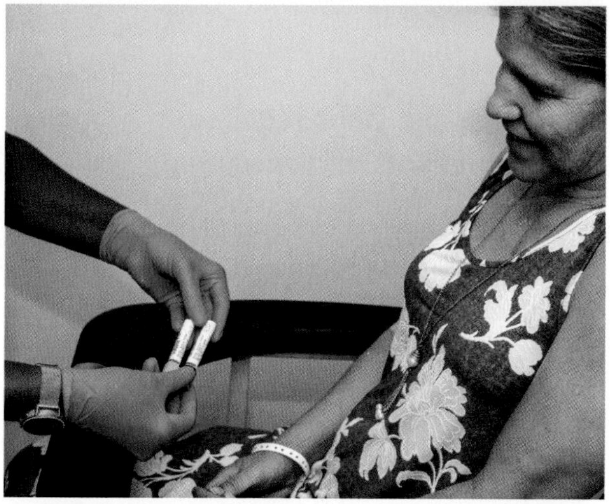

Fig. 8-16. *Tubes must be labeled and initialed immediately following the draw, and then confirmed by the patient. Failure to do so increases the chance that the tubes could become connected to the wrong patient.*

8. Describe preparations for the safe collection of blood specimens

Before collecting a blood specimen, the phlebotomy technician should ensure that he has the correct equipment to safely perform the procedure. This includes not only the needle assembly or lancet and collection tubes, bottles, or test strips/filter paper, but also the proper safety equipment. If the patient requires Transmission-Based Precautions, the PBT must don appropriate PPE, such as a mask, respirator, gown, and/or goggles/face shield.

Gloves must be worn for all patients, and the PBT should make sure that gloves are readily available should a pair need to be replaced (Fig. 8-17). The sharps receptacle should be within arm's reach of the drawing site and should not be overfilled. When a sharps receptacle is 3/4 full, it should no longer be used. A new receptacle should be acquired before another procedure is performed. All needles and lancets are equipped with engineering controls to reduce the risk of accidental needlesticks. Before starting a procedure, the PBT should make sure he is familiar with the equipment and understands how the safety mechanisms work. It can take some practice to master the use of new or unfamiliar devices.

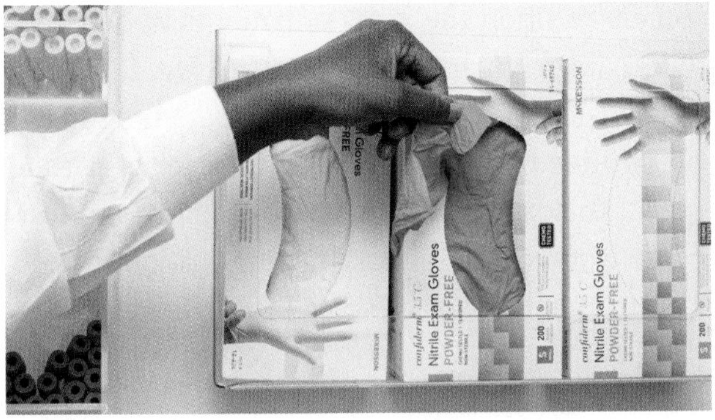

Fig. 8-17. An adequate supply of gloves ensures the phlebotomist is prepared to work safely.

Another aspect of safe blood collection is being mentally prepared for each procedure. A conscientious phlebotomist is prepared every time so that when an adverse reaction—such as a patient fainting or having a seizure—occurs, she is ready. Safety is about using the proper equipment and the proper procedures, but it is also about the technician's state of mind. Chapters 9 and 10 contain advice for dealing with common difficulties, but before any challenges arise, the most important step is for the phlebotomist to be alert, engaged, and prepared.

9. List preparations for protecting the integrity of specimens during collection and transportation

Most blood collection tubes are made of clear plastic or glass. Some microcollection tubes, however, are made of amber-colored plastic or glass. These tubes are used to collect specimens for tests that require the blood be protected from light (**bilirubin**, a substance associated with liver function, is a common light-sensitive analyte). If amber tubes are not available or a larger specimen is drawn for a light-sensitive analyte, it is possible to wrap a tube in foil or transport it in a specially tinted specimen bag or even a brown paper bag (within the proper transport container) (Fig. 8-18). Before drawing a specimen that requires light protection, the PBT should make sure to have some means of protecting it.

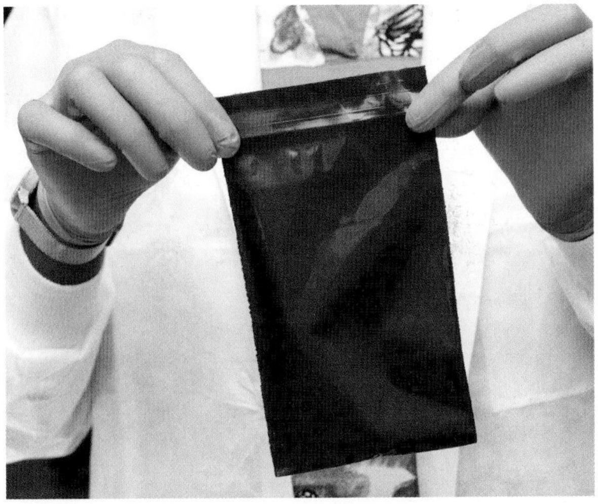

Fig. 8-18. Light protection is essential for certain analytes.

Some analytes require preservation at a particular temperature. Body temperature may need to be maintained for some specimens. Others may need to be chilled. Each facility will have its own procedures for maintaining required temperatures. The phlebotomist should know these procedures and where to find any necessary equipment. It is important to perform a procedure only after assuring that the required protections are available. Failure to maintain the proper temperature for a sensitive analyte will cause errors in the patient's results.

All specimens, regardless of any special handling requirements, must be treated with care and protected from any jostling or rough handling. Mishandling specimens can cause damage to the cells and alter test results. Phlebotomists should always follow facility policies regarding handling and transportation.

10. Discuss furniture and accessories necessary to a phlebotomy station

In addition to the equipment needed to access the patient's vein or capillaries and handle specimens, quality phlebotomy practice requires proper seating, positioning, and storage equipment. In outpatient laboratory settings, phlebotomy drawing stations are usually set up with a specialized chair for the patient and a cart or cabinet for supplies (Fig. 8-19). Trays may be available for organizing equipment prior to a procedure.

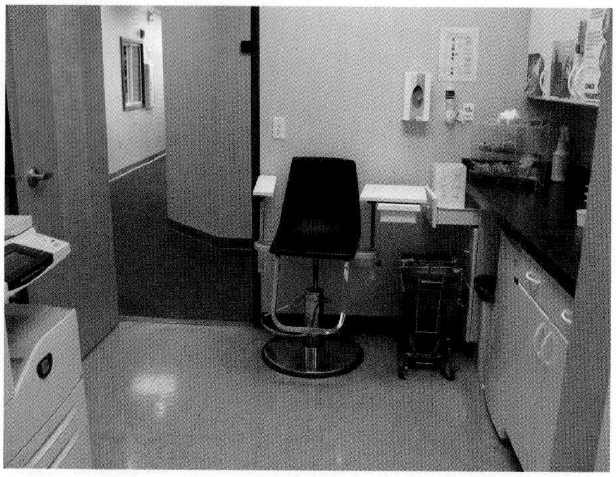

Fig. 8-19. *Typical drawing stations are equipped with adjustable chairs with armrests and a storage system for supplies.* (PHOTO COURTESY OF TRICORE REFERENCE LABORATORIES, WWW.TRICORE.ORG, 800-245-3296)

Some phlebotomy chairs are adjustable, and all have armrests to support the patient's extended arm for venipuncture. Chairs should adjust for height and should recline, or there should be a reclined or flat surface available for patients with a known tendency to faint during blood draws. Different chairs have different features. A phlebotomy technician should be familiar with the chairs at her facility. Phlebotomy is repetitive work and can cause strain to the technician's body if she is repeatedly leaning or bending. Work stations should be designed to allow for proper ergonomics.

Special equipment may be used for pediatric blood draws, especially at facilities where children are the primary or only patients, such as children's hospitals. Some pediatric tables have straps to hold a patient in place. It is always important to secure these straps prior to a draw. Pediatric drawing stations are scaled to a smaller size and may be decorated to appeal to children. PBTs should know their facility's accepted procedures for working with pediatric patients. Because most facilities do not have specialized stations for pediatric draws, parents or guardians usually help with positioning and holding the child.

Facilities may have foam wedges or other devices to help position the arms of patients in beds or wheelchairs during venipuncture (Fig. 8-20). Any device that is used between patients must be sanitized after use to avoid transfer of pathogens. This is true of phlebotomy chairs and other work surfaces in a drawing station. It is also true of portable devices like arm wedges.

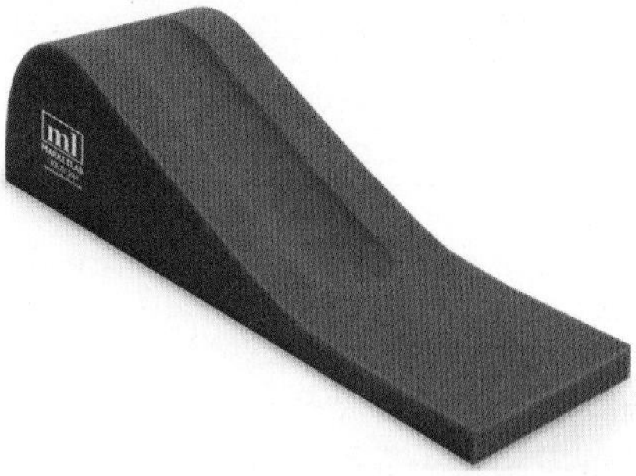

Fig. 8-20. *Positioning devices can help stabilize a patient's arm during venipuncture.* (PHOTO COURTESY OF MARKETLAB, INC., WWW.MARKETLAB.COM)

Bariatric equipment, such as a bariatric chair, may be available for patients who are obese. Phlebotomy technicians should know their facility's options for patients for whom a standard drawing chair is not comfortable (Fig. 8-21). If a standard disposable tourniquet is not comfortable or effective for a patient who is obese, a blood pressure cuff, inflated no higher than a point just below the patient's diastolic blood pressure (the second, lower number) can be used as a tourniquet instead. The diastolic blood pressure reading measures blood pressure during the resting phase of the heart, when it is not contracting and pumping out blood.

Inflating the cuff any higher than the patient's diastolic reading could prevent arterial flow to the limb. The goal of tourniquet use is to limit venous blood return while still allowing arterial flow. Previous standards indicated that the cuff should be inflated no higher than 40 mm Hg. PBTs should follow facility policy.

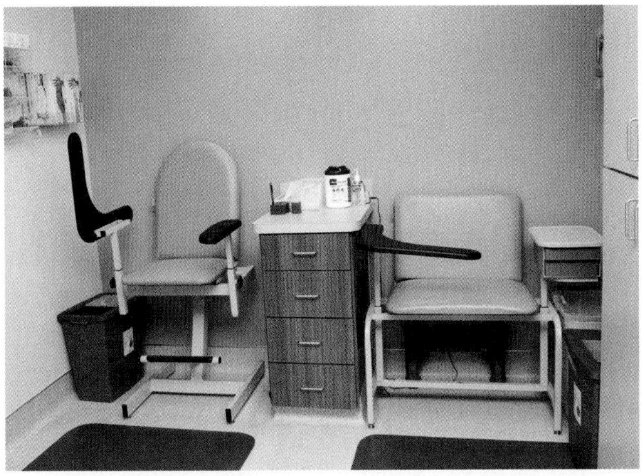

Fig. 8-21. This drawing station features a bariatric chair on the right and a standard chair on the left. The bariatric chair is wider and has additional legs for extra support.

Chapter Review

Multiple Choice

1. In which of the following cases is blood not collected in a tube?
   (A) When the requisition is marked *STAT*
   (B) When the patient is a toddler
   (C) When a point-of-care test requires the use of a test strip
   (D) When a glucose tolerance test is being conducted

2. Which of the following tubes is most likely to be the largest?
   (A) A tube to collect a capillary specimen from an infant
   (B) A tube to collect a venipuncture specimen from an adult
   (C) A tube to collect a capillary specimen from an elderly patient
   (D) A tube to collect a venipuncture specimen from a small child

3. An error that occurs before a blood specimen is tested is called a
   (A) Preliminary error
   (B) Preanalytical error
   (C) Phlebotomy error
   (D) Collection error

4. In which of the following cases should a phlebotomist contact the provider who ordered a test?
   (A) The phlebotomist does not think the patient looks sick enough to need the test ordered.
   (B) The requisition is marked *ASAP*.
   (C) It looks like the patient's veins might be hard to locate.
   (D) The writing on the requisition is not legible.

5. Assuming an 8:00 a.m. draw, *basal state* has not been achieved if the patient has
   (A) Attended a fitness class just before coming to the lab
   (B) Fasted since dinner the evening before
   (C) Slept for eight hours before coming in
   (D) Had a glass of water at bedtime and another just after waking up

6. A needle with a larger gauge number is
   (A) Narrower/thinner than one with a smaller gauge number
   (B) Wider/thicker than one with a smaller gauge number
   (C) Longer than one with a smaller gauge number
   (D) Shorter than one with a smaller gauge number

7. The angled tip of a phlebotomy needle is called the
   (A) Gauge
   (B) Hub
   (C) Point
   (D) Bevel

8. Which part of an evacuated tube system is placed in a sharps container after use?
   (A) The needle only, unscrewed from the holder
   (B) The holder only, unscrewed from the needle
   (C) The needle, holder, and collection tube
   (D) The needle and holder
9. What is the main risk of using an evacuated tube system on a patient with fragile veins?
   (A) The pressure on the vein may cause it to collapse.
   (B) The volume of the tubes is too great and it might cause anemia in the patient.
   (C) The slight movement of the needle during tube changes will cause too much pain.
   (D) The blood flows too quickly into the tubes and could cause the patient to faint.
10. Which antiseptic is most commonly used for routine venipuncture?
    (A) Povidone iodine
    (B) 70% isopropyl alcohol
    (C) ChloraPrep (chlorhexidine gluconate)
    (D) Tincture of iodine
11. Lancets used for heel sticks on premature infants puncture the skin to a depth of ______ mm.
    (A) 0.5
    (B) 0.85
    (C) 1.0
    (D) 2.2
12. What is accomplished by warming the site of a capillary puncture?
    (A) Decreased pain
    (B) Distraction of the patient
    (C) Increased blood flow
    (D) Better blood composition
13. Hematology studies are most often performed on specimens collected in
    (A) Tubes with light blue stoppers
    (B) Tubes with lavender stoppers
    (C) Tubes with yellow stoppers
    (D) Tubes with green stoppers
14. This sequence correctly follows the order of draw:
    (A) Light blue, blood culture, gray
    (B) Blood culture, gray, light blue
    (C) Blood culture, light blue, gray
    (D) Light blue, gray, blood culture
15. Which of these statements is correct?
    (A) Order of draw does not matter in capillary collections.
    (B) Order of draw for capillary collections is the same as for venous collections.
    (C) Order of draw for capillary collections is opposite that of venous collections.
    (D) Order of draw for capillary collections is based on different considerations than order of draw for venous collections.
16. A timed draw should be completed
    (A) Within five minutes of the designated time
    (B) Exactly at the designated time
    (C) Within 10 minutes of the designated time
    (D) Less than five minutes before the designated time
17. According to CLSI standards for patient identification, a patient must ______________ both first and last names.
    (A) Read and acknowledge
    (B) Hear and repeat
    (C) Record and initial
    (D) State and spell

18. In order to be used for patient identification, a wristband must be
    (A) Attached to the patient's body
    (B) Printed in black ink
    (C) Within three feet of the patient at the time of identification
    (D) Acknowledged by the patient as belonging to her

19. If a phlebotomy technician notices that the sharps receptacle is almost completely full before the first patient of the day, he should
    (A) Make a mental note to get a new container during his midmorning break
    (B) Take special care not to place his hand into the container when discarding needles
    (C) Carry used needles to his colleague's drawing station for disposal until a new container can be acquired
    (D) Acquire a new container before calling the first patient

20. Amber-colored plastic or glass tubes ensure that sensitive analytes are not overexposed to
    (A) Light
    (B) Heat
    (C) Movement
    (D) Cold

21. Phlebotomy chairs always feature
    (A) Straps to secure reluctant patients
    (B) The ability to spin a patient from side to side
    (C) A foot pump to adjust the height of the chair
    (D) An armrest for the patient

22. Which of these items needs to be sanitized after use?
    (A) A latex-free disposable tourniquet
    (B) A needle and holder assembly
    (C) A collection tube
    (D) An arm-positioning wedge

9 Collecting Blood Specimens by Venipuncture

1. Review how blood tests are ordered

Each facility has its own system for managing test requisitions. Often these systems are completely electronic: rather than using paper requisitions, the patient's electronic records indicate which tests are ordered. Many laboratories use software known as a **laboratory information system** (**LIS**). These systems integrate every part of the laboratory testing process, from orders and specimen collection through analysis and reports.

Each requisition is associated with a number, called an **accession number**, and that number is printed on all specimen labels related to the requisition. The accession number can be used to trace specimens and results through the LIS at each stage of the testing process. If an LIS is not in use, these tasks are performed manually. Accession numbers and patient identifiers are handwritten on specimen labels. LIS software can reduce the chance of identification errors in patient care, but only if it is used carefully. PBTs should always make sure that they are entering information for the correct patient.

Whether a requisition is on paper or in an electronic system, it must include the following information:

- Patient's name (first and last, sometimes with a middle name or initial)
- Patient's date of birth
- Patient's gender
- Name and contact information of the healthcare provider ordering the test
- Test or tests ordered and any special requirements, such as fasting, timed collection, etc.

Requisitions may also include diagnosis codes, identifiers such as phone number, address, or hospital record number, and insurance information. Phlebotomists should remember that all patient information is confidential and that giving advice about possible diagnoses is outside the PBT's scope of practice.

Most requisition forms are coded to indicate the type of collection tube required for each test (Fig. 9-1). The coding may be a reference to the color of stopper (e.g., light blue or lavender) or may be a reference to the required additive (e.g., citrate or EDTA). Some requisition forms include preprinted patient requirements such as fasting. In other cases, the ordering practitioner will make her own indications regarding patient preparation. PBTs should check each requisition closely to make sure the correct tubes are filled, all tubes needed for all tests are filled, and any preparation or timing requirements are met.

2. Identify the most common venipuncture blood tests

Blood tests are ordered either as part of routine medical care, to aid in diagnosis, or to monitor

HARTMAN MEDICAL CENTER
1313 IRON AVENUE SW | ALBUQUERQUE, NM 87102
505-291-1274 | HARTMANONLINE.COM

Hartman

LABORATORY REQUISITION

PATIENT NAME:	**REQUESTING PHYSICIAN:**
PATIENT MR#:	**PHYSICIAN PHONE NUMBER:**
PATIENT DATE OF BIRTH:	**FAX RESULTS TO:**
DATE COLLECTED:	**PROVIDER SIGNATURE:**
TIME: **AM/PM**	**FASTING:** **NON FASTING:**

ICD-10 DIAGNOSIS	CLINICAL NOTES OR OTHER TESTS

CHECK DEPARTMENT TESTING	CPT CODE		CHECK DEPARTMENT TESTING	CPT CODE		CHECK DEPARTMENT TESTING	CPT CODE	
PANEL			**HEMATOLOGY**			**CHEMISTRY**		
☐ Electrolyte Panel	80051	G	☐ CBC w/Auto Diff	85025	L	☐ Albumin	82040	G,S
☐ Basic Metabolic Panel	80048	G	☐ Reticulocyte Count	85044	L	☐ Alkaline Phosphatase	84075	G,S
☐ Hepatic Function Panel	80078	S,G	☐ Sedimentation Rate	85651	L	☐ ALT/SGPT	84450	G,S
☐ Comp Metabolic Panel	80053	S,G	☐ Platelet Count	85049	L	☐ Amylase	82150	G,S
☐ Lipid Panel	80061	S,G	☐ Body Fluid Cell Count	89051	L	☐ AST/SGOT	84460	G,S
☐ Renal Panel	80069	S,G	Source:			☐ Bilirubin, Total	82247	G,S
☐ Hepatitis Profile	80074	S,L	Total Volume:			☐ Bilirubin, Direct	82248	G,S
						☐ BUN	84520	G,S
COAGULATION			**MICROBIOLOGY**			☐ Calcium	82310	G,S
☐ PTT	85730	B	☐ Culture, Blood	87040		☐ Chloride	82435	G,S
☐ PT	85610	B	☐ Culture, Sputum	87045		☐ Cholesterol	82465	G,S
☐ Fibrinogen	85384	B	☐ Culture, Stool	87045		☐ CK, Total	82550	G,S
☐ D Dimer	85379	B	☐ Culture, Urine	87088		☐ Creatinine	82565	G,S
			☐ Culture, Other	87070		☐ Ferritin	82728	S
URINALYSIS			☐ Gram Stain	87205		☐ FSH	83001	G,S
☐ Urine Dip Reflex to Micro	81002	U	☐ Ova and Parasite	87177		☐ Glucose	82947	G,S
☐ UA Complete	81000	U	☐ Stool for WBC	87205		☐ HCG, Quantitative	84702	G,S
Source:			☐ Occult Blood	82270		☐ Hgb A1C	83636	G,S
						☐ HIV Ab Screen	86701	S,L
IMMUNOLOGY			**TUMOR MARKER**			☐ Iron	83540	S
☐ ANA	86038	S	☐ CA 27-29	86300	S	☐ Luteinizing Hormone (LH)	83002	S
☐ CRP	86140	S	☐ CA 125	86304	S	☐ Magnesium	83735	G,S
☐ C3	86160	S	☐ CEA	82378	S	☐ Phosphorous	84100	G,S
☐ Lyme Disease	86618	S	☐ PSA	84153	S	☐ Potassium	84132	G,S
						☐ Protein, Total	84155	G,S
HEPATITIS TESTS			**THYROID TESTS**			☐ Sodium	84295	G,S
☐ Hep A Ab	86709	S	☐ T4	86706	S	☐ TIBC	83550	S
☐ Hep B Core Ab	86707	S	☐ T3 Uptake	84479	S	☐ Triglycerides	84478	G,S
☐ Hep B Surface Ag	87340	S	☐ TSH	84443	S	☐ Uric Acid	84550	G,S
☐ Hep B Surface Ab	86706	S	☐ Free T4	84439	S			
☐ Hep B Ab	86707	S						
☐ Hep C Ab	96803	S						

Fig. 9-1. *Requisition forms often indicate tubes needed for collection. This form uses initials to designate the appropriate tube(s).*

a specific medication or condition. Most laboratory blood tests require venous blood. Specimens may be managed in different ways, depending on the analyte—or tested substance—involved. In some cases, such as complete blood count or erythrocyte sedimentation rate, the number or behavior of specific blood cells is observed. In other cases, specimens are tested for the presence or amount of specific substances.

Blood cultures detect bacterial or fungal infections in a patient's blood. **Electrolytes** are substances that affect the flow of nutrients and the removal of waste products in the blood. Electrolytes, enzymes, proteins (including antibodies), vitamins, and minerals can all be analytes. When monitoring therapeutic drugs, the levels of the drug in the blood are measured. In other situations, certain analytes are examined to make sure a medication is working and is not causing unintended damage. Blood may also be tested for the presence of illegal drugs or alcohol.

Venipuncture is used to collect blood specimens for most routine and diagnostic tests in adults and children over 1 year of age. A single specimen tube may be used to perform several different tests. Test **panels** are groups of tests either with related analytes (e.g., electrolyte panel, lipid panel) or related to a unifying condition or organ (e.g., renal panel, hepatic panel).

Table 9-1 lists blood tests often ordered as part of routine physical examinations.

TEST NAME	NOTES
Basic metabolic panel (BMP): • Glucose (blood sugar) • Calcium • Sodium (electrolyte) • Potassium (electrolyte) • Carbon dioxide (electrolyte) • Chloride (electrolyte) • Blood urea nitrogen (BUN; waste product related to kidney function) • Creatinine (waste product of muscles, related to kidney function)	• Serum separator tube (usually mottled red/gray or gold) • Heparin tube (green) may be used for stat testing • Fasting sometimes requested
Comprehensive metabolic panel (CMP): • All tests involved in basic metabolic panel • Albumin (protein produced in liver) • Total protein • Alkaline phosphatase (ALP; enzyme related to liver/bone health) • Alanine aminotransferase (ALT; enzyme related to the liver and kidneys) • Aspartate aminotransferase (AST; enzyme related to the liver and heart) • Total bilirubin (waste product generated in the liver)	• Serum separator tube • Heparin tube may be used for stat testing • Fasting sometimes requested
Lipid panel: • Total cholesterol • High-density lipoprotein (HDL) cholesterol • Low-density lipoprotein (LDL) cholesterol • Triglycerides	• Serum separator tube • Heparin tube may be used for stat testing • Usually requires fasting
Complete blood count (CBC): • White blood cell count (with or without differential) • Red blood cell count and measurements • Hemoglobin (Hgb; oxygen-carrying protein in the blood) • Hematocrit (Hct; ratio of RBCs to other components) • Platelet count	• EDTA tube (usually lavender) • Especially important to avoid rough handling

Table 9-1. *These test panels are often ordered as part of a routine physical.*

3. Describe appropriate tourniquet use

To aid in locating the best site for venipuncture the phlebotomist applies a tourniquet to the patient's arm, three to four inches above the puncture site. Since venipuncture is usually performed inside the elbow, the tourniquet is first applied to the patient's upper arm. Most laboratories use single-use (disposable), nonlatex tourniquets. For some patients, however, a blood pressure cuff inflated to a point just below the patient's diastolic blood pressure may be more comfortable and effective. (Follow facility policy regarding use of a blood pressure cuff in place of a tourniquet; the previous CLSI standard was to inflate the cuff no higher than 40 mm Hg.)

The constriction from the tourniquet causes the veins below to become fuller than usual, making them easier to see and feel. This is an essential tool in venipuncture, but care must be taken with its use. Thin or fragile skin may be damaged by a tourniquet. In these situations, the tourniquet may be placed over the patient's clothing, or gauze may first be wrapped around the arm as a protective barrier. In all cases the tourniquet should be applied so that it can be removed quickly and easily. This is accomplished by first crossing the ends, then forming a loop on one side and tucking it beneath the other. The loose end on the loop side can be pulled at any time and the tourniquet immediately released (Fig. 9-2).

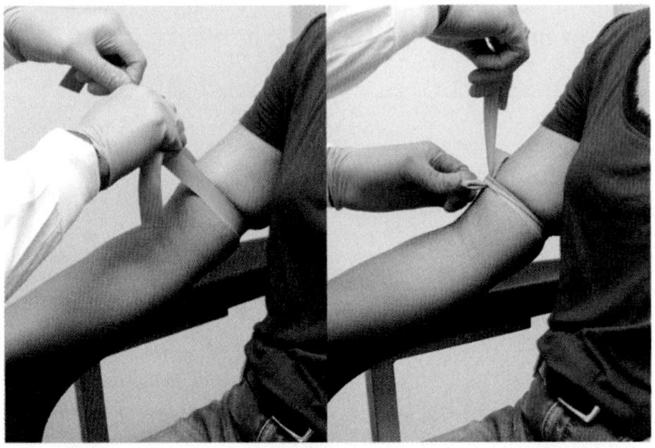

Fig. 9-2. *Making a tucked loop, rather than tying the tourniquet, allows for fast removal.*

A tourniquet is used to aid in vein location and selection and then released. It is applied again just prior to venipuncture and then removed once the vein is accessed and blood flow has begun. **The tourniquet must not be left in place longer than one minute.** Extended use not only causes discomfort for the patient but also can affect the results of tests. **Hemoconcentration** describes a buildup of blood cells (solid components) relative to the liquid components of the blood. This can occur when a tourniquet is left on too long and it falsely elevates blood cell counts. Tourniquet use beyond the one-minute mark can affect other analytes as well and can cause hemolysis. **Hemolysis** is the destruction of red blood cells. If a tourniquet must be released due to excessive time before completing a venipuncture procedure, **the PBT must wait at least two minutes before reapplying a tourniquet to the same arm.**

The tourniquet may also be applied to the area between the elbow and the wrist in preparation for venipuncture in the back of the hand. The tourniquet is applied in this location in the same way, leaving a loop for quick release (Fig. 9-3). The same time limits apply to tourniquet use above the hand.

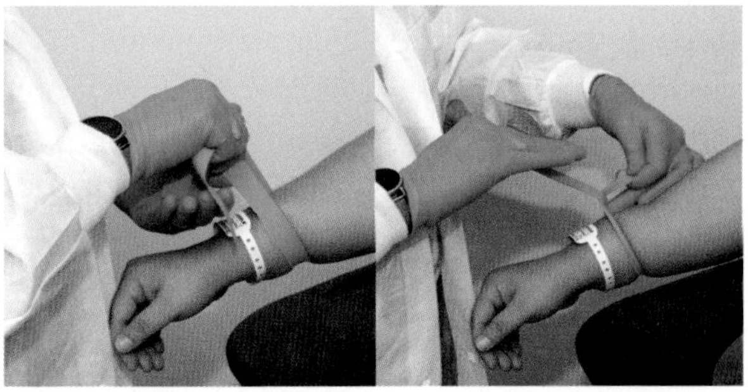

Fig. 9-3. *If the veins in the back of the hand must be used for venipuncture, the tourniquet is applied lower, 3–4 inches above the intended puncture site.*

Quality Counts

In addition to changing the results of a complete blood count due to hemoconcentration, extended use of a tourniquet can affect other analytes. The differences can be large enough to affect test results.

These analytes are especially likely to be affected: total protein, albumin, triglycerides, potassium, sodium, phosphate, calcium, alkaline phosphatase, magnesium, and glucose. Lactate is an analyte previously thought to be so sensitive to tourniquet use that some facility policies dictated not using a tourniquet at all when a specimen would be tested for lactate. More recent research indicates this is not the case. However, it is still important for PBTs to follow facility policy and always follow the one-minute rule and remove tourniquets promptly.

4. Identify appropriate sites for venipuncture

Venipuncture is most commonly performed in the area inside the elbow, called the **antecubital fossa**. Several veins are easily accessible here, but the first choice for the PBT should always be the **median cubital vein**. There are many advantages to selecting this site. Most importantly, the median cubital vein is usually well anchored (in other words, not likely to move back and forth). Using it poses the lowest risk of accidentally puncturing an artery or striking a nerve.

Puncturing or nicking a nerve can cause serious, sometimes permanent, damage, resulting in pain and/or loss of sensation. Arterial puncture is potentially dangerous, as blood flows through the arteries at higher pressure and bleeding from an arterial puncture can be more difficult to stop. Analytes are often present in different amounts in arterial blood. If a specimen of arterial blood is submitted and tests are completed assuming that the specimen is venous, the patient's doctor may receive inaccurate results.

Figure 9-4 shows two common configurations of veins in the antecubital area. In some patients the veins will form a slanted "H" shape and in some they will form an "M" shape. In the "H" formation, which is more common, the median cubital vein is the vein crossing between the **cephalic vein** and the **basilic vein**. In the "M" formation, the median cubital vein and the **median cephalic vein** form the inner, slanting portions of the letter "M." (**Note**: The median cubital vein is also known as the *median basilic vein*. In this book, however, it is always called the *median cubital vein*.)

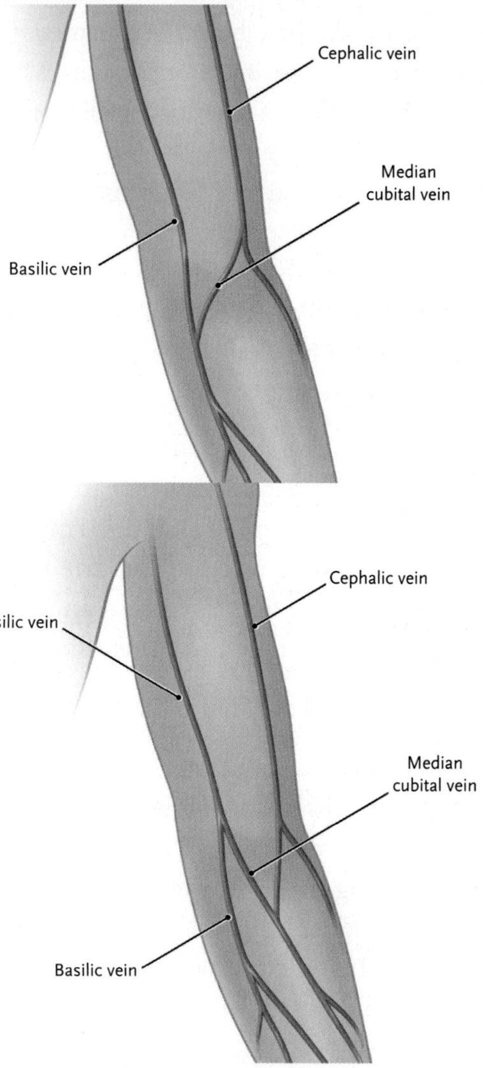

Fig. 9-4. *An illustration of the "H" formation is on top and an illustration of the "M" formation is on the bottom.*

Quality Counts

Accidental artery puncture or nerve contact is much less likely to happen when a PBT follows proper procedures. Taking every precaution possible to avoid these outcomes is the best approach. Still, it is important to know how to manage these situations if they occur. Arterial blood is easy to recognize due to its bright red color and noticeable pulsing as it enters the tube. If an artery is accidentally punctured, the PBT should make sure that bleeding has stopped after removing the needle. It will be necessary to hold pressure on the site for a longer period of time. Patients taking anticoagulation medications are especially likely to bleed from an arterial puncture. The patient should not be bandaged and allowed to leave until bleeding has stopped completely. The specimen should be clearly labeled as arterial blood. Shooting pain, tingling, numbness, or an "electric" feeling in the arm indicate contact with a nerve. The needle must be removed immediately if a patient reports these sensations. Nerve damage can be permanently disabling.

When selecting a site for venipuncture the primary consideration is promoting the patient's safety. This means avoiding locations where arteries and nerves may be easily hit. PBTs should also avoid sites where the vein is difficult to see or palpate. Unsuccessful attempts and patient discomfort are more likely at challenging sites. Figure 9-5 shows the veins of the antecubital fossa, along with the nerves and arteries. Although the nerves and arteries are located deeper than the veins, there is still a risk of missing a vein and striking the brachial artery or a nerve.

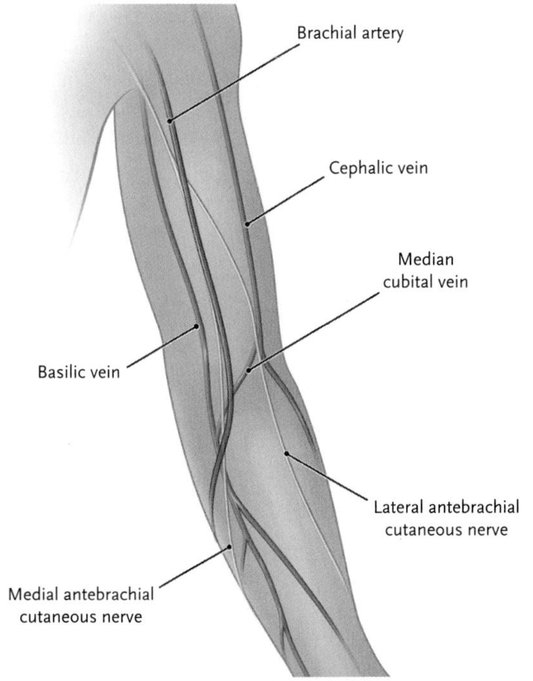

Fig. 9-5. *A number of nerves and arteries are present in the antecubital fossa, along with the veins used for venipuncture.*

In order of preference, the veins that a PBT should consider when selecting a venipuncture site are as follows:

1. Median cubital vein (also known as the median basilic vein)
2. Cephalic vein
3. Basilic vein

The basilic vein is considered to be the least favorable choice for venipuncture due to its location near the brachial artery and antebrachial cutaneous nerves. It is also the site most likely to cause pain for the patient. Before selecting this vein the PBT should first check both arms for a better choice. Veins should be examined by sight but also by palpation. People with different complexions, physical builds, and ages may have veins that are different in appearance (Fig. 9-6). Palpation is the most reliable way to locate the best vein for venipuncture.

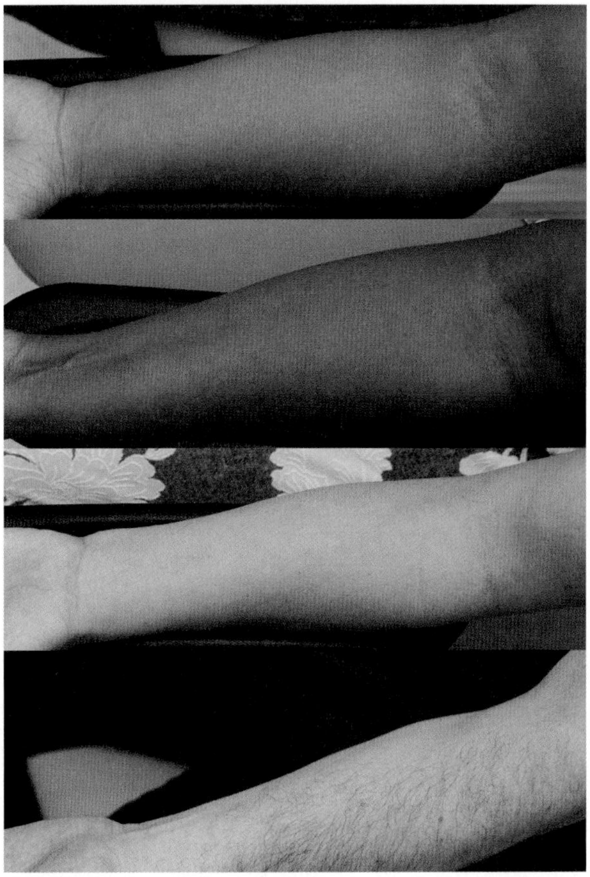

Fig. 9-6. *The antecubital area looks different in different individuals.*

When palpating a vein, the phlebotomist should line his finger up with the vein and judge, by touch, the following factors:

- **Vein health**. A healthy vein should feel springy and uniform and not hard or bumpy.
- **Vein depth**. Veins are located at different depths in different patients. The age and weight of a patient can influence vein depth. This is particularly important when palpating the veins of patients who are obese. The veins of these patients may not be easily visible. No matter the depth of the vein, the angle at which the needle is inserted remains the same for all patients. If, during palpation, the PBT discovers that a patient's veins are relatively deep under the skin, a longer needle should be used.
- **Anchoring of the vein**. Veins in the median antecubital area tend to be well anchored, meaning that they do not move or roll away easily. Some patients, however, have veins that tend to roll no matter where they are located. Palpation can help determine whether vein rolling is likely during venipuncture.
- **Diameter (width) of the vein**. Determining how wide the patient's vein is will help the PBT to select the appropriate gauge of needle and to insert the needle in the center of the vein.

Quality Counts

Patients who have been drinking plenty of water will have veins that are easier to locate and puncture. By the time a dehydrated patient reaches a phlebotomist's drawing station it is too late to address the situation. Drinking a glass of water at that moment will not result in an immediate change. The PBT can help the patient with future blood draws, however, by informing him that drinking plenty of water beforehand will make the procedure easier. Water is allowed and should be encouraged before both fasting and nonfasting blood draws.

When a patient's veins are difficult to locate, the PBT can try these techniques:

- The patient can be asked to hang her arm straight down for a few minutes. This causes blood to pool in the arm and may make finding a vein easier.
- A warm washcloth or a commercial heating pack can be applied to the area. The heat causes veins to dilate, or expand.
- The patient can form a fist, which will cause blood to temporarily surge. It is important *not* to allow the patient to pump her fist repeatedly. This can contribute to hemoconcentration and hemolysis.
- The phlebotomist should ask the patient where venipuncture has been successful in the past. Patients whose veins are difficult to access often know from experience where PBTs have drawn blood before. If, however, the patient indicates a vein that is considered unsuitable, the PBT should not attempt venipuncture at the site.
- **Phlebotomy technicians should *never* slap or flick the patient's skin to cause the veins to become more pronounced.** This was once considered a valid way to make veins more pronounced. Now it is seen as unprofessional. Patients may consider it abusive.

If, after visual inspection and palpation *of both arms*, the phlebotomist does not locate a suitable vein in the antecubital area, the veins on the back of the hand (also called the *dorsal aspect*) are possible alternate sites (Fig. 9-7). The veins in the wrist are *never* an acceptable site for venipuncture. Nerves, tendons, and arteries are all close to the surface of the skin in the wrist. The risk of accidental damage in this location is high. When collecting blood from a vein in the back of a hand, the PBT should be aware that this is usually more painful for the patient.

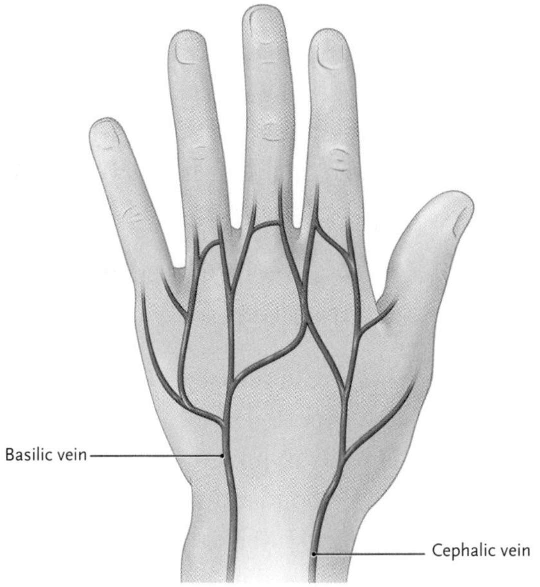

Fig. 9-7. *Veins on the back of the hand may be the best choice if the veins in the antecubital fossa cannot be located or cannot be used.*

In very rare instances, neither the veins in the antecubital area nor those in the back of the hand are acceptable for venipuncture. In these cases blood may be collected from the veins in the lower leg, ankle, or foot. Venipuncture in these areas can be risky, however, especially for patients with diabetes. These patients are prone to dangerous infections in the feet and legs due to problems with circulation and wound healing. Sites in the lower limbs are also dangerous in patients at an elevated risk for thrombosis. Because venipuncture in these areas can cause complications, blood may only be drawn from a leg, ankle, or foot with written approval from a physician.

Patients' Rights

Site selection

The first priority of a phlebotomist selecting a site for venipuncture should be the safety and health of the patient. Drawing blood from sites close to nerves or arteries, or from sites that are unsafe for other reasons, can harm or even permanently disable patients. A patient's comfort is also important. Venipuncture may cause some amount of pain no matter how carefully it is performed, but a phlebotomist should try to select the site that will cause the least discomfort.

5. Describe the proper cleaning of a venipuncture site

Once a site has been selected, it must be cleaned to reduce the risk of introducing harmful microorganisms either through the puncture wound or to the specimen collected. In most cases the antiseptic agent of choice is 70% isopropyl alcohol in the form of a commercially prepared disposable pad (Fig. 9-8). If commercial pads are not available, a gauze square can be moistened with 70% isopropyl alcohol and used to clean the site.

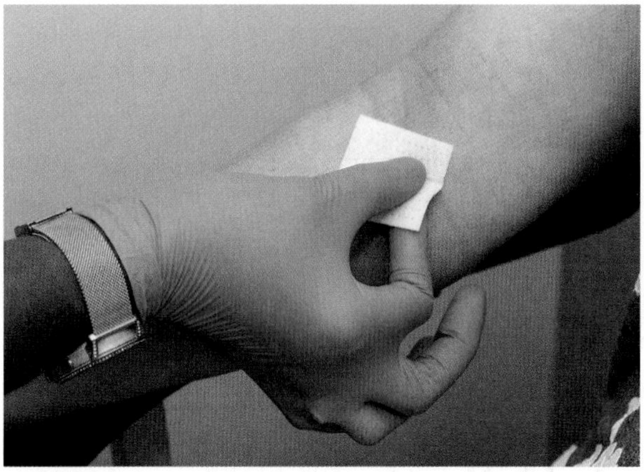

Fig. 9-8. *A commercially prepared alcohol pad or a gauze square soaked in alcohol is the most common instrument for cleaning a venipuncture site.*

Previous CLSI standards and many facilities' policies indicate that a venipuncture site should be cleaned in concentric circles, starting from the inside and working out. Research has not shown a clear benefit to this method, and the CLSI standard released in 2017 does not require this motion for site cleaning. There is no disadvantage to cleaning in circles; it is simply no longer considered superior. PBTs should follow facility policy.

The key to cleaning a site sufficiently is to create gentle friction while not damaging the patient's skin. The skin should then be allowed to air-dry before the venipuncture is performed. The alcohol must dry completely before the vein is punctured. This allows the alcohol sufficient time to act and destroy microorganisms. It prevents stinging at the puncture site, reducing pain for the patient. It is also said to reduce the chances that the specimen will suffer hemolysis, although some studies indicate it does not. Allow the alcohol to dry naturally for approximately 15 seconds, or until it is no longer shiny. Do not blow on the site to dry it, or fan the site, as this carries a risk of spreading pathogens. After the site has been cleaned, it must not be touched again. If the vein is palpated again prior to puncture, the site must then be cleaned once more.

In certain cases an antiseptic other than 70% isopropyl alcohol is required. When a blood culture is ordered, as many microorganisms as possible must be removed from the patient's skin to avoid contaminating the culture. Although it is possible to use isopropyl alcohol to prepare a site for a blood culture, the alcohol pad must remain in contact with the skin for a longer period. Facility procedures usually dictate that the site be cleaned with two or even three different pads for a total of 30–60 seconds.

More commonly, venipuncture sites for blood culture are prepared using a chlorhexidine gluconate product, such as ChloraPrep, or with a 2% tincture of iodine. When iodine is used, it is later removed from the skin with an alcohol prep pad. Otherwise it can pass through the skin and into the patient's bloodstream. It is important to note that some patients are allergic to iodine, and patients with a shellfish allergy are also likely to react to iodine-containing antiseptics. A phlebotomist should learn and follow the antiseptic procedure required for blood culture at her facility. Whatever antiseptic agent is used, it is important to follow the time requirements for cleaning and drying. Contamination of a blood culture produces inaccurate results and can affect patient outcomes.

When blood is being tested for alcohol content (as in a test requested by law enforcement personnel), the venipuncture site must be cleaned with an agent other than isopropyl alcohol or tincture of iodine. Both of these agents contain alcohol and may affect test results. Instead, povidone-iodine and antiseptic soap and water are commonly used. As with tincture of iodine, however, povidone-iodine should not be used on patients with iodine or shellfish allergies.

6. Identify techniques for proper needle placement and insertion

When the equipment is selected (see Chapter 8) and the best site located and cleaned, the phlebotomist is ready to puncture the vein. The thumb of the PBT's nondominant hand is used to pull down on the skin below the puncture site, anchoring the vein. The needle is placed at the selected site, bevel up, and inserted into the skin at an angle of 30 degrees or lower, then advanced gently until blood flow is established (Fig. 9-9). It is very important to insert the needle at the lowest angle possible. A deeper angle of insertion poses a much higher risk of penetrating an artery or hitting a nerve (Fig. 9-10). It also carries a risk of putting the needle straight through, rather than into, the patient's vein (this is often referred to as a *blown vein*).

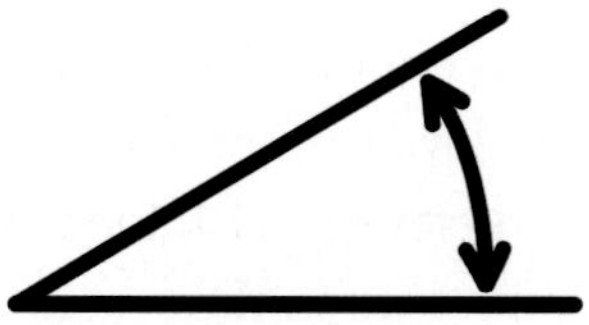

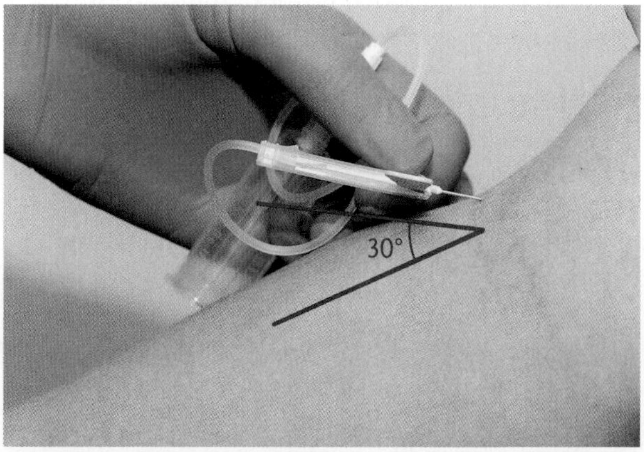

Fig. 9-9. *Inserting the needle at an angle of 30 degrees or lower reduces risk to the patient and improves the chance of a successful draw.*

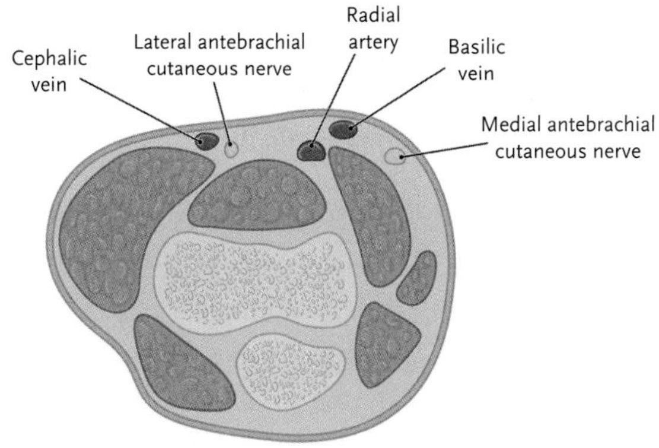

Fig. 9-10. *This cross-section of an arm at the elbow shows the depth of veins, arteries, and nerves. Puncturing the skin at a low angle is the safest way to ensure that a vein is punctured.*

Once the needle has been inserted, a number of problems can prevent blood flow. The patient's vein may have moved, or rolled. The needle may have gone through the entire vein. The bevel may not be fully inserted into the vein, or the vein may have collapsed against the bevel (Fig. 9-11).

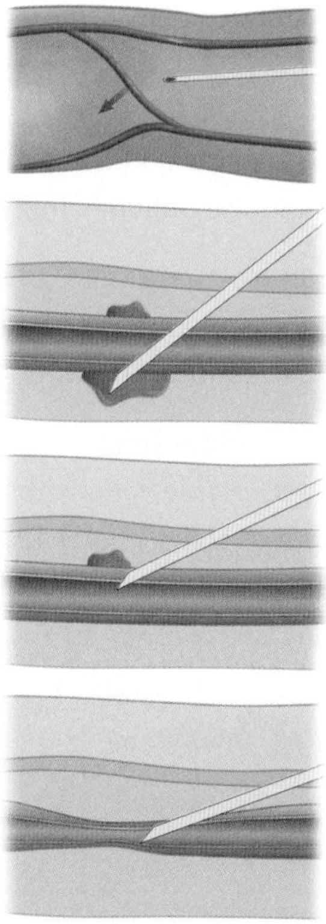

Fig. 9-11. *Veins may roll or may be punctured all the way through ("blown"). The bevel may not be situated completely inside the vein, or the vein may have collapsed onto it.*

If blood flow is not immediately established, it is very important that the PBT *not* move the needle around blindly, an action known as *probing for a vein.* This is painful for the patient and carries a high risk of creating a **hematoma**, or area of leaked blood beneath the patient's skin. Hematomas can develop even after the venipuncture procedure is complete and can place pressure on nerves, potentially causing damage. Blood drawn from a site within a hematoma may produce inaccurate test results.

After initially puncturing the patient's skin, the phlebotomist can gently adjust the needle slightly forward or slightly back (never side to side). If this does not result in blood flow, the tourniquet should be released, the needle removed, and another site selected. **A phlebotomist should not make more than two attempts at venipuncture on one patient**. If, after two attempts, blood flow cannot be established, the PBT should ask a supervisor for assistance.

7. Describe procedures for routine venipuncture

Most venipuncture procedures will be performed in the antecubital area of the arm with a straight, 21-gauge multisample needle and evacuated tubes. Changes to this equipment are usually based on the patient's age or condition. If there is no indication that a butterfly assembly is necessary for a particular patient, the PBT should select a straight multisample needle. These needles are easier to handle and pose less risk of accidental needlestick.

Prior to performing any venipuncture procedure the PBT should ask the patient if she has ever had difficulties with blood draws in the past. This will help the phlebotomist prepare appropriately. The PBT should also confirm that the patient has met any requirements—most commonly fasting—to prepare for the blood draw. She should make sure there is no gum or food in the patient's mouth. All equipment should be checked carefully for defects and, as applicable, for expiration dates. Expired or faulty equipment should be properly discarded.

Quality Counts

A tourniquet cannot remain in place for more than one minute without damaging the quality of a specimen. When a patient has veins that are easy to see, palpate, and puncture, a PBT who has his equipment prepared may be able to select and clean a site and access a vein all within a one-minute period. This creates a very tight timeline, though, and unnecessarily increases pressure to complete the collection quickly. It is better to release the tourniquet as soon as a site is selected and reapply it just prior to venipuncture. The tourniquet remains in place on the arm, but not tightened, while the PBT cleans the site and prepares the needle and holder. It is reapplied right before the vein is accessed. The loose ends of the tourniquet must not touch and contaminate the selected site. The tourniquet is released as soon as blood flow is established.

Note: This procedure instructs PBTs to don gloves at the beginning of patient contact. At some facilities, gloves are donned just prior to the actual venipuncture. If the patient has open sores on the arms or Contact Precautions are ordered, gloves must be donned before any contact takes place. Otherwise, the PBT should follow facility policy regarding when to don gloves.

Performing routine venipuncture with multisample needle and evacuated tube(s)

Equipment: Test requisition (paper or electronic); soap and water or alcohol-based hand sanitizer; gloves (additional PPE if required based on patient condition); tourniquet; 70% isopropyl alcohol pad (or other antiseptic agent); multisample needle of the correct gauge; needle holder; collection tubes required for ordered tests; specimen labels; 2"x2" gauze; adhesive or self-adhesive bandage; pen

1. Greet the patient. Identify yourself by name and title.
2. Identify the patient using two unique identifiers. Usually this means asking the patient to state and spell his first and last names and state his full date of birth. Check the information provided against the requisition form and against the patient's wristband if wristbands are used at your facility.
3. Explain the procedure to the patient. Allow the patient to ask questions, but refer questions regarding the purpose or interpretation of tests to her doctor. *If at any point the patient expresses that she does not consent to the procedure, do not continue until consent is given. If consent is not given, document the refusal according to facility policy and allow the patient to leave. Notify the ordering practitioner of the patient's refusal.*
4. Gather required equipment.
5. Wash (or sanitize) your hands. Don gloves and other PPE as required. (In the case of some Transmission-Based Precautions this will already have occurred outside the patient's room.)
6. Ask the patient to extend her arms for a visual inspection. Ask if, in her experience, one arm is better than the other for venipuncture. Choose an arm based on the appearance of the veins and the patient's input.
7. Apply the tourniquet to the selected arm, 3–4 inches above the bend in the elbow. Ask the patient to make (but not pump) a fist.
8. With a gloved index finger, palpate the arm to locate an acceptable vein, with a preference for the median veins (Fig. 9-12). If an acceptable site is not found, remove the tourniquet and apply it to the other arm.

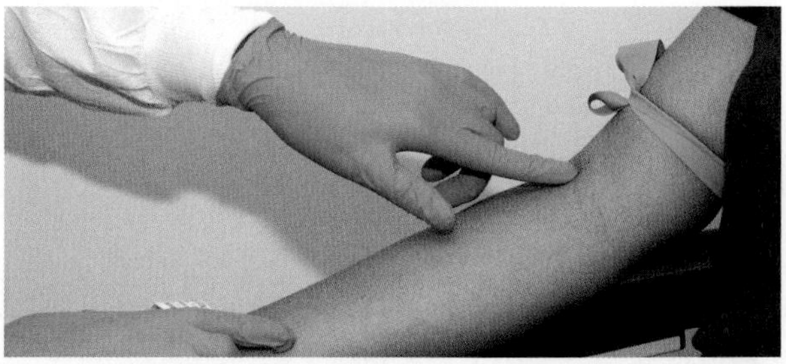

Fig. 9-12. *Palpate the arm with your index finger to find an acceptable vein.*

9. When a suitable site is located, release the tourniquet and clean the site thoroughly. Apply friction with the alcohol pad (or other antiseptic agent). It may be helpful to make a mental note of a physical marker associated with the site, such as a freckle or a crease in the skin.

10. Allow the alcohol to dry fully. Do not blow on, fan, or wipe the skin to speed drying, as this can recontaminate the site. While the alcohol dries, assemble the needle and holder (Fig. 9-13). The first tube may be inserted into the holder, but should not be advanced fully until the patient's vein is accessed.

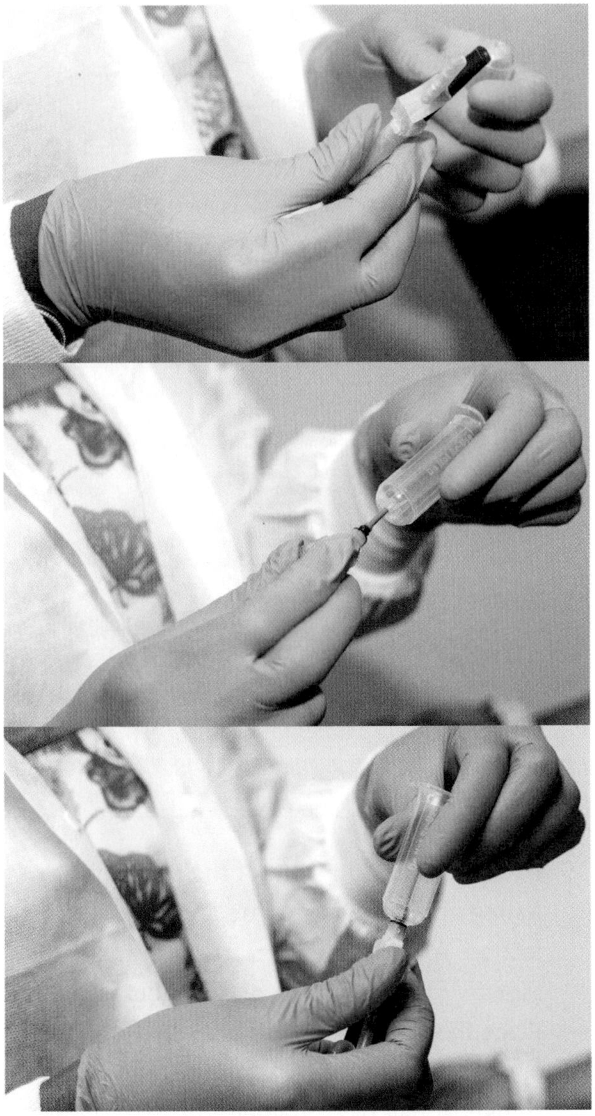

Fig. 9-13. *Assemble equipment while the patient's arm dries.*

11. Reapply the tourniquet.

12. Anchor the vein by grasping the patient's forearm with your nondominant hand. Use your thumb to apply pressure and pull the skin toward the wrist an inch or two below the venipuncture site. *Do not place an anchoring finger above the venipuncture site. This poses a needlestick risk.*

13. Inform the patient that she may feel brief pain as the needle enters the skin but that it will be over quickly. In a single, fluid motion, insert the needle into the skin to puncture the selected vein at an angle of 30 degrees or less (Fig. 9-14).

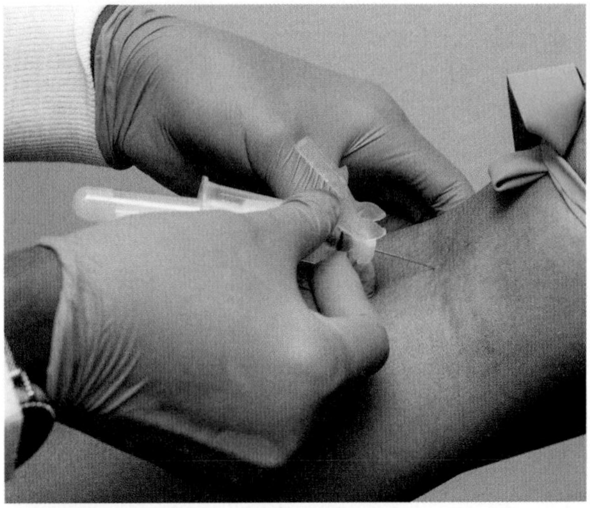

Fig. 9-14. *Be gentle but decisive when puncturing the patient's skin to access the vein.*

14. Insert the first collection tube, pressing it in to the point marked on the tube. As soon as blood flow is established, release the tourniquet, letting it hang loose. Allow the tube to fill completely. The vacuum should draw in exactly the right amount of blood.

15. If multiple tubes are required, replace the first filled tube with the next tube according to proper order of draw. Continue until all necessary tubes are filled. Remove the last tube from the holder.

16. Place a piece of gauze, folded into quarters, over the needle.

17. Withdraw the needle from the patient's arm, engaging the safety device before or after, as appropriate to the style of needle. Dispose of the needle and holder in an appropriate sharps receptacle. Maintain pressure on the gauze, asking the patient to assist as she is able (Fig. 9-15). Do not allow the patient to bend her arm up, as this can create a hematoma.

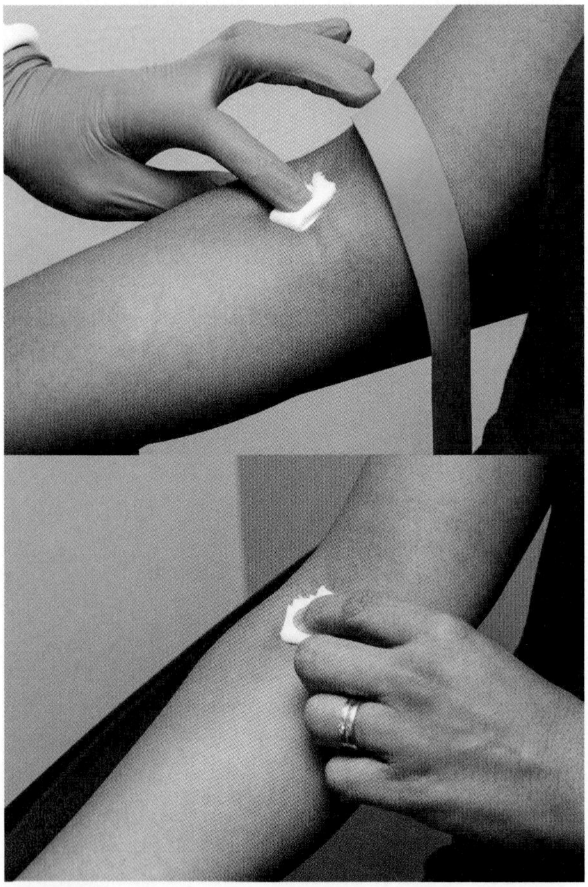

Fig. 9-15. *Apply pressure to the gauze immediately after the needle is withdrawn. The patient can then hold pressure if she is able.*

18. Mix tubes as indicated by the manufacturer. Most citrate and serum tubes require 3–5 inversions; most other tubes require 8–10. This is accomplished by gently turning the tube upside down and then right side up again (Fig. 9-16). This counts as one inversion. Mix tubes promptly. If multiple tubes are required, the tube collected first can be mixed while the next tube fills.

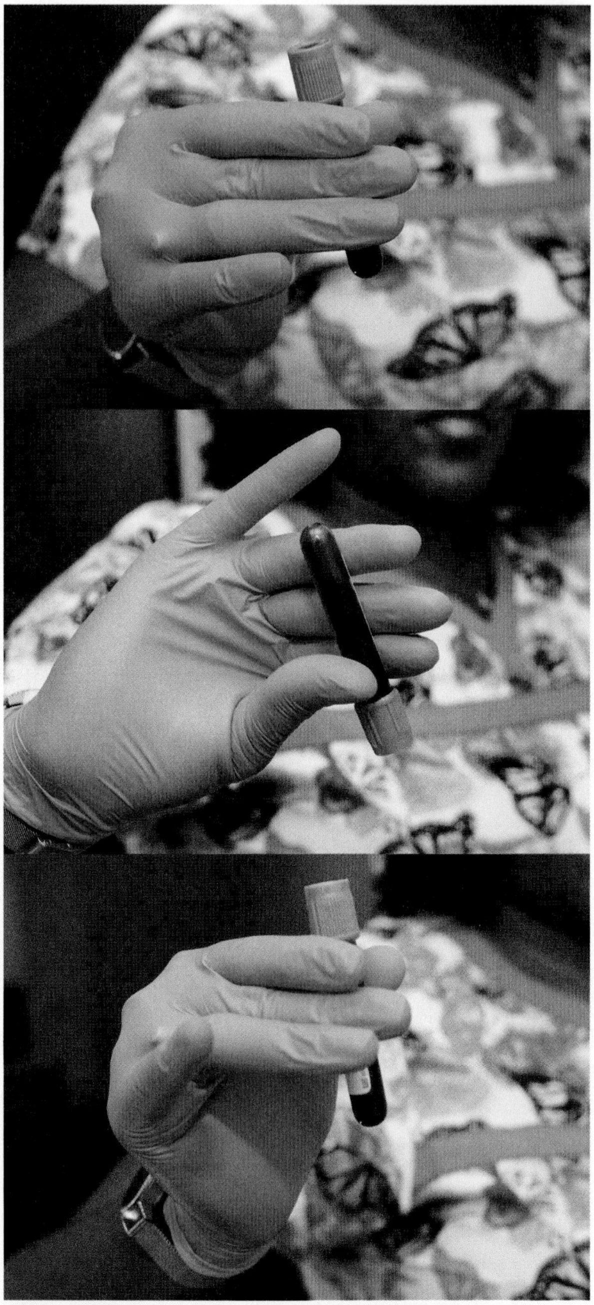

Fig. 9-16. *Never shake tubes to mix them. Smooth, gentle inversions ensure adequate mixing while preventing hemolysis.*

19. Label the tubes in front of the patient, initialing and noting the time and date of collection. Ask the patient to confirm that the identifying information on the label is correct. Place the specimens and the requisition or any required paperwork in the appropriate transport bag or container. Properly discard any waste.

20. Check to make sure that the patient is no longer bleeding. In the case of patients on anticoagulant medication, this can take as long as five minutes.

21. Place a bandage over the gauze on the patient's arm. Self-adhesive bandages are less likely to damage skin and may be better suited to patients with fragile skin (Fig. 9-17). Advise the patient to leave the bandage in place for the next 15 minutes.

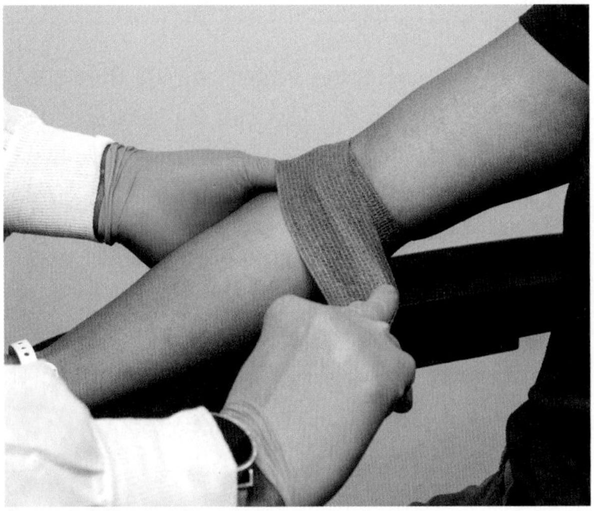

Fig. 9-17. *Self-adhesive bandages are convenient and often more comfortable for the patient.*

22. Observe the patient for any signs of dizziness or discomfort. Do not allow the patient to stand if she seems unsteady or says that she feels faint.

23. Thank the patient and tell her she may leave and will receive results from the ordering practitioner.

24. Remove gloves and wash your hands.

25. Document the procedure according to facility policy.

If a suitable location cannot be found in the patient's arm or if the arms are not accessible, the back of the hand may be a good alternative. Because the veins of the hand are smaller and thinner, a winged collection system is generally used for venipuncture at this site. Winged collection sets feature a length of flexible tubing between the needle and the tube holder. Because this tubing is initially filled with air, some tests may require that a discard tube be drawn before tubes are filled for testing. This ensures that the proper amount of blood is collected in the tubes and that the ratio of blood to tube additive is correct. The discard tube must either be a citrate tube or a tube without any additive to avoid contamination of the specimens collected afterward. It does not have to be filled completely as it will not be tested. It can be removed as soon as it begins to fill. This reduces the chance of confusing a discard tube with a tube for testing.

Performing venipuncture in the hand with winged collection system and evacuated tube(s)

Equipment: Test requisition (paper or electronic); soap and water or alcohol-based hand sanitizer; gloves (additional PPE if required based on patient condition); tourniquet; 70% isopropyl alcohol pad (or other antiseptic agent); winged collection set with needle of correct gauge; medical tape for securing needle (optional); collection tubes required for ordered tests, including citrate or additive-free discard tube if needed; specimen labels; 2"x2" gauze; adhesive or self-adhesive bandage; pen

1. Greet the patient. Identify yourself by name and title.

2. Identify the patient using two unique identifiers. Usually this means asking the patient to state and spell her first and last names and state her full date of birth. Check the information provided against the requisition form and against the patient's wristband if wristbands are used at your facility.

3. Explain the procedure to the patient. Allow the patient to ask questions, but refer questions regarding the purpose or interpretation of tests to her doctor. *If at any point the patient expresses that she does not consent to the procedure, do not continue until consent is given. If consent is not given, document the*

refusal according to facility policy and allow the patient to leave. Notify the ordering practitioner of the patient's refusal.

4. Gather required equipment (Fig. 9-18).

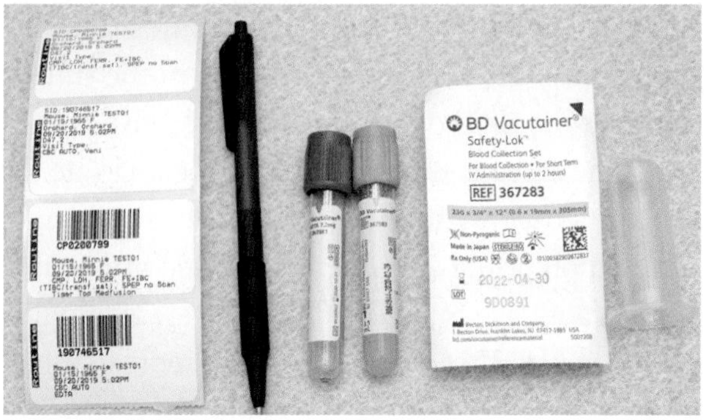

Fig. 9-18. *Having equipment organized neatly can reassure the patient and help the procedure run more smoothly.*

5. Wash (or sanitize) your hands (Fig. 9-19). Don gloves and other PPE as required. (In the case of some Transmission-Based Precautions this will already have occurred outside the patient's room.)

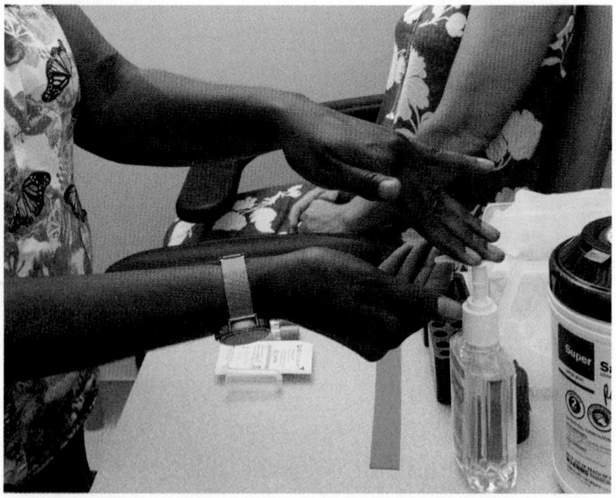

Fig. 9-19. *Hand hygiene must be performed before every venipuncture procedure.*

6. Ask the patient to extend her hands, palms down, for a visual inspection. Choose a hand based on the appearance of the veins.

7. Apply the tourniquet to the forearm above the selected hand, 3–4 inches above the intended puncture site. Ask the patient to make (but not pump) a fist (Fig. 9-20).

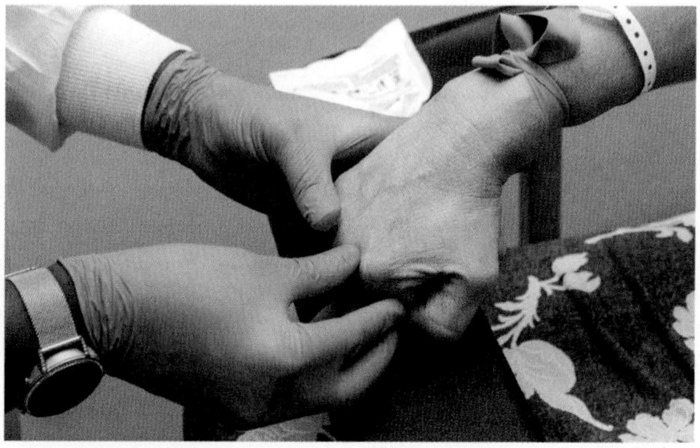

Fig. 9-20. *Veins may appear more prominently when the patient forms a fist.*

8. With a gloved index finger, palpate the vein and determine the best site for puncture. If an acceptable site is not found, remove the tourniquet and apply it to the other forearm.

9. When a suitable site is located, release the tourniquet and clean the site thoroughly. Apply friction with the alcohol pad or other antiseptic agent (Fig. 9-21). It may be helpful to make a mental note of a physical marker associated with the site, such as a freckle or a crease in the skin.

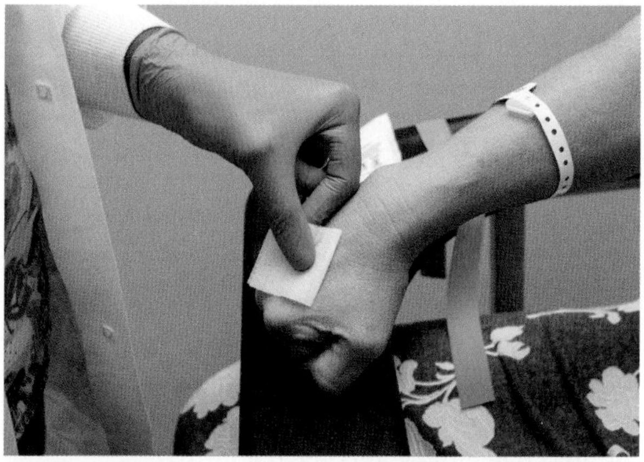

Fig. 9-21. *Clean the puncture site with gentle friction.*

10. Allow the alcohol to dry fully. Do not blow on, fan, or wipe the skin to speed drying, as this can recontaminate the site. While the alcohol dries, prepare the winged collection set and holder (Fig. 9-22). The first tube may be inserted into the holder but should not be advanced fully until the patient's vein is accessed.

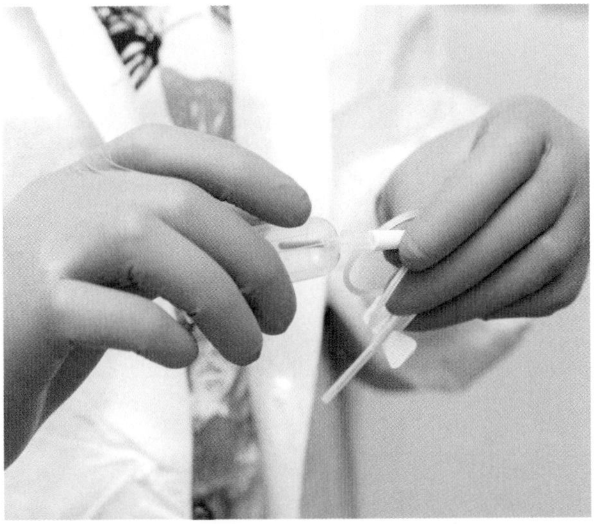

Fig. 9-22. *The butterfly and holder can be assembled while the antiseptic dries.*

11. Reapply the tourniquet.
12. Anchor the vein by grasping the patient's hand with your nondominant hand. Use your thumb to apply pressure and pull the skin toward the knuckles below the venipuncture site (Fig. 9-23). *Do not place an anchoring finger above the venipuncture site. This poses a needlestick risk.*

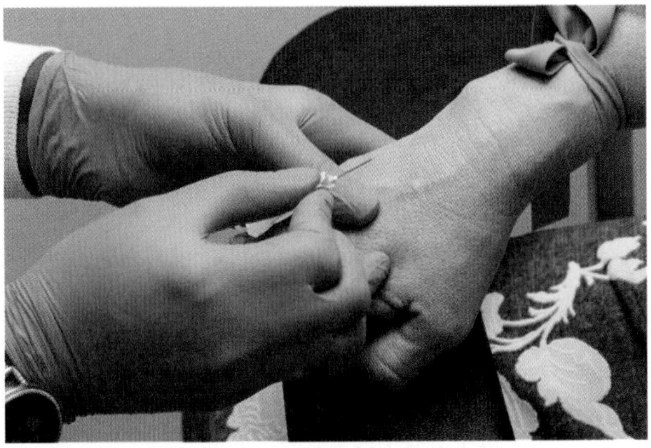

Fig. 9-23. *Veins in the hand may be more difficult to access, so proper anchoring is important.*

13. Inform the patient that she may feel brief pain as the needle enters the skin but that it will be over quickly. In a single, fluid motion, insert the needle into the skin to puncture the selected vein (Fig. 9-24). As soon as blood flow is established, release the tourniquet, letting it hang loose.

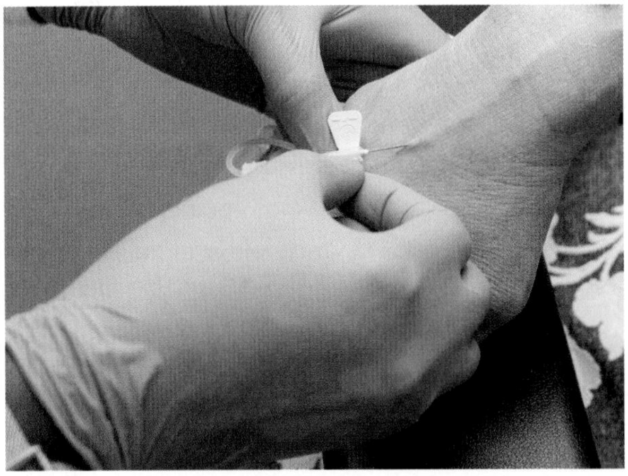

Fig. 9-24. *Hold the "wings" to guide the needle as it is inserted.*

14. Secure the needle of a winged collection set throughout the draw, following CLSI standards. Either hold the needle with one hand and insert/change tubes with the other, or tape the needle in place (Fig. 9-25).

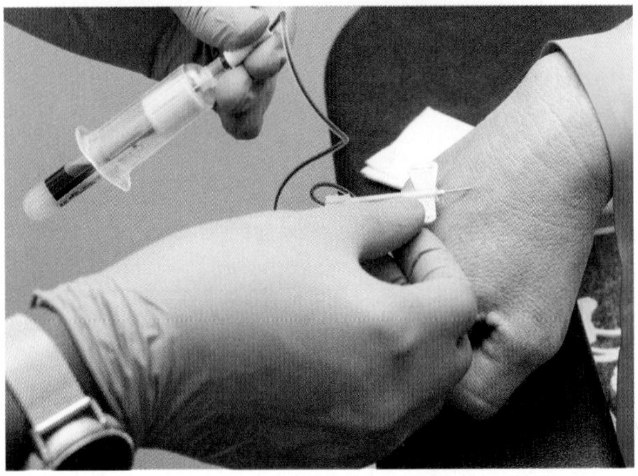

Fig. 9-25. *Secure the needle by holding it or taping it in place.*

15. If a discard tube is needed, insert it first. It can be removed and discarded in the sharps container as soon as blood enters it. Insert the first collection tube. Allow it to fill completely. (The vacuum should draw in exactly the right amount of blood.)
16. If multiple tubes are required, replace the first filled tube with the next tube according to proper order of draw. Continue until all necessary tubes are filled. Remove the last tube from the holder.

17. Place a piece of gauze, folded into quarters, over the needle.

18. Withdraw the needle from the patient's hand, engaging the safety device before or after, as appropriate to the style of needle. Discard the needle, tubing, and holder in an appropriate sharps receptacle (Fig. 9-26). Maintain pressure on the gauze, asking the patient to assist as she is able.

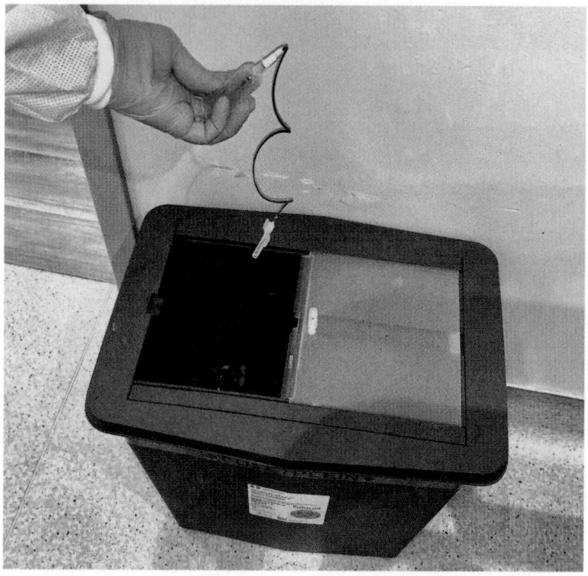

Fig. 9-26. *The assembled winged set is discarded in one piece.*

19. Mix tube(s) as indicated by the manufacturer. Most citrate and serum tubes require 3–5 inversions; most other tubes require 8–10. This is accomplished by gently turning the tube upside down and then right side up again. This counts as one inversion. Mix tubes promptly. If multiple tubes are required, the tube collected first can be mixed while the next tube fills.

20. Label the tubes in front of the patient, initialing and noting the time and date of collection (Fig. 9-27). Ask the patient to confirm that the identifying information on the label is correct. Place the specimens and the requisition or any required paperwork in the appropriate transport bag or container. Properly discard any waste.

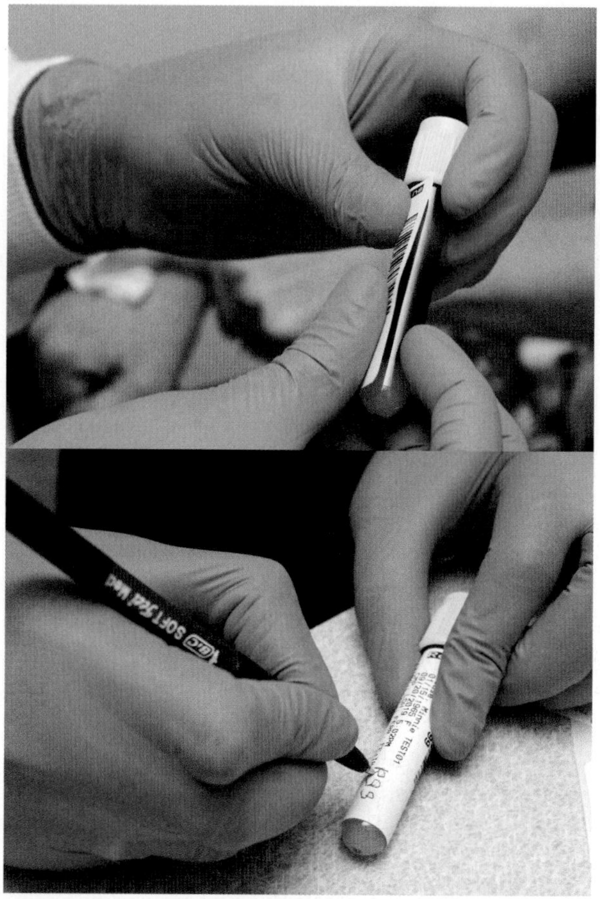

Fig. 9-27. *Carefully place the patient's label on the specimen, then mark the label with your initials and the time/date.*

21. Check to make sure that the patient is no longer bleeding. In the case of patients on anticoagulant medication, this can take as long as five minutes.

22. Place a bandage over the gauze on the patient's hand. Self-adhesive bandages are less likely to damage skin and may be better suited to patients with fragile skin. Advise the patient to leave the bandage in place for the next 15 minutes.

23. Observe the patient for any signs of dizziness or discomfort. Do not allow the patient to stand if she seems unsteady or says that she feels faint.

24. Thank the patient and tell her she may leave and will receive results from the ordering practitioner.

25. Remove gloves and wash your hands.
26. Document the procedure according to facility policy.

A winged collection set may also be used for venipuncture in the antecubital area (Fig. 9-28). While there are certain advantages to butterfly assemblies, they are also associated with a higher number of needlestick incidents. Care should be taken with all needles, but extra awareness is required when using a butterfly set.

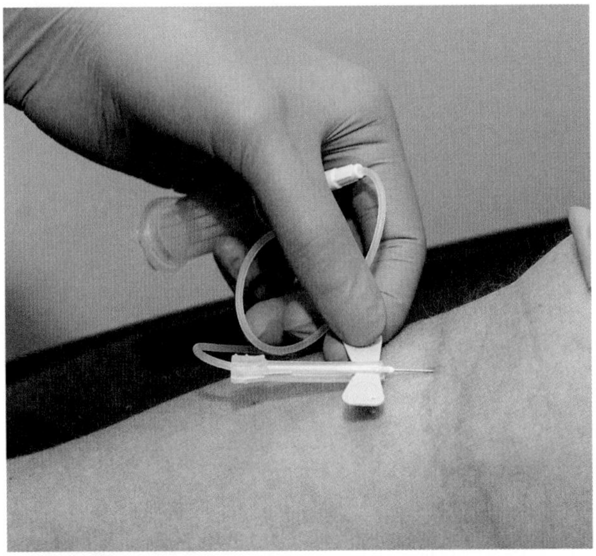

Fig. 9-28. *Winged collection sets may be used for venipuncture at any acceptable site.*

8. Discuss adaptations to routine venipuncture for special populations and conditions

Pediatric and elderly patients, as well as patients undergoing chemotherapy or other long-term medical treatments, may have small and/or fragile veins. In some cases, the pressure placed on the veins by the vacuum in evacuated tubes is too great and causes veins to collapse, stopping the flow of blood. Smaller collection tubes place less pressure on the veins, and may be appropriate for pediatric, elderly, or medically fragile patients.

In these situations, another option is to use a winged collection system and a syringe. This procedure can be performed either in the antecubital area or in the dorsal aspect of the hand (as shown in the procedure below). After completing a blood draw using a syringe, the blood must be transferred to the appropriate evacuated tubes using a syringe transfer device. Because blood may be transferred to multiple tubes, the PBT should select a syringe that can draw enough blood for all ordered tubes. Phlebotomists must never use the venipuncture needle to puncture an evacuated tube and transfer blood from a syringe. This poses a needlestick risk and can damage or contaminate the specimen. The needle should be removed and deposited in a sharps receptacle immediately after it is taken out of the patient's skin.

Collecting a blood specimen using a syringe and transfer device

Equipment: Test requisition (paper or electronic); soap and water or alcohol-based hand sanitizer; gloves (additional PPE if required based on patient condition); tourniquet; warming pack or washcloth soaked in warm water (as needed for vein location); 70% isopropyl alcohol pad (or other antiseptic agent); winged needle of correct gauge; syringe; medical tape for securing needle (optional); specimen labels; 2"x2" gauze; adhesive or self-adhesive bandage; collection tubes required for ordered tests; syringe transfer device; pen

1. Greet the patient. Identify yourself by name and title.
2. Identify the patient using two unique identifiers. Usually this means asking the patient to state and spell her first and last names and state her full date of birth. Check the information provided against the requisition form and against the patient's wristband if one is worn.
3. Explain the procedure to the patient. Allow the patient to ask questions, but refer questions regarding the purpose or interpretation

of tests to her doctor. *If at any point the patient expresses that she does not consent to the procedure, do not continue until consent is given. If consent is not given, document the refusal according to facility policy and allow the patient to leave. Notify the ordering practitioner of the patient's refusal.*

4. Gather required equipment.

5. Wash (or sanitize) your hands. Don gloves and other PPE as required. (In the case of some Transmission-Based Precautions this will already have occurred outside the patient's room.)

6. Ask the patient to extend her hands, palms down, for a visual inspection. Choose a hand based on the appearance of the veins. (If drawing from the antecubital fossa, see vein selection steps, 6–9, in the procedure *Performing routine venipuncture with multisample needle and evacuated tube(s)*). Application of a warming pack to the area can make veins more prominent.

7. Apply the tourniquet 3–4 inches above the selected area. Ask the patient to make (but not pump) a fist.

8. With a gloved index finger, palpate the vein and determine the best site for puncture. If an acceptable site is not found, remove the tourniquet and apply it to the other side.

9. When a suitable site is located, release the tourniquet and clean the site thoroughly. Apply friction with the alcohol pad (or other antiseptic agent). It may be helpful to make a mental note of a physical marker associated with the site, such as a freckle or a crease in the skin.

10. Allow the alcohol to dry fully. Do not blow on, fan, or wipe the skin to speed drying, as this can recontaminate the site. While the alcohol dries, assemble the needle and syringe (Fig. 9-29).

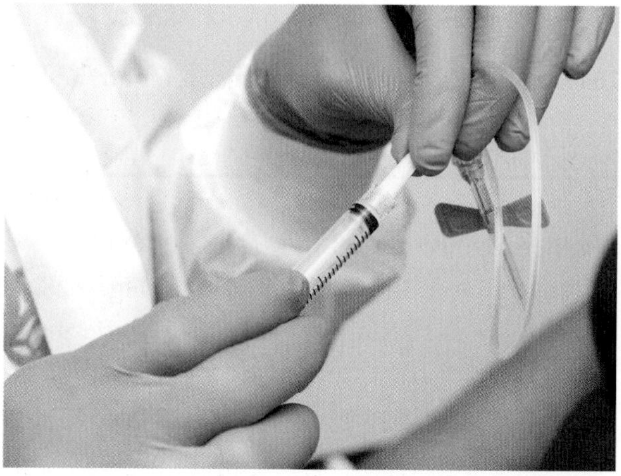

Fig. 9-29. *The tubing of a winged needle can be screwed on to a syringe just as it is screwed on to an evacuated tube holder.*

11. Follow facility guidance and manufacturer instructions to prepare the syringe for use. This may involve drawing the plunger back to break a seal and then pressing it back in to push air out of the barrel (Fig. 9-30).

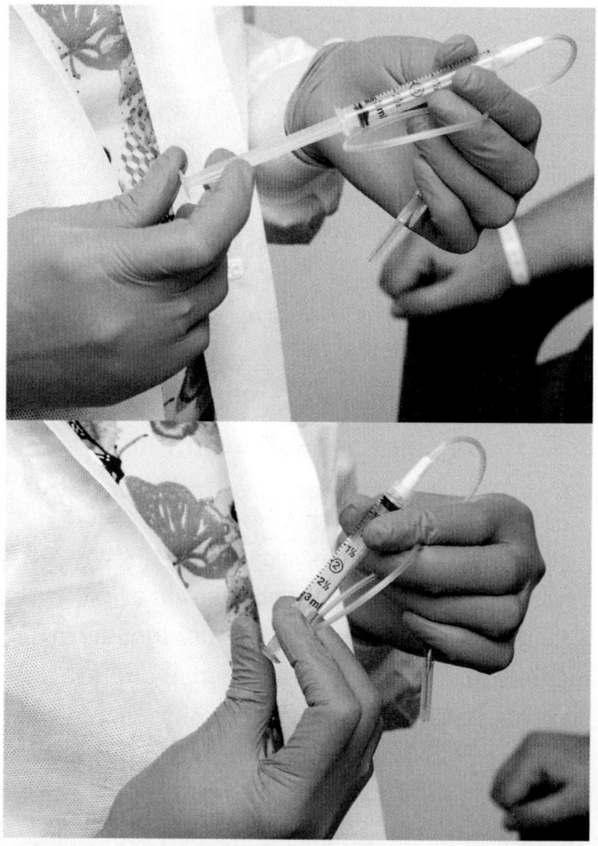

Fig. 9-30. *In most cases the plunger of the syringe should be pulled out and pushed back in before it is used to draw blood.*

12. Reapply the tourniquet.

13. Anchor the vein by grasping the patient's hand (or arm) with your nondominant hand. Use your thumb to apply pressure and pull the skin toward you, below the venipuncture site. *Do not place an anchoring finger above the venipuncture site. This poses a needlestick risk.*

14. Inform the patient that she may feel brief pain as the needle enters the skin but that it will be over quickly. In a single, fluid motion, insert the needle into the skin to puncture the selected vein (Fig. 9-31). As soon as blood flow is established, release the tourniquet, letting it hang loose.

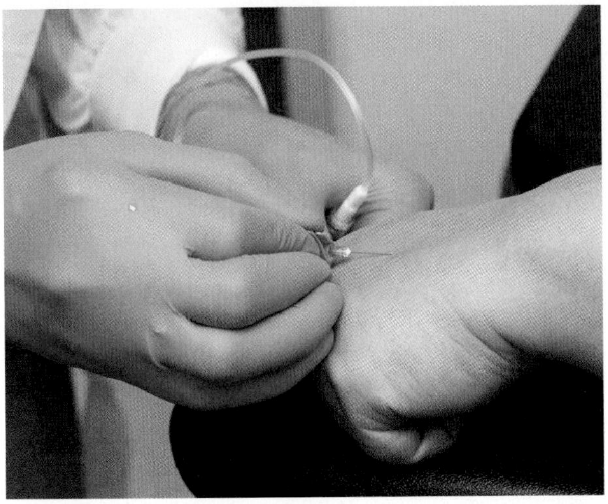

Fig. 9-31. *A low angle of insertion, as shown here, is safest and most effective. Angle of insertion is important no matter the venipuncture site, but a high angle of insertion in the hand can be especially painful.*

15. Secure the needle of a winged collection set throughout the draw, following CLSI standards. Either hold the needle with one hand and insert/change tubes with the other, or tape the needle in place.

16. Pull back gently and steadily on the syringe plunger until the necessary volume of blood is collected (Fig. 9-32). Do not pull the plunger back forcefully, as this can cause the vein to collapse and can also damage the specimen.

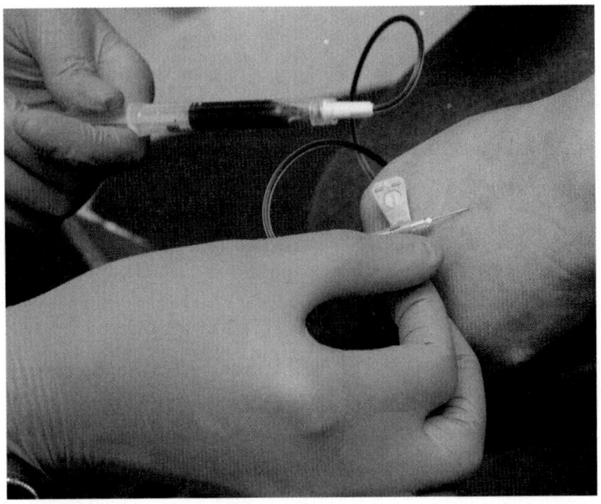

Fig. 9-32. *The needle can be secured with one hand and the plunger gently pulled back with the other. Alternately, the needle may be taped in place.*

17. Place a piece of gauze, folded into quarters, over the needle.

18. Withdraw the needle from the patient's body, engaging the safety device before or after, as appropriate to the style of needle. Maintain pressure on the gauze, asking the patient to assist as she is able.

19. Remove flexible tubing from the syringe and place the needle and tubing in a sharps disposal container.

20. Immediately screw the syringe onto the syringe transfer device (Fig. 9-33).

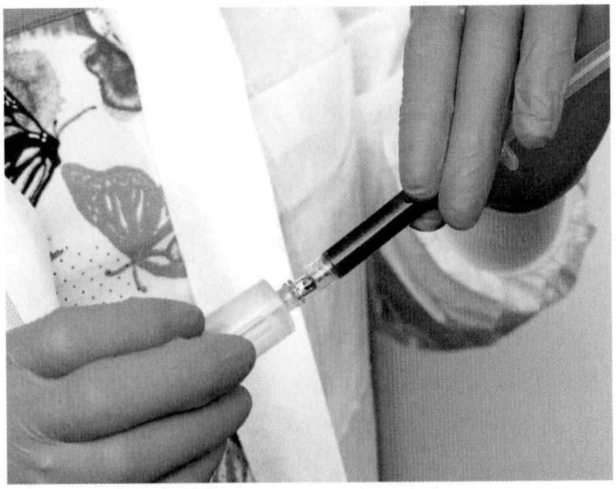

Fig. 9-33. *A syringe transfer device looks very much like an evacuated tube holder but is designed to attach securely to a syringe.*

21. Insert appropriate collection tube(s), according to order of draw. Do not press on the syringe plunger as the blood transfers. The vacuum in the tube will draw the blood in to the required level (Fig. 9-34).

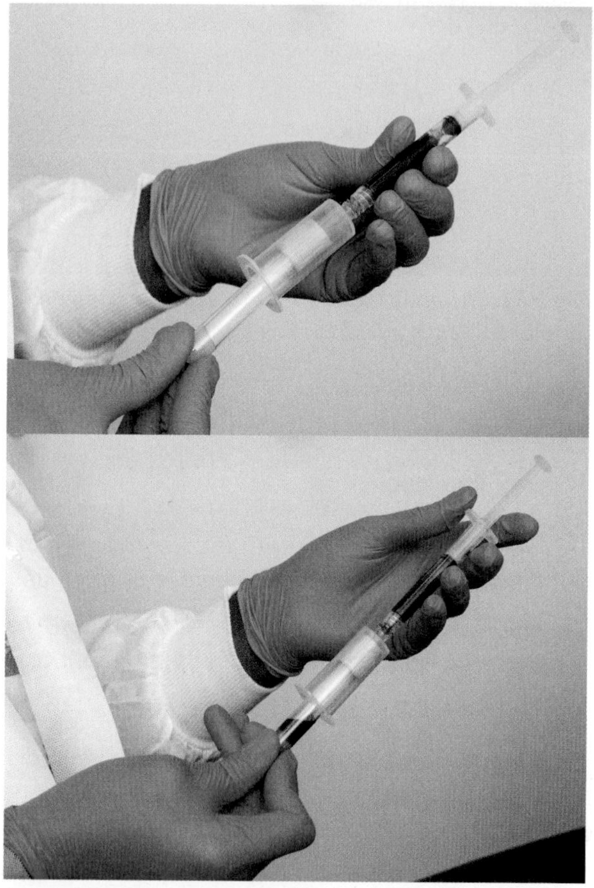

Fig. 9-34. *Tubes are inserted in syringe transfer devices just as in evacuated tube holders. Pressing on the plunger increases hemolysis risk, so allow the vacuum to draw the blood in.*

22. Dispose of the syringe and transfer device in the sharps container.

23. Mix tube(s) as indicated by the manufacturer. Most citrate and serum tubes require 3–5 inversions; most other tubes require 8–10. This is accomplished by gently turning the tube upside down and then right side up again. This counts as one inversion.

24. Label the tubes in front of the patient, initialing and noting the time and date of collection. Ask the patient to confirm that the identifying information on the label is correct. Place the specimens and the requisition or any required paperwork in the appropriate transport bag or container. Properly discard any waste.

25. Check to make sure that the patient is no longer bleeding. In the case of patients on anticoagulant medication, this can take as long as five minutes.

26. Place a bandage over the gauze on the patient's hand (Fig. 9-35). Advise the patient to leave the bandage in place for the next 15 minutes.

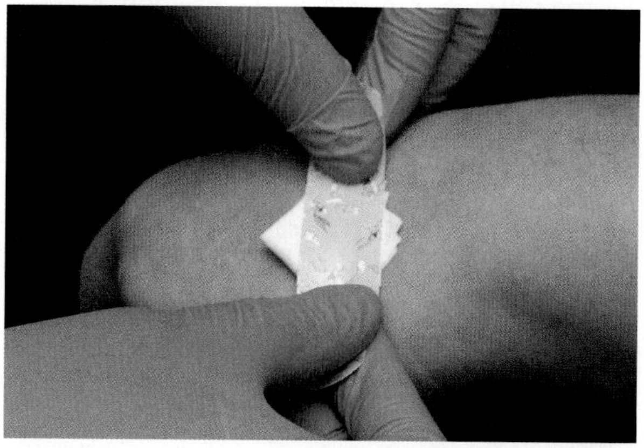

Fig. 9-35. *Secure the bandage over the gauze after bleeding has stopped.*

27. Observe the patient for any signs of dizziness or discomfort. Do not allow the patient to stand if she seems unsteady or says that she feels faint.

28. Thank the patient and tell her she may leave and will receive results from the ordering practitioner.

29. Remove gloves and wash your hands.

30. Document the procedure according to facility policy.

In addition to selecting appropriate equipment for pediatric patients, PBTs should alter their approach to these patients. Using age-appropriate vocabulary, getting down on the physical level of the child while still respecting his personal space, providing a distraction, and ensuring that he is kept still during the procedure can all help the procedure pass quickly and with minimal trauma. Some facilities may use devices that chill and/or vibrate above the puncture site. This has been shown to diminish the child's perception of pain during venipuncture. Facilities using these devices or other methods of pain management will train PBTs in their use.

Pediatric patients and patients who are hospitalized and undergoing frequent blood testing—especially those in intensive care units—are at increased risk for a condition called **iatrogenic anemia**. *Iatrogenic* means *medically caused*, and this form of anemia results from excessive removal of the patient's blood. No more than 2.5% of a patient's blood volume should be drawn in any single day, and no more than 5% in a 30-day period. PBTs should be aware of these concerns. It is beyond the scope of practice for phlebotomists to limit blood collection volumes. PBTs can help by performing their jobs carefully: not collecting more tubes than required, and avoiding the need to repeat a collection. They should also follow any orders regarding collection tube volume. Some facilities use smaller-volume tubes for patients who are at risk of developing iatrogenic anemia.

Routine venipuncture technique applies to patients who are obese, but vein location can be challenging. Allowing the arm to dangle, applying a warm pack, and asking the patient for site guidance based on previous successful procedures can all aid in locating an acceptable site. A blood pressure cuff inflated to a point just below the patient's diastolic blood pressure (the second, smaller number) is generally more effective as a tourniquet. Veins in patients who are obese are located deeper beneath the skin, but the phlebotomist must still insert the needle at an angle of 30 degrees or lower, so a longer needle is helpful. Veins should be anchored firmly (but not painfully) before the needle is inserted. A phlebotomist should not make more than two attempts to access a vein before seeking assistance.

Cognitive impairment and *mental health disorders* are different terms that can cover a wide variety of conditions and symptoms. Both can cause a patient to behave unpredictably in some situations. Phlebotomists should keep supplies out of reach of these patients during the blood draw. It may be best to have help from another staff member or to ask for guidance from the patient's physician. Having a family member or caregiver there may be calming for the patient. The phlebotomist should be prepared to release the tourniquet and remove the needle quickly if a patient becomes combative.

Patients who suffer seizures will usually know of their condition and can alert phlebotomists to the possibility of a seizure. If a seizure occurs during a blood draw, the tourniquet should be released and the needle removed, sheathed, and discarded immediately. A PBT should never place anything in the mouth of a patient experiencing a seizure. The priorities are keeping the patient safe from head injury and protecting both the patient and the PBT from accidental needlesticks.

Feeling faint or losing consciousness (the medical term for this is *syncope*) during a blood draw is a relatively common reaction. It can happen with little or no warning. Many patients who are prone to syncope know that it is a risk and can inform the phlebotomist. In these cases, the draw should take place with the patient in a reclining or supine position. If syncope occurs with the patient already lying down, the tourniquet can be released and the needle removed with little risk of harm to the patient or the phlebotomy technician. If a patient faints unexpectedly, the PBT should first release the tourniquet and remove, sheath, and discard the needle. The next priority is to keep the patient safe from falling and, particularly, from head injury. Facilities should have a staff member who is trained to respond to situations like seizures or fainting.

After the patient is no longer in immediate danger, the PBT can call this person to assist.

If a patient indicates before a blood draw that she is feeling faint, a cool washcloth can be applied to the forehead or neck (Fig. 9-36). The patient should be allowed to rest, and juice or snacks can be offered (if the patient is not fasting). After the patient has rested, the blood draw should be performed with the patient in a reclined or supine position.

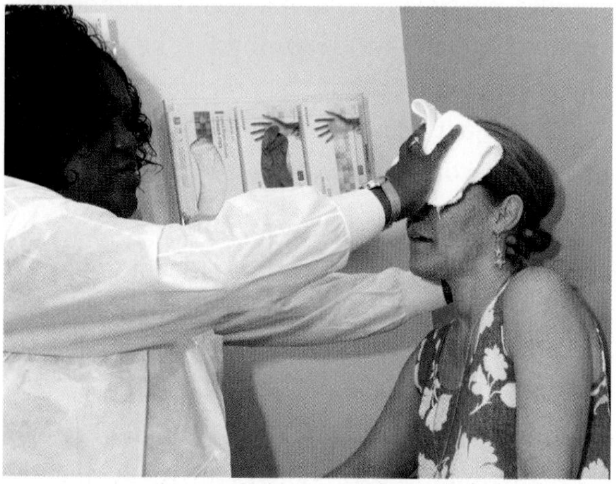

Fig. 9-36. *A cool washcloth can help ease discomfort when a patient is feeling faint or lightheaded.*

Patients' Rights

Phobias are real

A significant number of people, children and adults alike, have **phobias**, or strong fears, about needles and/or blood. Although phobias are often described as *illogical* or *irrational*, the fears are very real for the people who experience them. Telling a phobic patient that there is nothing to be afraid of will not help the patient overcome his fear and is not consistent with respecting patients' rights. PBTs can support phobic patients by treating them with dignity. When a patient verbally or nonverbally communicates a fear of needles or blood, a PBT should acknowledge the fear and not dismiss it. The phlebotomist can suggest that the patient look away during preparation of the equipment and during the procedure, but should still inform the patient prior to inserting the needle. The PBT should never try to "trick" a patient, performing venipuncture when it is not expected. This can increase, rather than remove, anxiety and fear.

There are some situations in which site selection must be modified due to patient conditions. Patients who have had a mastectomy should never have blood drawn on the mastectomy side without a doctor's written permission. This rule applies no matter how long ago the operation took place. In many mastectomies some or all of the lymph nodes are removed, putting the patient at greater risk for a condition called **lymphedema** if blood flow is constricted (as with a tourniquet or blood pressure cuff). In the case of a bilateral (double) mastectomy, blood should never be drawn from either arm or hand without written permission from the patient's physician.

Patients who are receiving medications or other fluids intravenously require special consideration of venipuncture sites. Venipuncture should not be performed in an arm with an IV. This risks contamination of the specimen with the IV fluids. If a specimen must be collected from an arm with an IV (for example, the right arm is in a cast and the left has an IV), the phlebotomist should request that the nurse stop the IV for two minutes. He should then draw the specimen from a location *below* the IV, meaning a location farther from the heart than the point at which the IV needle is inserted. In medical terminology, blood is drawn from a site *distal* to the IV. The PBT should also document that the specimen was taken from an arm with an IV.

Patients who have suffered a stroke or have diminished sensation on one side of the body should not have blood drawn on the affected side. During the venipuncture procedure, a PBT relies on the patient to communicate sensations like shooting pain or tingling that would indicate a nerve has been hit. If a patient has lost sensation in both sides (e.g., a patient who is quadriplegic, or paralyzed from the neck down), extreme care must be taken in drawing blood. The PBT should follow the CLSI standard precisely to minimize risk to the patient.

An **arteriovenous (AV) fistula** is a connection between a vein and an artery. It may be a naturally occurring defect or it may be surgically created in patients receiving dialysis, a treatment for kidney failure. A **graft** is a place where a person's vein has been redirected to a surgically implanted vein. Arms with fistulas or grafts should not be used for venipuncture.

PBTs must also avoid sites with the following conditions:

- Burns
- Bruising
- Scarring
- Hematoma
- **Phlebitis** (inflamed superficial veins) or thrombosis
- Swelling (edema)
- Recent tattoos
- Open wounds
- Skin infections

Phlebotomy technicians should be aware that some patients may develop a rash-like condition known as **petechiae** after a tourniquet is applied. These small, flat red or purple dots are created by the leaking of blood from capillaries. Petechiae may be associated with a number of different health conditions. Their appearance is not a cause for discontinuing tourniquet use or stopping venipuncture. It is important, though, that the PBT watch carefully after the procedure is finished to ensure that bleeding has stopped completely before dismissing the patient. Patients prone to petechiae may also be prone to prolonged bleeding.

9. Identify guidelines for ensuring specimen integrity

The primary responsibility of a phlebotomist is to obtain a high-quality specimen while treating the patient with courtesy, dignity, and respect. Following procedures carefully and making adaptations based on patient needs will help ensure that these goals are achieved. Most problems with blood testing are caused by preanalytical errors. The following are common errors and ways to avoid them and preserve the **integrity**, or high quality and reliability, of specimens.

Guidelines: Venipuncture Specimen Integrity

G **Identification errors**. Always strictly follow facility policy regarding patient and specimen identification. Never label and initial a tube before collection, as this creates the possibility that the tube will be accidentally used for the wrong patient. Always label and initial tubes after a blood draw and in front of the patient. Confirm with the patient that the information on the label is accurate and then initial it, adding the time and date of collection.

G **Additive-related errors**. Always check and double-check that correct, unexpired tubes are gathered before accessing the patient's vein. Always insert collection tubes according to the proper order of draw. Never remove stoppers and share specimens between tubes, even if the tubes have the same additive. If a tube was forgotten, call the patient back rather than using blood collected in the incorrect tube. Follow manufacturer guidance regarding the number of inversions required for each tube. Failure to follow these directions can result in **microclotting** and make testing less accurate.

G **Hemoconcentration**. Remove the tourniquet after site selection, and then again as soon as blood starts to flow. If a tourniquet is left on the arm for longer than a minute prior to venipuncture, release it and do not reapply it until at least two minutes have passed. Hemoconcentration can also occur if a patient has just sat up straight from a supine position (as may occur in an inpatient setting), or if a patient pumps his fist prior to venipuncture. Patients may believe that fist-pumping is helpful, and in fact it may be encouraged when blood is collected for donation. For routine phlebotomy, however, the resulting hemoconcentration can cause inaccurate test results.

- **Hemolysis**. Red blood cells can be destroyed during the process of a blood draw, resulting in unusable specimens. Any action that places too much pressure on the cells can cause hemolysis. Do not use a needle with too small a gauge, pull too forcefully on a syringe plunger, or handle collection tubes roughly. Do not overtighten a tourniquet or leave it in place for longer than one minute. Mix additives by gently inverting tubes, not by shaking them. Use a safe syringe transfer device to transfer blood to tubes from a syringe. Never use the collection needle to transfer blood from a syringe to evacuated tubes. This is a hemolysis risk, a needlestick risk, and can contaminate the specimen.

- **Insufficient quantity**. The initials **QNS** stand for *quantity not sufficient* and commonly mark specimens that are rejected for testing. Fill collection tubes to the level indicated on the label. This ensures that there is enough blood for testing and that the relationship between the amount of blood and any tube additive is correct. If a tube stops filling partway through a draw, adjust the needle gently (forward or back only, never side to side) to see if flow can be reestablished. Try a different tube, as the vacuum may have been inadequate. Be careful with these techniques, as even gentle movement of the needle can cause hemolysis. If blood flow cannot be reestablished, a new puncture in the other arm may be required.

10. Describe special collections

Some common tests require adjustments or additions to routine venipuncture procedures. These include blood culture, glucose challenge and glucose tolerance tests, and blood alcohol tests.

Blood Culture

A blood culture is ordered when a patient may have a bacterial or fungal infection in her blood. This can occur when a smaller, localized infection spreads to the blood. It is especially dangerous for people whose immune systems are compromised. When a blood culture is ordered, blood is introduced, or *inoculated*, into two bottles prepared with a liquid (called a *broth*) designed to encourage the growth of any bacteria or fungi in the blood. One is called the **aerobic bottle** and the other is the **anaerobic bottle** (Fig. 9-37). Each bottle encourages the growth of a different type of infectious agent. Aerobic microorganisms require oxygen and anaerobic microorganisms do not. The bottles are left to develop for a set period of time, after which they are studied to see if infectious microorganisms are present.

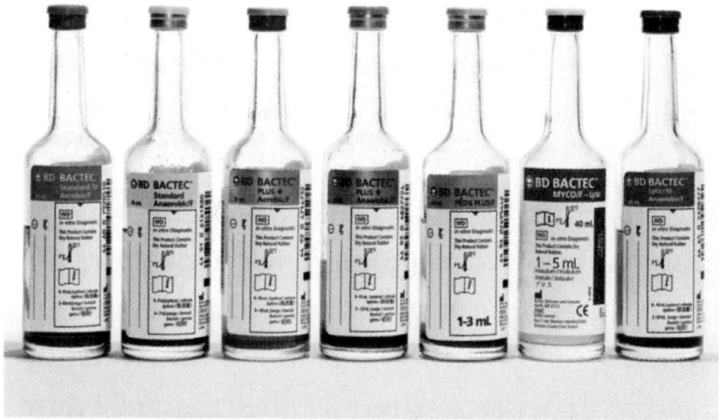

Fig. 9-37. *Aerobic and anaerobic bottles are inoculated with a patient's blood to determine the presence of infection. This photo shows several types of blood culture bottles from one manufacturer.* (COURTESY AND ©BECTON, DICKINSON AND COMPANY)

The following adjustments are made to routine venipuncture procedure when collecting specimens for a blood culture:

- A winged collection set is used in most cases. Using the butterfly set, with its flexible tubing, allows the bottle to be kept upright as it fills. This prevents the broth from entering the patient's blood. It also allows the PBT to see clearly when the bottle is completely filled.

- The site is cleaned more thoroughly. In many cases an initial cleaning with a 70% isopropyl alcohol pad is followed (after drying) by cleaning with a chlorhexidine gluconate swab. The second cleaning is generally timed and must last at least 30 seconds. Length of time will vary according to manufacturer instructions. The second antiseptic must also be allowed to dry fully before venipuncture is performed.
- Some blood culture bottles compatible with evacuated tube systems can be inserted in a holder just as any tube would be. Other systems require that blood be collected using a syringe and transfer device. Blood cultures may also be collected in tubes containing the anticoagulant additive sodium polyethanol sulfonate (SPS), and later transferred to culture bottles. PBTs should collect blood for culturing according to facility policy. Each transfer increases the risk of specimen contamination. PBTs should follow facility procedures and avoid transfers whenever possible.
- The rubber stoppers on both blood culture bottles must be cleaned, each with a new alcohol swab, and allowed to dry just prior to collection. If blood is collected in an SPS tube, the tube stopper must be cleaned and dried prior to collection.
- In most cases, the aerobic bottle should be filled first and the anaerobic bottle filled second. This avoids introducing air into the anaerobic bottle.
- Sometimes blood cultures are ordered to be collected at two different venipuncture sites, with both aerobic and anaerobic bottles filled from each site. This increases the chance of accurately detecting the presence of pathogens in the blood.
- Blood culture specimens are always drawn before any other tubes are filled, if additional tests are ordered.

Glucose Tests

There are several related tests used to determine how well a person's body is able to process glucose (sugar). These may be ordered during pregnancy to screen for gestational diabetes or when a diagnosis of diabetes is being considered.

Phlebotomists should know these details about glucose testing:

- Glucose deteriorates quickly after blood is collected (this is called glycolysis). Gray-topped tubes contain sodium fluoride to prevent glycolysis and are used in glucose testing.
- A **glucose challenge test** is routinely performed during every pregnancy. It does not require fasting. The patient drinks a very sweet liquid and blood is drawn an hour later to check glucose levels. If the levels are high, the patient will usually be scheduled for further testing.
- Glucose tolerance tests (GTTs) are longer than the challenge test and require that the patient fast for 8–12 hours prior.
- For all GTTs an initial specimen is drawn before the patient drinks the glucose beverage.
- The amount of glucose consumed may vary from 50 to 100 grams.
- Blood is drawn at varying intervals after the beverage has been consumed. The most typical intervals are hourly tests that take place after one and two hours or after one, two, and three hours. It is important to follow the draw schedule closely and to document the time at which each specimen is drawn.

Blood Alcohol Testing

Ethanol, sometimes abbreviated *EtOH*, is the intoxicating ingredient in alcoholic beverages. When a person is suspected of driving under the influence of alcohol, or if for any other reason a determination must be made of the amount of alcohol in a person's body, a blood test may be ordered. In many states, simply applying for a driver's license constitutes consent to blood alcohol testing if a police officer suspects that a driver is intoxicated.

In most ways venipuncture for blood alcohol testing is like any routine collection. Possible exceptions include the following:

- Depending on state law, a specimen might be drawn even over the objection of the patient if she is suspected of drunk driving.
- When drawing blood for a blood alcohol determination, many facilities use an antiseptic agent other than isopropyl alcohol to avoid any possible risk that the alcohol used for cleaning will cause inaccurate results. PBTs should use whatever agent they are directed to use.
- Because this test may be performed as part of a legal action, the specimen may require **chain of custody** documentation. This documentation notes the exact path a specimen takes from collection to analysis and it provides legal proof that the specimen has not been changed or tampered with.

Blood donation

There is a high need for donated blood. Donated blood may be transfused into patients who have certain illnesses, are undergoing surgery, or have lost blood due to trauma (serious injury). In many ways blood collection for donation is identical to venipuncture for diagnostic testing. PPE use, site selection, and venipuncture technique are all the same. A larger needle, usually 16- or 18-gauge, is used and the site is cleaned as for blood culture. The needle is part of a collection set that includes tubing and a bag treated with an anticoagulant additive. Potential donors must read educational materials, provide informed consent, complete a questionnaire about medical and social history, and have a brief medical examination. Blood pressure, temperature, weight, and hematocrit/hemoglobin levels are checked before donation takes place. Donated blood is tested for blood type and screened for bloodborne pathogens after collection. Donors are informed of any positive results. Some people have health conditions that require therapeutic phlebotomy, or the regular removal of blood. Collection for therapeutic phlebotomy is similar to blood donation, but there is no screening process involved.

11. Discuss the processing and transportation of blood specimens

Each work setting for phlebotomists has different procedures for specimen processing and transport. Depending on the workplace, a PBT may only collect, label, and package specimens for transportation. She may collect and label specimens and also perform any or all of these preanalytical steps:

- Spinning samples in a centrifuge (centrifugation) (Fig. 9-38)
- Using a **pipette**, or narrow tube with a suction bulb, to remove the liquid portion from the solid portion of the centrifuged specimen
- Dividing the specimen or the serum/plasma portion of the specimen into **aliquots**, or smaller amounts for testing

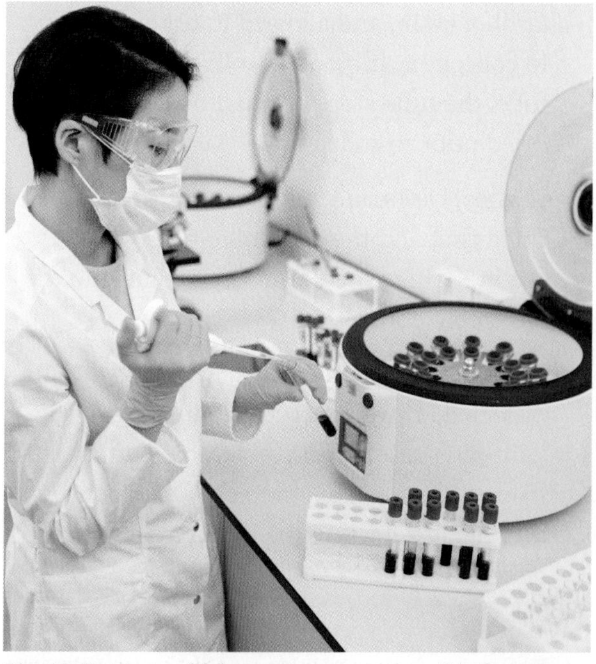

Fig. 9-38. *Many phlebotomists are responsible for centrifuging specimens before sending them for testing.*

If a PBT is expected to process specimens, he will be trained to do so. Centrifuges differ by type and manufacturer, but there are two main types of centrifuge: fixed angle and swing bucket. Tubes placed in a fixed angle centrifuge stay oriented at the same angle while spinning. Swing bucket centrifuges allow the tubes to swing into a horizontal (sideways) orientation as they spin. Specimens appear differently based on the type of centrifuge used. A fixed angle centrifuge will leave layers of cells, gel, and liquid at an angle inside the tube. A swing bucket centrifuge will leave layers straight across the tube. PBTs should follow these guidelines when centrifuging specimens:

Guidelines: Centrifuge Use

- **G** Wear appropriate PPE during centrifugation. This typically includes gloves, a face shield or goggles and mask, and a gown or lab coat. Sometimes centrifuges are located beneath a shield that offers face protection. Other facilities consider the centrifuge lid adequate protection against splashing or spraying and do not require face protection. Follow facility policy.
- **G** Centrifuge anticoagulated tubes immediately if time allows.
- **G** Allow serum tubes (with or without separator gel) to clot fully before they are centrifuged. Clotting usually takes 30–60 minutes. Keep the tubes upright during clotting.
- **G** Only operate the centrifuge with the lid closed and the load balanced. The tubes should be placed evenly within the centrifuge.
- **G** Specimens collected for whole blood testing are not centrifuged.
- **G** Do not centrifuge specimens more than once.
- **G** Do not remove tube stoppers before a specimen is centrifuged.
- **G** Follow manufacturer and facility instructions regarding centrifuge timing and speed. Specimens are usually centrifuged for 10–15 minutes. Different tube additives may require different centrifuge times.
- **G** Special care is required for specimens affected by temperature. Because the action of the centrifuge creates heat, centrifuges with cooling mechanisms may be necessary for some specimens. Follow facility procedures.
- **G** CLSI standards require centrifugation within two hours of specimen collection. Some specimens may need to be centrifuged within a shorter timeframe (e.g., coagulation tests for patients taking the anticoagulant heparin).

After centrifugation, the phlebotomy technician should check the separated specimen. If the tube contains a separator gel it should have produced a complete barrier between the liquid and cellular components. This is especially important to check when using a fixed angle centrifuge. The plasma or serum should be clear and straw-colored. The following alterations are signs of possible problems with the specimen and should be documented before the specimen is transported to the lab:

- Hemolysis will result in a liquid blood portion tinged pink or red. Mild cases of hemolysis may cause an orange tint. Hemolyzed specimens do not provide accurate results for many analytes.
- The liquid portion of a **lipemic** specimen will look cloudy or milky. The word *lipemic* is related to *lipid*, which is a scientific term for fats and related substances. Most frequently a lipemic specimen results when a patient has consumed meat, cheese, or other fatty foods before having blood drawn. Lipemia should be noted and documented, but if the test to be performed did not require fasting, a lipemic specimen is unlikely to cause problems.

- **Icteric** specimens have a liquid component with a deeper yellow color than the straw color of normal serum or plasma. This indicates a high level of bilirubin in the blood. The word *icteric* comes from the Latin term for jaundice. Icteric specimens relate to the health condition of the patient and are not within the control of the phlebotomy technician (Fig. 9-39).

Once a specimen without a separator gel is centrifuged, the liquid portion should be removed quickly to preserve its integrity. In tubes with a separator gel this is not as immediate a concern, and centrifuged gel tubes may be sent on for testing as they are. Each laboratory will have procedures for each test, and PBTs will be trained to process specimens according to these procedures. Removing serum or plasma, whether in its entirely or into smaller aliquots, requires special care.

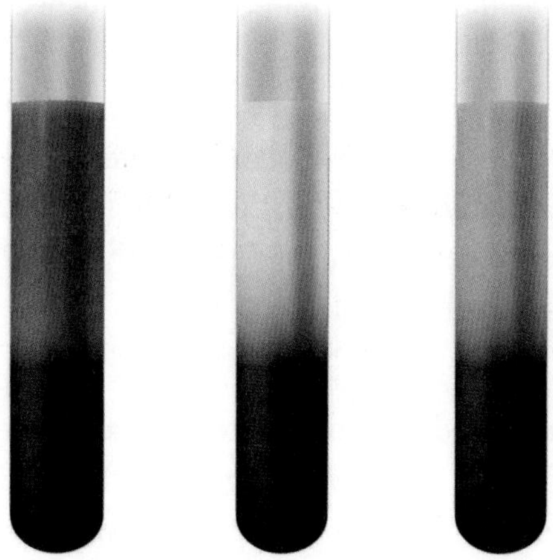

Fig. 9-39. *Hemolyzed, lipemic, and icteric specimens will not have the typical clear, straw-colored liquid layer.*

Guidelines: Separating Serum or Plasma

G Wear appropriate PPE during any specimen handling.

G Label the containers into which aliquots are moved with the patient's identifying information and the accession number associated with the blood draw.

G Take care in removing stoppers. Some types of stoppers are removed using opening tools. Others may be removed by hand, but should never be "popped off" with a thumb. This greatly increases the chance that the contents will be aerosolized or spilled.

G Use standard pipettes or serum filters designed to fit into collection tubes when removing liquid from tubes, according to facility policy. Serum filters are especially helpful when removing liquid from tubes without a separator gel. The filter has a straw-like attachment and is inserted into the tube to prevent the solid materials from contaminating the serum or plasma (Fig. 9-40). The liquid collects in the straw-like tube. Depending on the design of the tube, the liquid may be poured out while the filter is in place, or the filter may retain the liquid so it can be removed, labeled, and stored in the device until testing.

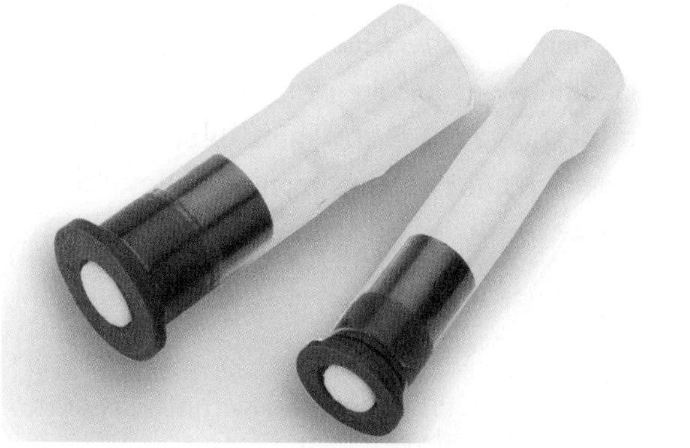

Fig. 9-40. *Serum filters simplify the process of separating the liquid portion of a centrifuged blood specimen.*
(PHOTO COURTESY OF MARKETLAB, INC., WWW.MARKETLAB.COM)

G When using a pipette, do not to touch the tip of the pipette to the solid matter below (buffy coat or separator gel).

G A new filter or pipette should be used for each collection tube.

G Always follow instructions for handling of serum or plasma.

At some point, whether immediately after collection or after processing, blood/serum/plasma specimens are transported from the phlebotomist to the laboratory where they will be tested. All specimens should be transported in biohazard containers that are clearly marked. Each facility will have its own procedures for transporting specimens. Here are some of the most common arrangements for specimen transport:

- The phlebotomist personally delivers specimens (processed or not) to the laboratory where technicians will perform testing.
- Specimens are placed in a box or other container and are collected by a courier or by laboratory personnel for testing.
- Specimens are sent through a **pneumatic tube system** or other automated system from the area where they are drawn to the testing area. Pneumatic tube systems may not be appropriate for all specimens. Facilities will train PBTs regarding the use of any automated systems.

As noted in Chapter 8, some analytes are sensitive to temperature and/or light and must be handled with special care. Bilirubin is an example of a light-sensitive analyte. Amber collection tubes may be used for tests of light-sensitive analytes, or tubes may be wrapped in aluminum foil. Special containers may be used for transportation of these specimens, but any container that blocks light is adequate.

While most analytes are stable at room temperature for at least a certain period after collection, some specimens must be kept cold or warm in order to produce accurate results. Facilities have equipment available to aid in maintaining correct specimen temperatures. This equipment may include **heating blocks**, or racks designed to hold tubes in an upright position while maintaining a specific temperature, cooling or warming packs to wrap around specimens, and refrigerators/freezers. The following guidelines are important to managing specimen temperature:

Guidelines: Handling Temperature-Sensitive Specimens

- G For specimens that must be kept at body temperature (98.6°F/37°C), collect the specimen in a prewarmed tube and then place it in a heating block (Fig. 9-41).

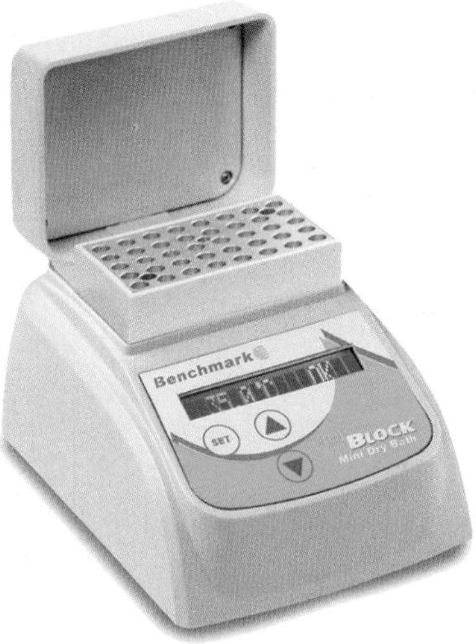

***Fig. 9-41.** Heating blocks can be set to maintain specimens at an exact temperature.* (PHOTO COURTESY OF BENCHMARK SCIENTIFIC, WWW.BENCHMARKSCIENTIFIC.COM)

- G When handling temperature-specific specimens, ensure that they remain at the target temperature until they are delivered for testing. Follow facility procedures. Some facilities use color-coded transport bags indicating the temperature required.
- G When a specimen must be kept cold, do not pack it with cubed ice. This will chill the tube unevenly. Store and transport chilled specimens in an **ice slurry**, which is a mixture of crushed ice and water, or in a specially designed cold pack.
- G If samples are to be frozen, do not place them in a frost-free freezer. The temperatures in frost-free freezers change frequently and the specimen may be partially thawed and refrozen. This can damage the specimen.
- G When temperature-sensitive specimens must be transported to a different facility for

testing, carefully follow facility procedures for packing and delivering or arranging for delivery. Because blood specimens are a biological hazard, there are very strict guidelines regarding their handling. Always follow facility policies carefully.

Quality Counts

PBTs should remember these common analytes that require light protection or maintenance at a specific temperature. This list is not complete, and it is always essential to check requisitions and employers' procedures for any special instructions.

Protect from light

- Bilirubin
- Many vitamins
- Carotene
- Folate

Keep cold (ice slurry)

- Ammonia
- Gastrin
- Lactate/lactic acid
- pH

Keep at body temperature (98.6°F/37°C)

- Cold agglutinins
- Cryoglobulin
- Cryofibrinogen

After processing and preparing specimens for transport, the phlebotomist can remove and discard PPE and wash his hands (or use a hand rub if his hands are not visibly soiled). Surfaces in the area where specimens were processed must also be disinfected. PBTs should follow facility policy for regular cleaning of equipment such as centrifuges and heating blocks.

Chapter Review

Multiple Choice

1. Which of the following information on the requisition form relates to an essential part of the phlebotomist's job?
   (A) The patient's insurance details
   (B) The patient's full name and date of birth
   (C) The reason the patient's doctor ordered the test
   (D) The symptoms the patient has been experiencing

2. A *test panel* is
   (A) The complete list of tests a laboratory can perform
   (B) A chart describing each test and the required tubes
   (C) The full list of tests ordered for a specific patient
   (D) A group of tests related to the same system or type of analyte

3. Which of the following is a common complication of extended tourniquet use?
   (A) Hemoglobin
   (B) Hemostasis
   (C) Hemophilia
   (D) Hemoconcentration

4. What is the scientific term for the inside of the elbow?
   (A) Antechamber
   (B) Anterior fossa
   (C) Cephalic fossa
   (D) Antecubital fossa

5. The basilic vein is the last choice among veins in the antecubital fossa because
   (A) It is not present in all patients
   (B) It carries less blood than other veins
   (C) It is located near nerves and an artery
   (D) It is very difficult to find

6. Patients who are allergic to shellfish may have a reaction to antiseptics containing
   (A) Isopropyl alcohol
   (B) Chlorhexidine gluconate
   (C) Iodine
   (D) Hydrogen peroxide
7. Which of these techniques is an acceptable way to make a patient's veins easier to see and palpate?
   (A) Lightly slap the antecubital area
   (B) Ask the patient to pump his fist
   (C) Leave the tourniquet in place for at least a minute before palpating
   (D) Direct the patient to dangle his arm downward for a few minutes before applying the tourniquet
8. Why should a needle not be inserted into a patient's vein at an angle greater than 30 degrees?
   (A) Because angles greater than 30 degrees do not result in adequate blood flow.
   (B) Because angles greater than 30 degrees pose a greater risk of striking an artery or nerve.
   (C) Because angles greater than 30 degrees will cause hemolysis.
   (D) Because angles greater than 30 degrees affect sensitive analytes like potassium.
9. Which of the following needle movements is acceptable if blood flow is not established after needle insertion?
   (A) Gentle forward and backward motion
   (B) Gentle circling motion
   (C) Slow side-to-side motion
   (D) Quick needle removal and repuncturing of the skin
10. This is the *only* situation in which a citrate tube does not have to be filled to the fill line:
    (A) When it is used as a discard tube
    (B) When it is drawn for testing on a pediatric patient
    (C) When it is drawn on a patient who is at risk for iatrogenic anemia
    (D) When there are more than five tubes required for testing
11. Which patient is most likely to require the use of a syringe and transfer device?
    (A) A healthy middle-aged adult
    (B) A teenager
    (C) An elderly person
    (D) A pregnant woman
12. A patient reports that she had a right-sided mastectomy ten years ago. She has an IV in her left arm. What will the phlebotomy technician probably need to do?
    (A) Draw from the right arm
    (B) Draw from the IV site
    (C) Ask the nurse to stop the IV and draw below the IV
    (D) Ask the nurse to stop the IV and draw above the IV
13. Which scenario is most likely to cause hemolysis?
    (A) The phlebotomist leaves a tourniquet on a patient's arm for 45 seconds prior to drawing blood.
    (B) A patient makes a fist while the PBT looks for a suitable vein.
    (C) While transferring a specimen from a syringe to a tube, the PBT speeds the process by pressing the syringe plunger.
    (D) The phlebotomist forgets to mix an EDTA tube after collection.

14. Blood cultures are commonly performed to detect the presence of ________________ infection in the patient's blood.
    (A) Bacterial or fungal
    (B) Viral or bacterial
    (C) Viral or fungal
    (D) Bloodborne pathogen
15. How long after collection should most blood specimens be centrifuged?
    (A) Within two hours
    (B) Within a 24-hour day
    (C) Within a workday
    (D) Within an hour
16. A patient who had bacon and eggs right before a blood draw is likely to have a serum specimen that is
    (A) Lipemic
    (B) Icteric
    (C) Hemoconcentrated
    (D) Hemolyzed

10 Collecting Blood Specimens by Capillary (Dermal) Puncture

Note: Information regarding requisitions/orders and specimen handling, processing, and transportation is included in Chapter 9 and not repeated in this chapter.

1. List the most common situations in which capillary puncture is required

Blood collection by capillary puncture is commonly performed for certain tests. It is also the best way to collect blood for some patients. Point-of-care tests are conducted using blood from capillary puncture. Monitoring glucose for patients with diabetes and blood clotting times for patients taking the anticoagulant drug warfarin are among the most common point-of-care tests. Hemoglobin/hematocrit can also be tested using a point-of-care device, as can hemoglobin A1c (HbA1c), another measure of health for patients with diabetes. Some facilities may have point-of-care devices for testing electrolytes, measuring blood gases, or performing a complete blood count on capillary specimens. The number of tests that can be performed in this way is growing.

The following patients may have blood collected by capillary puncture:

- Patients who are obese
- Patients whose arms are burned, heavily scarred, or otherwise not accessible (e.g., due to a body cast)
- Patients predisposed to blood clots in the veins (venous thrombosis)
- Patients whose veins must be used only for specialized treatments such as chemotherapy
- Patients whose veins are extremely fragile or damaged
- Patients whose veins are difficult to access

Not all tests performed on venipuncture specimens can be performed on the small volume of blood collected by capillary puncture. Erythrocyte sedimentation rate, which is a test that measures the time it takes for red blood cells to settle to the bottom of a container, requires more blood than can be collected by capillary puncture. So do coagulation studies. Some analytes are significantly different in capillary blood, which is a mixture of venous and arterial blood and tissue fluids. The type of specimen collected should always be documented clearly.

A capillary specimen is closer than a venous specimen to the nature of arterial blood, so blood gases are sometimes measured from a capillary specimen. Capillary blood may also be used to create a peripheral blood smear, sometimes simply called a *blood smear*. This is often ordered to follow up on abnormal results in a complete blood count. The blood smear allows for examination of the different blood cells under a microscope (more in Learning Objective 7).

Quality Counts

As noted in Chapter 9, the guideline for preventing iatrogenic anemia is to draw no more than 2.5% of a patient's blood volume in 24 hours and no more than 5% in 30 days. The blood volume of infants (in milliliters) can be estimated by multiplying weight (in kilograms) by 80. A kilogram equals 2.2 pounds. An eight-pound baby weighs just over 3.5 kilograms. Multiplying 3.5 by 80 gives a total blood volume of around 280 mL. This is only about 2/3 the volume of a typical beverage can. Taking 2.5% of 280 mL gives the maximum daily draw amount of 7 mL. The monthly draw limit would be 14 mL. Amounts higher than these could cause iatrogenic anemia and require blood transfusion. PBTs do not order blood draws, but they can be careful to reduce the need for redraws. They can also speak to a supervisor if multiple practitioners order draws on the same child. All of the orders may be necessary, but it is also possible that lack of communication caused duplicate orders.

Blood specimens for children under 1 year of age are typically collected by capillary puncture of the heel. Iatrogenic anemia is an important concern when drawing blood from small children. The small volume of blood required to complete a capillary puncture specimen is safer to remove than a larger venipuncture specimen. Newborns often experience **jaundice**, or an excess of bilirubin in the blood. This occurs because their livers are not yet mature enough to clear bilirubin effectively. Specimens for testing bilirubin levels in infants are collected by capillary puncture. Newborns also have a series of screening tests for possibly dangerous conditions that can be treated if they are detected early. The blood for these tests is accessed by capillary puncture and allowed to drip onto a special type of filter paper (more in Learning Objective 7).

2. Discuss the selection of an appropriate site for capillary puncture

In most cases capillary specimens are collected from the middle or ring finger of an adult's or child's nondominant hand, or from the side of an infant's heel. Capillary blood used to be collected from the earlobe or from the first toe (the "big toe"). The earlobe is no longer considered appropriate. The big toe is not a preferred site but is allowed if other sites cannot be used.

These points are important to consider when selecting a fingerstick site:

- The fingers on a person's dominant hand are more likely to be calloused. This makes puncturing the skin more difficult and potentially more painful.
- The index finger (also called the *second finger*) of either hand may be calloused, and this finger contains more nerve endings, which makes it more sensitive to pain.
- The bones of the smallest finger (the *pinky finger* or *fifth finger*) are closer to the skin than the bones of the other fingers. This makes it a poor choice for capillary collection.
- There is a pulse point in the thumb (considered the *first finger*). The risk of excessive bleeding eliminates the thumb as a collection site.
- If a patient is undergoing frequent testing by capillary puncture, the selected finger/site should be rotated. The same site should not be used twice in a row.
- A finger stick may only be performed on an infant over 6 months of age weighing 10 kilograms (22 pounds) or more. Heel stick is required for younger infants and infants who weigh less.

Once a finger is selected, the best area for performing the puncture is the fleshy part near the tip, toward either side of the finger, but not completely on the side (Fig. 10-1). The medical term for this site is the *palmar surface* of the distal segment of the finger. The very tip should be avoided. The bone is closer to the surface here, which poses a greater chance of injury. A fingertip puncture may also be more painful and more likely to reopen and bleed after the procedure is complete.

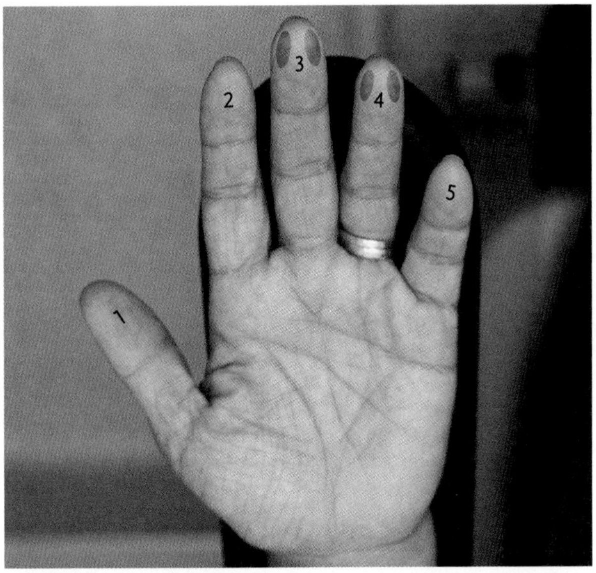

Fig. 10-1. *The third and fourth fingers of the nondominant hand are best for capillary puncture. The best sites are near the fingertip on the palm side of the hand, toward one side or the other.*

The following situations may cause difficulties with a capillary puncture site:

- Cyanotic—blue- or gray-tinged—fingernail beds indicate poor circulation. Poor circulation makes capillary collection difficult or impossible.
- Patients with **edema**, or swelling, of the hands are not good candidates for capillary puncture. Their capillary blood is likely to contain a high volume of fluid.
- Patients whose fingers are burned, injured, scarred, bruised, or covered with a rash are not good candidates for capillary puncture.
- Capillary puncture should not be performed on the same side as a mastectomy. Patients who have had a bilateral (double) mastectomy require written physician permission for either a capillary or venous draw on either side. This is true no matter how long ago the surgery took place.
- Dehydration makes any type of blood collection more difficult. It may not be possible to collect an adequate amount of capillary blood from a dehydrated patient.

If capillary collection is ordered for patients in these situations, the PBT should discuss alternatives with a supervisor or with the ordering practitioner.

When performing a heel stick to collect capillary blood from an infant, great care must be taken to avoid locations at which the bone is very close to the surface of the skin. Striking the heel bone, or **calcaneus**, with the lancet can cause a bone infection called **osteomyelitis**. The arch of the foot, the bottom surface of the heel, and the very back of the heel must be avoided. The sole of the foot is called the **plantar surface**. The *medial* (inside) and *lateral* (outside) plantar surfaces of the heel are allowable sites for infant heel stick (Fig. 10-2). The lateral plantar surface is that part of the heel roughly in line with the smallest toe. The medial plantar surface is roughly in line with the outer half of the big toe.

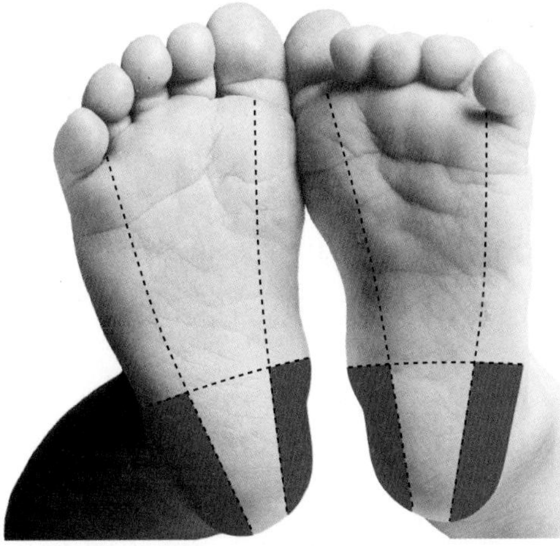

Fig. 10-2. *The sides of the bottom surface of the heel (shaded in this picture) are the sites where infants' heel bones are located deep enough beneath the skin to allow capillary puncture.*

3. Describe the proper cleaning of a capillary puncture site

Isopropyl alcohol pads are most commonly used to clean a site for capillary puncture. Some facilities may use a different antiseptic for newborn or premature infants, as isopropyl alcohol can sometimes irritate or damage very sensitive skin. Phlebotomists should follow facility policies. Povidone iodine is not used during the process of capillary puncture because it can interfere with some analytes.

Fingers are more likely to be visibly dirty or to harbor larger numbers of bacteria than venipuncture sites such as the antecubital fossa or the back of the hand. If a patient's hands are visibly dirty, the PBT can request that she wash her hands with soap and water prior to the procedure. The site must then be dried and cleaned thoroughly with the antiseptic of choice. The antiseptic agent must also be allowed to dry completely. Allowing the antiseptic to dry fully accomplishes several things. It is required for complete disinfecting action. It minimizes pain for the patient. It also reduces the risk of antiseptic entering the specimen and causing contamination. Infant heels must be allowed to dry thoroughly after cleaning with the facility-designated agent as well.

The key for complete, effective cleaning is to use friction, rubbing firmly but not painfully. Special care must be taken when cleaning infants' heels and the skin of pediatric and elderly patients.

4. Identify techniques for proper preparation and puncture of the skin

Warming a capillary puncture site prior to collecting blood can result in as much as seven times greater blood flow. Warming the site has other effects as well. It serves to **arterialize** the blood, meaning that the blood collected after warming will resemble arterial blood more closely than it would otherwise. This is especially important when collecting specimens for blood gas analysis.

Capillary puncture sites should be warmed before cleaning, either by holding a warm, damp cloth to the site or by using a commercially prepared warming pack (Fig. 10-3). When warming the site, the PBT should not use a cloth that is warmer than 105°F. This temperature is warm but not hot to the touch. Higher temperatures can damage a patient's skin. Instructions on commercial heating packs will describe how to activate the pack and how long it should be applied. Typically capillary puncture sites are warmed for 3–5 minutes.

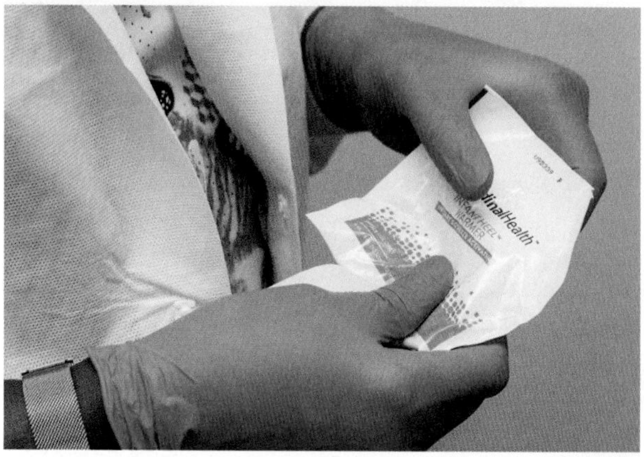

Fig. 10-3. *Warming the site before capillary puncture will make it easier to collect the required amount of blood.*

A wide variety of single-use, retractable lancets is available. Each is suited to a particular patient or test requirement. Some lancets puncture the skin with a needle-like spike (Fig. 10-4). These are available in different gauges and create different-sized punctures. Larger punctures are more appropriate for collecting higher volumes of blood. For example, a lancet with a 30-gauge needle may be used when a single drop of blood is needed. A 21-gauge lancet may be used for filling a small microcollection tube. The most commonly used lancet for collecting larger capillary specimens is one with a small retractable blade. The blade measures between 1.5 and 2.5 mm across. This device makes a tiny incision in the patient's skin rather than a puncture.

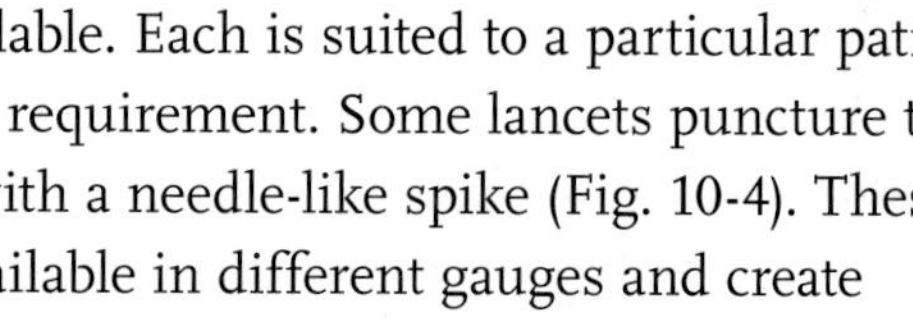

Fig. 10-4. *This photo shows the inside of a needle lancet. The needle is spring-loaded so it can puncture the skin and then retract, reducing the risk of accidental needlesticks.* (PHOTO COURTESY OF GREINER BIO-ONE, WWW.GBO.COM)

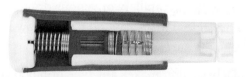

The depth to which a lancet punctures is an important consideration. Lancet depth for infant heel stick cannot be greater than 2.0 mm; 1.5 mm for infant finger stick. Manufacturers of lancets typically have a product line especially for use in infant heelstick procedures. These are usually blade-style lancets that puncture at a depth of 0.85 mm for premature infants or 1.0 mm for full-term infants. As a general guideline, the phlebotomist should use the smallest lancet that will successfully draw the amount of blood needed. It is not necessary to use a high-flow lancet to collect one drop of blood. Conversely, using a narrow-gauge needle lancet when 500 µL of blood must be collected will result in an unsuccessful procedure. Choosing the right lancet for the draw will reduce pain for the patient and increase the chances of a high-quality draw.

When puncturing the patient's skin, the angle at which a blade-style lancet is placed can affect the success of the collection. Fingerprints can create channels for blood to run into, making it more complicated to get the blood to flow and drip into the collection device. This is less likely to happen if the lancet is placed perpendicular to (across, rather than in line with) the fingerprint lines (Fig. 10-5).

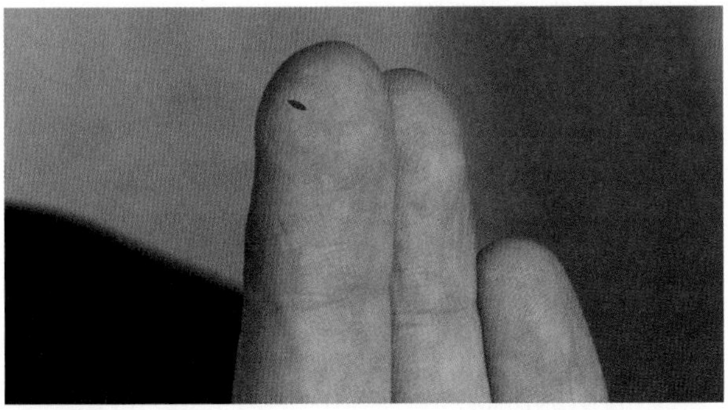

***Fig. 10-5.** Cutting across, rather than along, fingerprint lines will make capillary collection easier and more efficient.*

Similarly, using the lancet at a 90-degree angle to the length of the baby's foot will allow the phlebotomist to squeeze the heel gently and open the incision slightly to increase blood flow.

Lancets are designed either to activate automatically when they are pressed to the patient's skin or to activate at the press of a button. When using the button-activated style, a PBT should not press the lancet too forcefully into the patient's skin. This can result in an incision that is deeper than intended.

Prior to activating a lancet for a capillary collection, the PBT should have all equipment assembled and within easy reach. Capillary collections must be completed quickly and efficiently. The longer the procedure takes, the greater the likelihood the specimen will begin to clump due to platelet accumulation or the blood flow will stop altogether. Squeezing the puncture site excessively to keep blood flowing can hemolyze the specimen and cause discomfort for the patient. The best solution is to use an appropriate lancet and to be prepared to collect the blood right away.

After cleaning the puncture site and preparing the lancet, the PBT should have these items close by:

- **Gauze.** In most cases the first drop of blood from a capillary puncture is wiped away before collection begins. This serves two purposes. First, it reduces dilution of the specimen with tissue fluid, which is concentrated more heavily in the first drop of blood. Second, it disturbs the clotting process and promotes blood flow. For point-of-care tests this step may not be required. PBTs should follow manufacturer instructions and facility protocol.
- **Collection device.** This may include microcollection tubes with or without an additive, thin plastic capillary tubes (heparinized or untreated), or filter paper for newborn screening. Light-blocking amber microcollection tubes are often used for bilirubin tests on infants. When conducting point-of-care tests, the collection device may be a test strip inserted into a machine. It may be

helpful to have extra tubes or strips ready in case a puncture must be repeated.

- **Appropriate seal for tubes.** Microcollection tubes may have lids that screw or snap on. Capillary tubes are usually sealed with caps or with clay. Tubes with additives need to be capped and mixed immediately after collection, according to manufacturer instructions.
- **Bandage appropriate to the patient.** An adhesive bandage is usually placed over a capillary puncture site in children and adults. If the patient is sensitive to latex, a nonlatex bandage must be used. Adhesive bandages pose a choking hazard for infants and toddlers. They should not be used on children under 2 years of age. PBTs should follow facility policy for bandaging puncture sites for these patients.
- **Specimen labels and pen.** Microcollection tubes often have hollow extensions that allow for a full-sized specimen label to be affixed to them (Fig. 10-6). Others may require smaller labels. The specimen must be labeled in front of the patient, and the patient must confirm that he is identified correctly on the label. Follow facility guidance regarding patient identification when completing newborn screening. The filter paper may have identification fields to be filled out by hand, the form may be preprinted with the child's information, or a label may be placed on the paper.

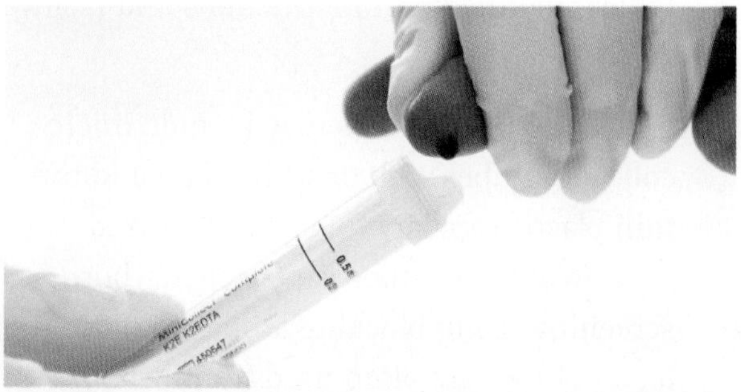

Fig. 10-6. The smaller blood collection chamber of this collection tube is nested inside a larger tube that allows for an easier grip and will accommodate a full-sized specimen label. (PHOTO COURTESY OF GREINER BIO-ONE, WWW.GBO.COM)

5. Describe procedures for routine capillary puncture in the finger and the heel

The fingerstick procedure for capillary blood collection is performed on children over 1 year of age and on adults of all ages. The PBT should follow these guidelines:

Guidelines: Fingerstick Collections

- **G** Always review the test requisition carefully. Capillary puncture should only be used when it is ordered and not as a replacement for venipuncture. Check with the ordering physician if venipuncture is ordered but capillary puncture seems better suited to the patient. Contact a supervisor or the ordering physician with any questions.
- **G** Select a lancet according to the size and age of the patient and the amount of blood required for testing. Puncture/incision depth varies by manufacturer. Facility policy may also vary, but a 1.0 mm lancet is often used for children under 3, 1.5 mm for school-aged children, and 1.8 mm or 2.0 mm for adults. Also consider the needle gauge or incision width. These factors affect the amount of blood that can be acquired from a single puncture.
- **G** Confirm that the patient has met any fasting, medication timing, or other pretest requirements.
- **G** Ensure there is no food or gum in the patient's mouth.
- **G** Check equipment carefully for defects and, as applicable, for expiration dates. Discard expired or faulty equipment.
- **G** Follow the order of draw for capillary collections. EDTA microcollection tubes are filled first, followed by tubes with other additives, and finally tubes without additives. (Learning Objective 7 describes special collections that

may be performed before filling standard tubes.)

- G Always select a new finger if a second puncture is necessary. Take any questions about the volume of blood required to a supervisor.
- G Position the patient with her arm supported and slanting slightly downward. The chair must have safety features to protect a patient who faints or falls. Patients who have experienced syncope or felt faint during previous blood draws should be reclined or supine.
- G If the patient is a young child, request that the parent or guardian hold the child during the procedure (Fig. 10-7). This will comfort the child and also help ensure that she is still while the collection takes place.

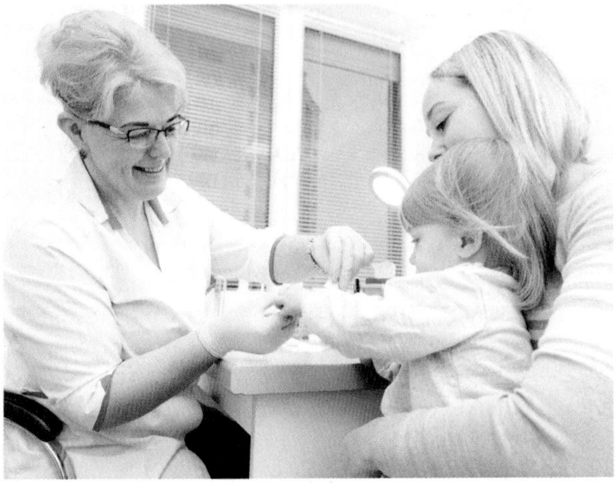

Fig. 10-7. *Pediatric collections are usually easier when the child is sitting in the lap of a parent or trusted adult.*

Performing routine capillary puncture by finger stick

Equipment: Test requisition (paper or electronic); soap and water or alcohol-based hand sanitizer; gloves (additional PPE if required based on patient condition); 70% isopropyl alcohol pad; retractable, single-use lancet appropriate to the patient and specimen requirements; collection device(s) required for ordered test(s); specimen labels; 2 pieces of 2"x2" gauze; adhesive bandage; pen

1. Greet the patient. Identify yourself by name and title.
2. Identify the patient using two unique identifiers. Usually this means asking the patient to state and spell her first and last names and state her full date of birth. Check the information provided against the requisition form and against the patient's wristband if wristbands are used at your facility (Fig. 10-8).

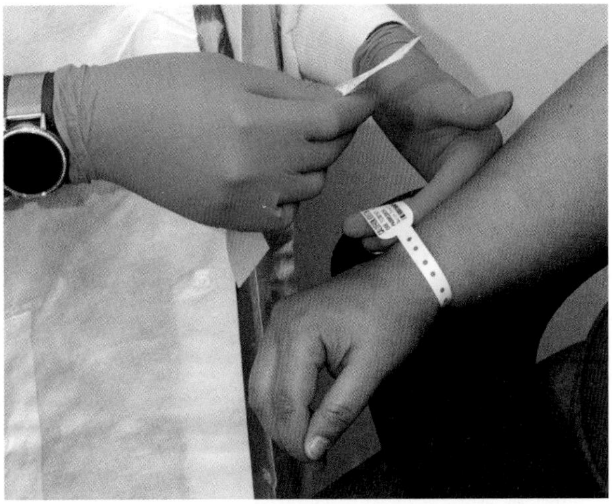

Fig. 10-8. *Confirming the patient's identification is an essential part of all blood collection procedures.*

3. Explain the procedure to the patient. Allow the patient to ask questions, but refer questions regarding the purpose or interpretation of tests to her doctor. *If at any point the patient expresses that she does not consent to the procedure, do not continue until consent is given. If consent is not given, document the refusal according to facility policy and allow the patient to leave. Notify the ordering practitioner of the patient's refusal.*
4. Gather required equipment.
5. Wash (or sanitize) your hands. Don gloves and other PPE as required. (In the case of some Transmission-Based Precautions this will already have occurred outside the patient's room.)
6. Ask the patient to extend her hands, palms up, for a visual inspection. Choose a puncture site free of bruising, rashes, broken skin (including recent capillary puncture), swelling, and cyanosis.

7. Warm the site for up to 5 minutes using a warm, damp cloth or a commercial warming pack to improve blood flow, following facility policy. Asking the patient to wash her hands in warm water can also warm the finger.

8. Clean the selected puncture site thoroughly with the alcohol pad, creating gentle friction (Fig. 10-9). Allow the site to dry fully.

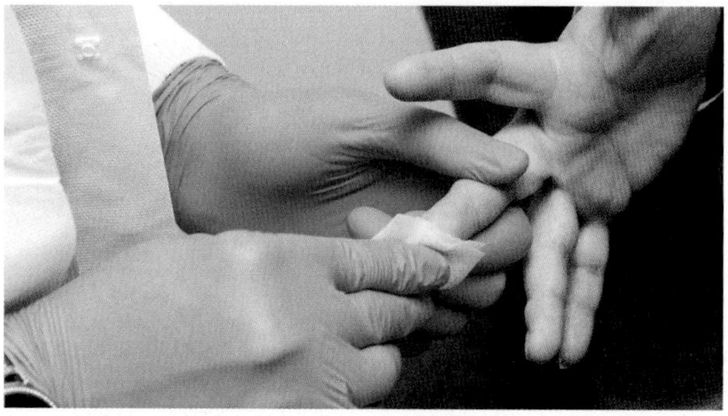

Fig. 10-9. *The puncture site should be cleaned carefully and allowed to air-dry completely without blowing on or wiping the site.*

9. Prepare the selected lancet and collection devices for use. Remove packaging or remove the safety device on the lancet (Fig. 10-10). Once the lancet is prepared, use it immediately or discard it. If the lancet is put down, it is considered to be contaminated.

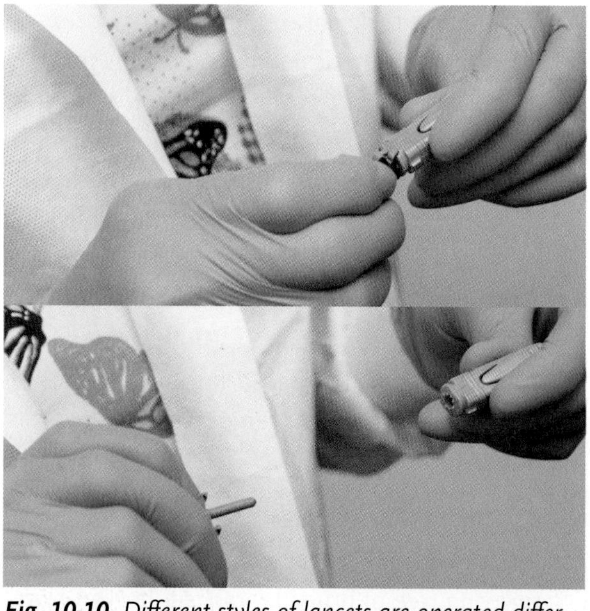

Fig. 10-10. *Different styles of lancets are operated differently. This lancet has a safety cap that must be removed before use.*

10. Inform the patient that she may experience brief pain when the lancet is engaged. Press the lancet gently against the patient's skin at the selected puncture site and activate the lancet to puncture the skin (Fig. 10-11).

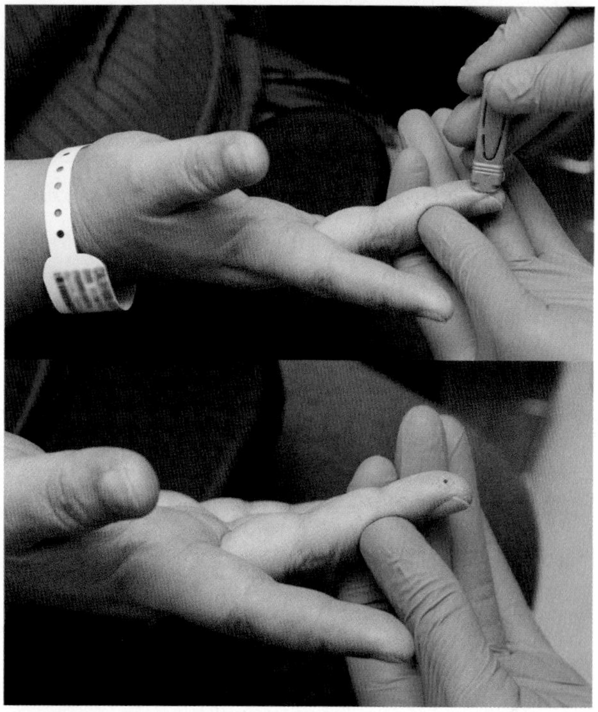

Fig. 10-11. *The retractable needle or blade of a lancet will create blood flow quickly and with minimal pain.*

11. Discard the used lancet in an appropriate sharps receptacle.

12. Use a gauze square to wipe away the first drop of blood if the ordered test does not indicate otherwise (Fig. 10-12).

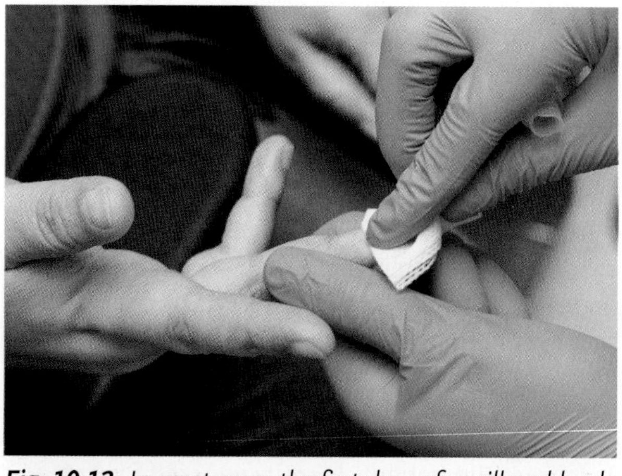

Fig. 10-12. *In most cases the first drop of capillary blood is wiped away before a specimen is collected.*

13. Collect the patient's blood in the required container(s). Apply gentle pressure. Do not squeeze or "milk" the finger. Gently apply and then release pressure to facilitate blood flow. Do not touch the spout or any part of the collection device to the patient's skin. Instead, allow the blood to drip into the tube and create a channel down the side of the collection tube (Fig. 10-13). Scraping the skin can cause hemolysis and can also prompt platelet activation. This can slow collection and compromise the specimen. Gently tapping the collection tube as the blood enters will help mix the specimen with the anticoagulant. It will ensure continued flow.

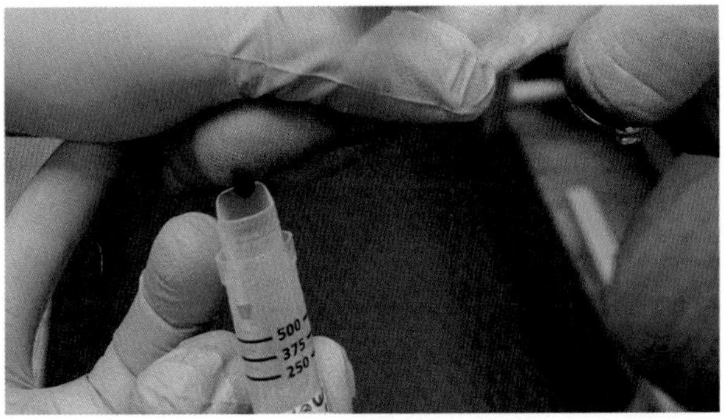

Fig. 10-13. *Allow blood to enter the collection container without scraping, scooping, or excessive squeezing of the finger.*

14. Continue to hold the patient's finger and the collection device in place until the container is filled to the appropriate level (Fig. 10-14). After filling, cap/seal the specimens appropriately, following manufacturer and facility instructions, and mix them promptly.

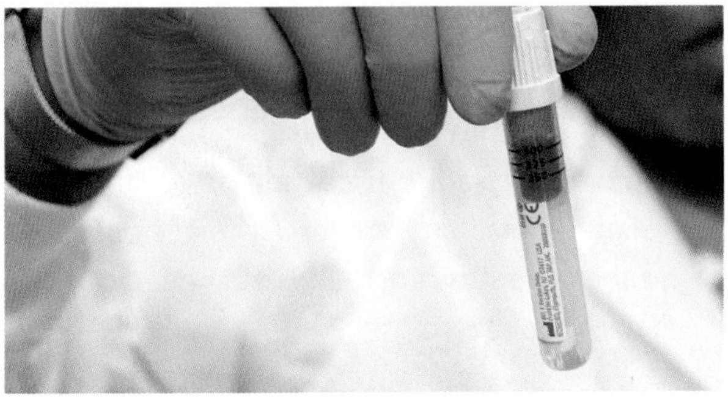

Fig. 10-14. *Fill containers to the proper level to ensure sufficient blood for testing and an appropriate balance of blood to additive.*

15. After all required containers are filled, place gauze over the puncture site and apply pressure. The patient can hold pressure if she is able.

16. Label the tube(s) in front of the patient, initialing and noting the time and date of collection. Ask the patient to confirm that the identifying information on the label is correct (Fig. 10-15). Place the specimens and the requisition or any required paperwork in the appropriate transport bag or container. Properly discard any waste.

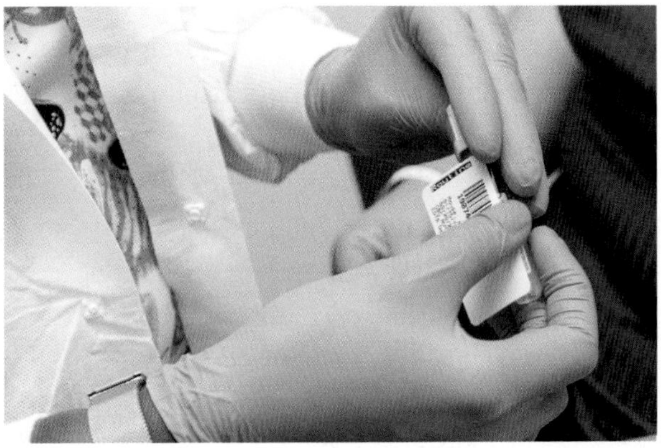

Fig. 10-15. *Always label specimens in front of the patient and confirm that the identification details are correct.*

17. Check to make sure that the patient is no longer bleeding. In the case of patients on anticoagulant medication, this can take as long as five minutes.

18. Place a bandage over the puncture site if the patient is over 2 years old (Fig. 10-16). Advise the patient to leave the bandage in place for the next 15 minutes.

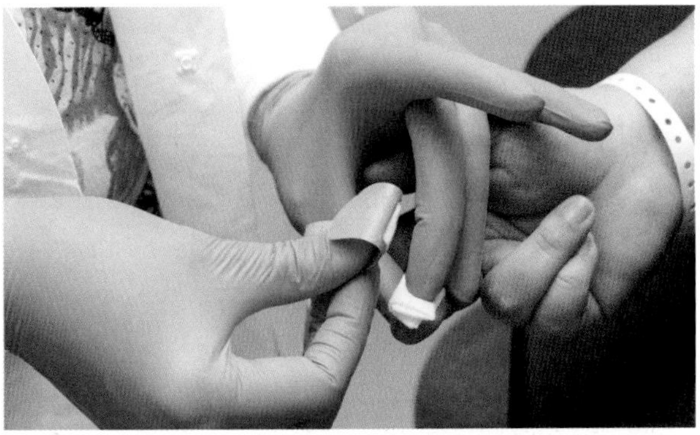

Fig. 10-16. *Apply a bandage after bleeding has stopped.*

19. Observe the patient for any signs of dizziness or discomfort. Do not allow the patient to stand if she seems unsteady or says that she feels faint.

20. Thank the patient and tell her she may leave and will receive results from the ordering practitioner.

21. Remove gloves and wash your hands.

22. Document the procedure according to facility policy.

Babies under 6 months of age and weighing less than 10 kilograms (22 pounds) do not have enough flesh on their fingers to protect against striking bone during a finger stick. Blood is collected from small infants using a heelstick procedure. In addition to certain screening tests (see Learning Objective 7), bilirubin tests are frequently ordered for newborns. If newborn screening tests indicate the need for any further investigation, other blood tests may be ordered. PBTs should remember these guidelines when collecting blood from an infant heel stick:

Guidelines: Heelstick Collections

G Many healthcare facilities have special PPE requirements for workers entering a nursery. Be aware of these requirements and follow them carefully. Newborns, particularly if they are premature or small at birth, may become much sicker from common illnesses than older children or adults.

G Most lancet manufacturers produce lancets meant for use in heelstick procedures. They are generally available in two varieties: one for premature infants and one for full-term infants. Follow any manufacturer or facility guidelines regarding use of these devices.

G Follow facility protocol regarding positioning of the baby during the procedure. Babies held and/or breastfed by their mothers during a heel stick may experience less pain. Swaddling and providing a sugar-treated pacifier may also reduce pain. Ideally, the infant's heel should be slightly lower than the body. Follow facility procedures.

G Infants have very sensitive skin and some antiseptics may cause irritation. Follow facility policy regarding antiseptic use.

G Although parents can be a comfort to the child, allow parents to exit the room if they are distressed by the procedure.

G Babies who are jaundiced may be placed under special lights to help clear bilirubin from their bodies (Fig. 10-17). When testing an infant for bilirubin, ensure that the specimen is protected from light at all times. Turn off treatment lights prior to the heel stick and use light-blocking or foil-wrapped collection devices.

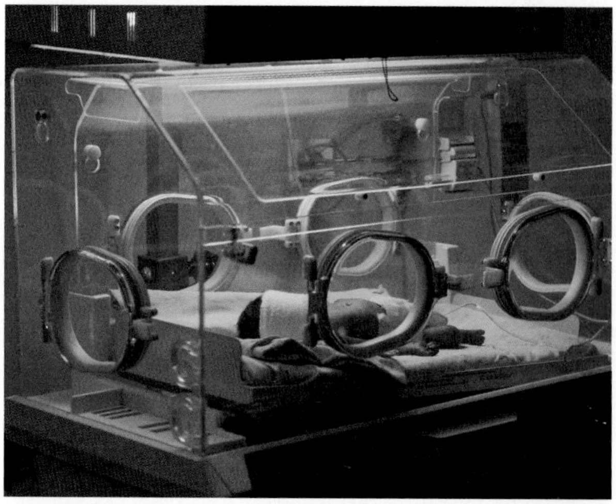

Fig. 10-17. *Newborns, and especially premature newborns, often experience jaundice. Light treatment can help these infants process bilirubin.*

G Do not place adhesive bandages on an infant. Babies often reflexively place objects in their mouths, and a loose bandage can be a choking hazard.

G See Learning Objective 7 for details on newborn metabolic screening (PKU).

Performing routine capillary puncture by heel stick

Equipment: Test requisition (paper or electronic); soap and water or alcohol-based hand sanitizer; gloves (additional PPE if required based on patient condition or facility protocols); 70% isopropyl alcohol pad or facility's preferred antiseptic; retractable, single-use heelstick lancet; collection device(s) required for ordered test(s); specimen labels; 2 pieces of 2"x2" gauze; rolled gauze or other facility-approved bandage (not adhesive); pen

1. Greet the patient's parent(s) or guardian(s). Identify yourself by name and title.
2. Identify the patient using two unique identifiers. Usually this means asking the patient's parent/guardian to state and spell the child's first and last names and state his full date of birth. Document the name and relationship of the person who identifies the patient. Check the information provided against the requisition form and against the patient's identification band if identification bands are used at your facility. Infant bands may be placed on the ankle rather than the wrist.
3. Explain the procedure to the parent/guardian. Allow the parent/guardian to ask questions, but refer questions regarding the purpose or interpretation of tests to the child's doctor. *If at any point the parent/guardian expresses that she does not consent to the procedure, do not continue until consent is given. If consent is not given, document the refusal according to facility policy and discontinue the procedure. Notify the ordering practitioner of the parent/guardian's refusal.*
4. Gather required equipment.
5. Wash (or sanitize) your hands. Don gloves and other PPE as required (this may have occurred outside the room/nursery, based on facility policies).
6. If facility policy allows and the parent wishes to hold the baby during the procedure, place the baby in the parent's arms (Fig. 10-18).

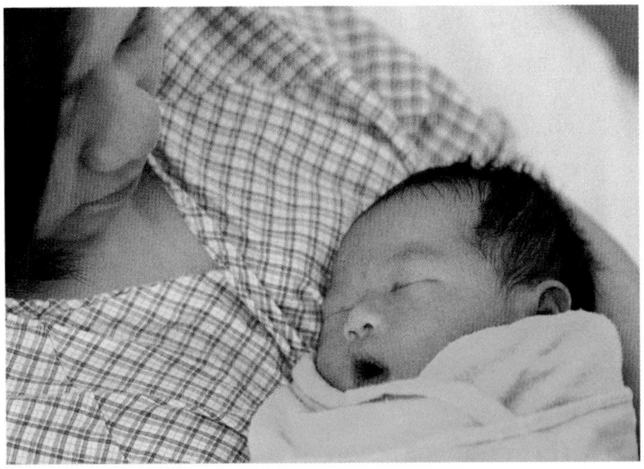

Fig. 10-18. *A baby may experience less pain from a heel stick if she is held by a parent.*

7. Warm the site for up to 5 minutes using a warm, damp cloth or a commercial warming pack to improve blood flow, following facility policy.
8. Clean the selected puncture site (medial or lateral plantar surface of either heel) thoroughly with the antiseptic pad, creating gentle friction. Allow the site to dry fully.
9. Prepare the lancet and collection devices for use. Remove packaging or remove the safety device on the lancet and remove the lid of the collection device.
10. Inform the parent/guardian that the infant may experience brief pain when the lancet is engaged. Press the lancet gently against the patient's skin at the selected puncture site and activate the lancet to puncture the skin (Fig. 10-19).

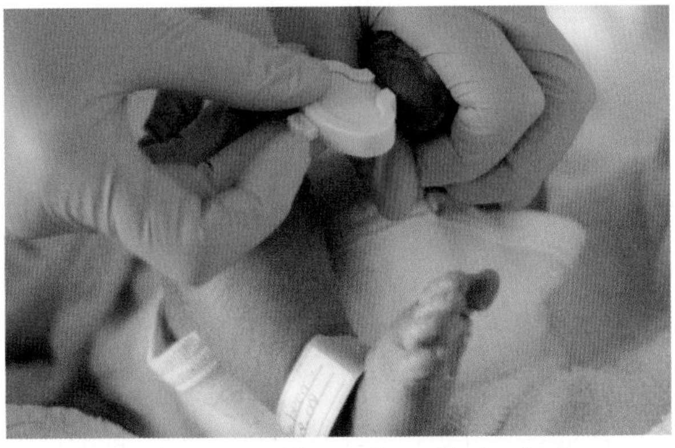

Fig. 10-19. *The retractable needle or blade of a lancet will create blood flow quickly and with minimal pain.*

11. Discard the used lancet in an appropriate sharps receptacle.

12. Use a gauze square to wipe away the first drop of blood if the ordered test does not indicate otherwise.

13. Collect the patient's blood in the required container(s). Alternately apply and release gentle pressure to the sides of the baby's heel (Fig. 10-20). Do not touch the spout or any part of the collection device to the infant's skin. Instead, allow the blood to drip into the tube and create a channel down the side of the collection tube. Scraping the skin can cause hemolysis and can also prompt platelet activation. This can slow collection and compromise the specimen. Gently tapping the collection tube as the blood enters will help mix the specimen with the anticoagulant and ensure continued flow.

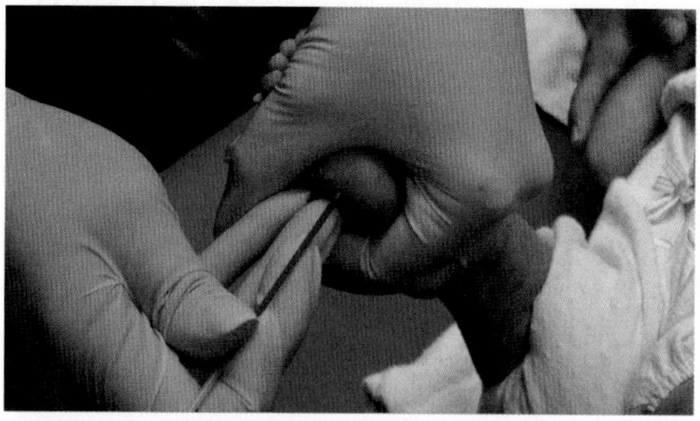

Fig. 10-20. *Fill the collection container without scraping it against the baby's skin.* (SAFE-T-FILL® CAPILLARY BLOOD GAS TUBES, RAM SCIENTIFIC, NASHVILLE, TN)

14. Continue to hold the baby's heel and the collection device in place until the container is filled to the appropriate level. After filling, cap/seal the specimens appropriately, following manufacturer and facility instructions, and mix them promptly.

15. After all required containers are filled, place gauze over the puncture site and apply pressure.

16. When the puncture site is no longer bleeding, bandage the heel according to facility policy (do not use adhesive bandages).

17. Label the tube(s) in front of the patient's parent(s) or guardian(s), initialing and noting the time and date of collection. Confirm that the identifying information on the label is correct. Place the specimens and the requisition or any required paperwork in the appropriate transport bag or container. Properly discard any waste.

18. Thank the patient's parent or guardian and tell her she will receive results from the ordering practitioner.

19. Remove gloves and wash your hands.

20. Document the procedure according to facility policy.

6. Identify guidelines for ensuring the integrity of capillary puncture specimens

Capillary puncture specimens can be affected by the technique used by the phlebotomist. Following procedures carefully will ensure the best quality specimens and the most accurate results for patients.

Guidelines: Capillary Puncture Specimen Integrity

- G Do not collect specimens from sites that are swollen (*edematous*). The blood will be diluted with excessive amounts of tissue fluid. This can cause inaccurate test results.
- G Do not collect specimens from patients with poor circulation to the extremities. This may be indicated by cyanosis, often seen as a blue tinge to the nail beds.
- G Avoid sites where bruising, rash, burns, calluses, or broken skin is present.
- G Warm the site for 3–5 minutes prior to puncture to improve blood flow. This can help reduce the chance of hemolysis, which can be caused by excessive squeezing of the finger/heel.

G Allow the antiseptic agent to dry completely before collecting blood.

G Work quickly but carefully once the puncture has been performed. As time goes by, platelets will gather and the quality of the specimen will decline.

G Do not scrape the collection device against the patient's skin, squeeze the finger/heel forcefully, or "milk" the finger/heel. A pattern of gently squeezing and releasing will produce the best flow.

G Always fill containers to the appropriate volumes. If a tube is not sufficiently filled before blood flow stops, a second puncture and a new collection tube may be required. Ask a supervisor for guidance.

G Carefully follow manufacturer instructions regarding specimen mixing.

7. Describe special capillary puncture collections

Some tests run on capillary blood require adjustments to routine procedures. These include capillary blood gas testing, newborn metabolic screening, and preparation of a peripheral blood smear.

Capillary Blood Gas Testing

Blood gas determinations are most commonly performed using arterial blood. Collecting arterial blood is beyond the scope of practice for phlebotomy technicians, and this procedure is usually performed by a respiratory therapist. Due to the risk involved in acquiring arterial blood from an infant, however, capillary blood is sometimes used for blood gas testing in babies.

When collecting a specimen for capillary blood gas testing, these adjustments are made:

- The specimen for blood gas testing is taken first. Any other specimens are collected according to the order of draw.
- The specimen is collected in a heparinized capillary tube and must be collected carefully so as not to create air bubbles.
- Every effort must be made to minimize contact between the blood and room air.
- Processing a capillary blood gas specimen may involve inserting a small piece of metal (called a *flea*) into the tube, capping it, and mixing the specimen by using a magnet to move the flea back and forth within the tube (Fig. 10-21).

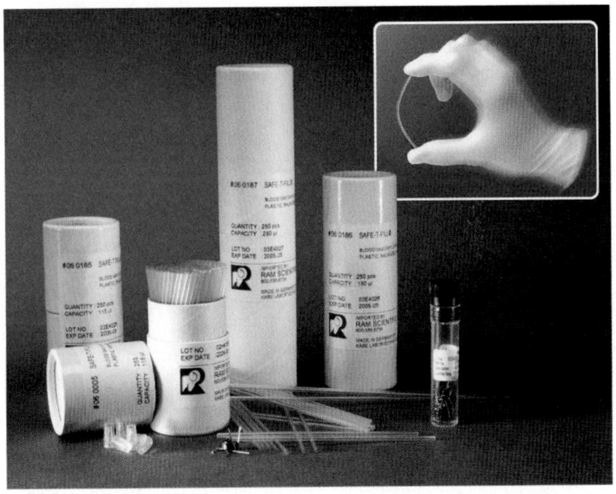

Fig. 10-21. *Capillary blood gas specimens are collected in heparinized tubes and then capped and mixed before testing.* (SAFE-T-FILL® CAPILLARY BLOOD GAS TUBES, RAM SCIENTIFIC, NASHVILLE, TN)

- After mixing, the tube must be delivered for testing right away.

Newborn Metabolic Screening

All US states either strongly encourage or require by law that newborn babies be tested early in life for certain illnesses. If detected early, these illnesses can be treated before serious damage is done to the child's health. All states test for **phenylketonuria**, or **PKU**, a rare condition that can cause brain damage if left untreated. Many other tests are performed at the same time. Because these conditions relate to the body's ability to generate or process hormones and enzymes, the screening is called *metabolic screening*, but it is often simply referred to as *PKU*. The capillary puncture procedure is performed as a heel stick as with any capillary collection in an infant, but the test differs in these ways:

- Rather than collecting blood in a capillary tube or microcollection device, the blood is dripped onto specialized filter paper. The paper is marked with circles for each blood drop required (Fig. 10-22).

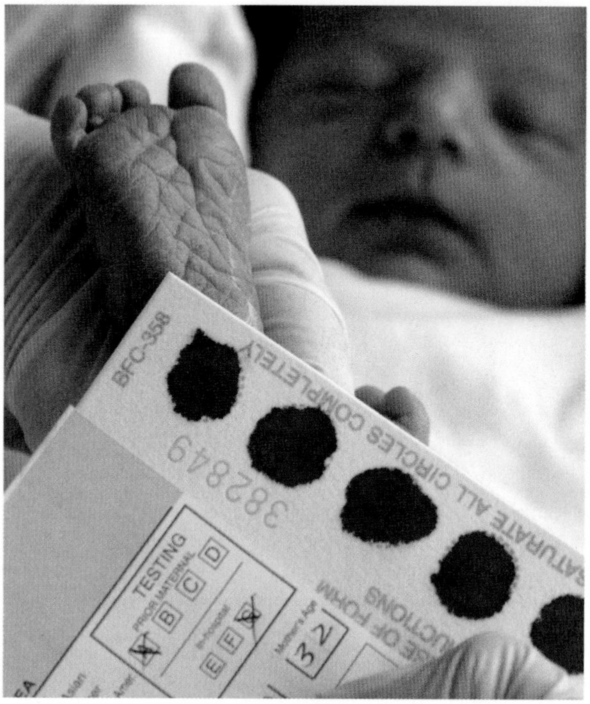

Fig. 10-22. *Newborn metabolic screening is conducted using blood collected on filter paper sheets.* (PHOTO COURTESY OF MARCH OF DIMES, MARCHOFDIMES.ORG, 571-257-2307)

- When collecting this specimen, the paper is not touched to the baby's foot. Instead, the blood is allowed to drip onto each circle.
- Each circle should be fully covered and soaked through, with the blood visible on both the front and back of the paper.
- The blood should only be dripped onto the front side of the filter paper.
- Only one drop should be placed in each circle.
- Filter paper collection forms vary, but all information must be either preprinted or completed by the technician before the form is sent for testing.

Blood Smear

When a complete blood count reveals possible problems with a patient's blood cells, a blood smear (sometimes called *peripheral blood smear* or *blood film*) may be ordered. Blood smears may also be used to detect bloodborne parasites or for other purposes. When blood is required for a smear, the following steps are taken:

- A blood smear is made on a microscope slide. A second clean, unused slide or a blood smear tool is also needed to spread the blood for the smear.
- The blood smear is created using a drop of blood. This blood may be from an EDTA tube or it may be allowed to drip directly onto the slide from a capillary puncture site.
- The blood drop should be placed about 1/3 of the way from the edge of the slide.
- The spreading slide or blood smear tool is placed at a 30-degree angle to the slide and pulled into the drop of blood (Fig. 10-23).

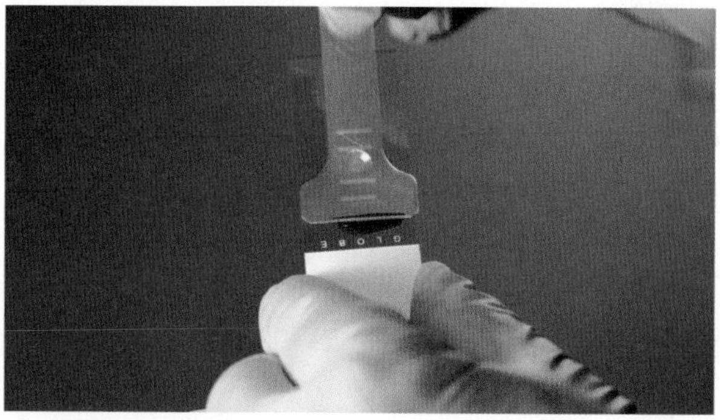

Fig. 10-23. *The spreading tool or second slide will collect blood along its edge.* (PHOTO COURTESY OF GLOBE SCIENTIFIC, INC., WWW.GLOBESCIENTIFIC.COM)

- Once blood has collected along the edge of the spreader or slide, it is pulled across the center of the slide (Fig. 10-24).
- The smear should have a "feathered" appearance at the edge.
- Blood smears must be allowed to dry fully. Further processing steps will vary based on facility procedures and the purpose of the test.

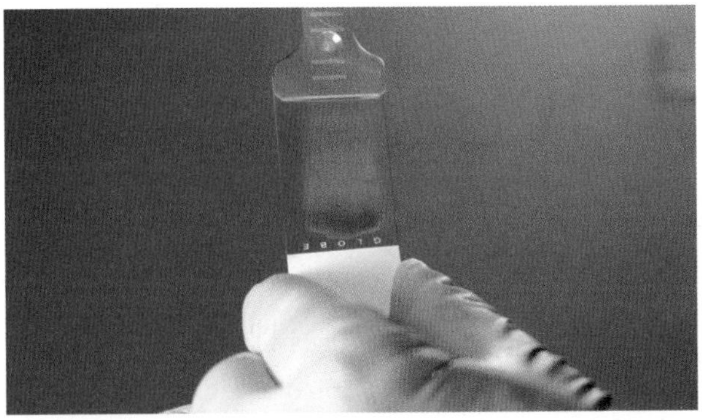

Fig. 10-24. The blood should be spread out across the slide. (PHOTO COURTESY OF GLOBE SCIENTIFIC, INC., WWW.GLOBESCIENTIFIC.COM)

- Procedures regarding labeling and transporting blood smear slides will vary by facility, and PBTs who are expected to perform peripheral blood smears will be trained in processing the finished slides.

8. Describe guidelines for performing point-of-care tests on capillary blood

Many people are most familiar with capillary puncture as a means of testing glucose levels. Patients with diabetes are often trained to use home glucose meters, which allow them to monitor their blood sugar levels without frequent trips to a doctor's office. These meters generally require a finger stick and are completed using a single drop of blood placed directly on a test strip that is inserted in the machine. Similar home-use machines exist for conducting **PT/INR** testing, or tests of a patient's *prothrombin time* and *international normalized ratio*. These are measurements of the time it takes for a person's blood to clot, and PT/INR is monitored closely in patients who take the anticoagulant medication warfarin.

Home-based point-of-care tests are convenient and useful for patients who must monitor ongoing health concerns. Professional models of these same point-of-care devices are also used in doctor's offices, hospitals, long-term care facilities, and other healthcare settings (Fig. 10-25). CLIA waived tests such as point-of-care glucose or PT/INR can be performed by any trained healthcare worker. They require only a small specimen—usually a single drop of blood—and can be performed quickly, usually with near-immediate results.

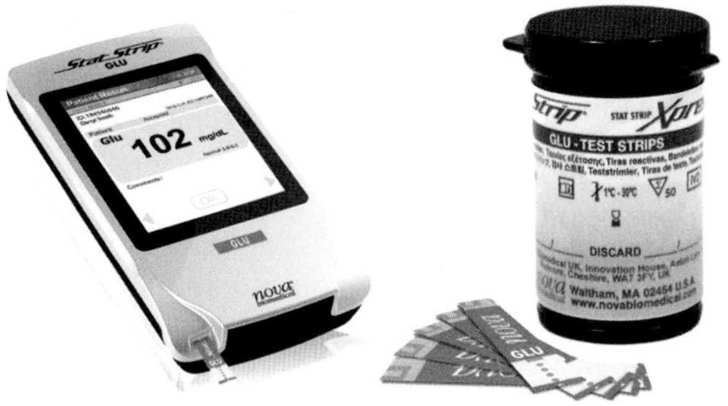

Fig. 10-25. Point-of-care tests make routine testing quicker and simpler for patients and healthcare workers. (PHOTOS COURTESY OF NOVA BIOMEDICAL, NOVABIOMEDICAL.COM, 781-894-0800)

Point-of-care blood tests may also include tests for HbA1c (also useful in the management of diabetes) or for hemoglobin/hematocrit, measurements related to a patient's red blood cell quantities. Hemoglobin/hematocrit tests are performed prior to blood donation to ensure that the donor does not have anemia.

All of the procedures listed in this chapter apply to capillary puncture for point-of-care testing as well, but the process of collecting the specimen may differ. In most cases, a test strip is placed into a testing machine and a single drop of blood is allowed to drip directly from the puncture site onto the test strip. Manufacturer instructions outline whether the first drop of blood can be used or whether, as with most capillary collections, it should be wiped away. Some point-of-care tests require that blood be collected in a small container or receptacle, which is then inserted into the machine for analysis.

Phlebotomy technicians who conduct point-of-care testing should be aware of these guidelines:

Guidelines: Point-of-Care Blood Tests

G Follow all facility procedures regarding patient identification and infection prevention.

- Do not perform a point-of-care test using a testing device you do not know how to operate. If you are asked to use a machine that is unfamiliar to you, ask a supervisor for training.
- Follow all manufacturer instructions regarding the use of point-of-care testing devices. This may include performing a quality control procedure before testing.
- Check expiration dates on test strips or any other supplies required for the testing device. Ensure that the strips have been stored properly. Out-of-date or damaged test strips can produce inaccurate results.
- Only touch test strips with clean gloves. Change gloves if a test is repeated or if a second strip is needed for any reason. Do not touch fresh strips with dirty gloves.
- Confirm that the patient has met any conditions regarding diet or medication.
- Document any changes the patient reports regarding medication or diet (e.g., if a patient being tested for PT/INR reports missing a dose of warfarin).
- Follow facility procedures for communicating and documenting test results.
- Even though point-of-care testing will give immediate or nearly immediate results, remember that PBTs are not permitted to discuss diagnosis or treatment with patients. The patient's doctor or other healthcare practitioner will discuss the results with the patient.
- Many point-of-care tests have **critical values**, or ranges for results that require intervention and must be reported to a supervisor or physician immediately. Facilities usually require that point-of-care tests be repeated if results are in critical ranges. This confirms that the first result was not an error. Know critical values for any tests performed. Report critical value results right away even if a second test is within normal range. Report both test results.
- Dispose of test strips or containers properly. These items must be discarded in a biohazard waste receptacle.
- Follow facility procedures for cleaning and conducting quality control checks on point-of-care testing devices. The machines must be cleaned thoroughly after every use if they are not dedicated to a single patient. Quality control checks are usually performed and documented on a daily basis.

Chapter Review

Multiple Choice

1. Capillary puncture is the most common way of collecting blood specimens from
   (A) Infants
   (B) Toddlers
   (C) Adolescents
   (D) All children
2. What is the name of the infection that may be caused if a lancet strikes bone?
   (A) Osteomyelitis
   (B) Osteopathy
   (C) Osteoporosis
   (D) Osteonia
3. When cleaning a site prior to capillary puncture,
   (A) The site should be wiped with dry gauze after cleaning
   (B) The favored antiseptic agent is povidone iodine
   (C) Less thorough cleaning is required than for venipuncture
   (D) It may first be necessary to ask the patient to wash her hands

4. What is one reason capillary collections should be completed quickly?
   (A) Because patients will not tolerate the pain for very long
   (B) Because platelet clumping will begin to interfere with the procedure
   (C) Because supervisors expect them to take less time than venipuncture
   (D) Because they are usually ordered for very urgent testing

5. What usually happens to the first drop of blood in a capillary collection?
   (A) It is wiped away.
   (B) It is collected in a separate capillary tube.
   (C) It is allowed to drip into a biohazard waste container.
   (D) It is collected with the rest of the specimen.

6. "Milking" the finger during a capillary collection can cause
   (A) Decreased blood flow
   (B) Hemolysis
   (C) Hemoconcentration
   (D) Numbness in the patient's finger

7. Why may additional PPE be required when conducting a capillary collection on an infant?
   (A) Because infants often carry dangerous illnesses
   (B) Because infants will usually kick and squirm during the procedure, which poses a greater risk of an accidental lancet stick
   (C) Because babies may become very ill from sicknesses that are not dangerous to adults
   (D) Because it will cause the parents to view the PBT as more of a professional

8. The edge of a blood smear should appear
   (A) Rough
   (B) Smooth
   (C) Thick
   (D) Feathered

9. Which of the following sentences reflects correct procedure in conducting a newborn metabolic screening?
   (A) A small drop of blood should be within each circle, with a white border between the drop and the circle's edge.
   (B) Each circle should be completely filled with a drop of blood.
   (C) Blood may be dripped onto the paper from either side.
   (D) The filter paper should be pressed against the baby's heel.

10. What should a PBT do if the test strips for a glucose meter are out of date?
   (A) Document the expiration date when reporting results
   (B) Ask the patient if he minds using the expired strips
   (C) Request that the patient reschedule the test
   (D) Acquire a new container of unexpired test strips

11 Nonblood Specimens

1. Identify nonblood specimens collected for laboratory testing

Diagnostic tests performed on a patient's blood can provide doctors with a wide range of information. Tests are also routinely performed on other body fluids and specimens. After blood, urine is the most commonly tested specimen. It can be collected easily, usually without invasive procedures, because urination is a natural process. Other specimens that may be collected and tested easily include the following:

- Stool (feces)
- Saliva
- Sputum
- Sweat
- Breath (exhaled into a bag)
- Semen
- Hair
- Fingernail clippings

Other specimens can be collected with only minimal discomfort for the patient. These include specimens collected using **swabs** or pads of synthetic material at the end of a stick or wire (Fig. 11-1). Swabs are often used to collect specimens to determine whether bacteria or other pathogens are present. They may also be used to collect cells for analysis. This analysis could include DNA testing or the evaluation of cells for abnormalities. Swabs are frequently used to collect specimens from these areas of the body:

- Throat
- Cheek (buccal)
- Nose and nasal cavities (nasal and nasopharyngeal)

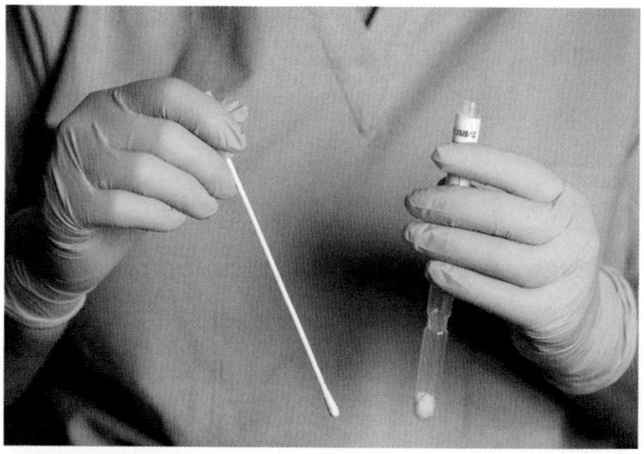

Fig. 11-1. *Swabs can be used for throat cultures, influenza (flu) testing, and a number of different types of specimen collection.*

Testing is also performed on body tissues and internal substances. These specimens must be removed through more invasive or even surgical processes. In many cases they are **aspirated**, or drawn out by suction, usually through a needle inserted into the body. These specimens include the following:

- Tissues for *biopsy*, or examination for abnormalities (removed surgically or by aspiration)
- Bone marrow

- Fluid surrounding a fetus in the mother's uterus (amniotic fluid)
- Fluid surrounding the brain and spinal column (cerebrospinal fluid)
- Fluid from the joints (synovial fluid)
- Fluid from the lining of the lungs (pleural fluid)
- Fluid from the lining of the heart (pericardial fluid)
- Fluid from the abdominal cavity (peritoneal fluid)

Only physicians or other specially trained healthcare professionals collect these specimens. In some settings, a phlebotomist might handle or transport this type of specimen. These specimens are always hand-delivered and never transported in automated systems. Healthcare workers should follow facility procedures. Some of these collection processes involve risk to the patient that makes repeating the process impossible. Even if the process can be repeated, collection is often difficult for the patient, and replacing a damaged specimen can be stressful, painful, and costly.

2. Describe types of urine specimens and demonstrate how to collect a clean-catch urine specimen

Urine testing may be conducted on a routine basis, as part of a physical exam, or to aid in diagnosis of a particular illness or condition. Urine is examined in several different ways. It is observed for color, clarity, and the presence of any visible solid substances (Fig. 11-2). Its odor may be noted, as a sweet or especially unpleasant odor may indicate illness. It may be strained to remove and examine any solid particles, such as kidney stones.

Urine is also tested for a number of different chemical components or qualities. This testing may be done by dipping a test strip treated with chemical reagents into the urine. Urine specimens are sometimes centrifuged. Then the concentrated portion at the bottom of the tube is examined under a microscope by a medical technician. If a patient has had repeated or severe urinary tract infections, a **culture and sensitivity test** may be performed. This test can identify microorganisms in the urine and help the physician choose an appropriate antibiotic if one is needed.

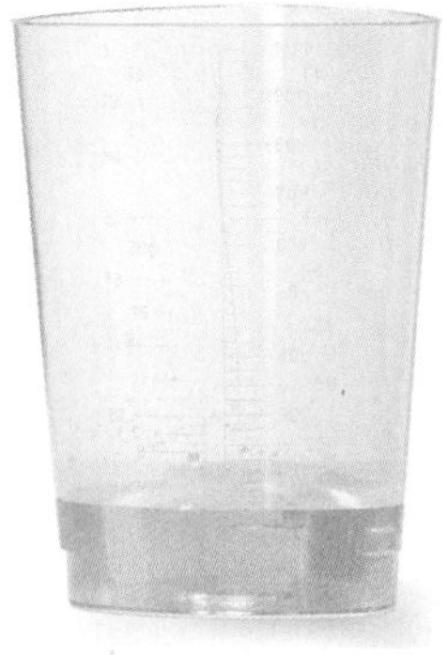

Fig. 11-2. *Normal urine is light or pale yellow (straw-colored). It should be clear, not cloudy.*

Collection of urine is performed in several different ways:

- **Routine urine specimens** can be collected any time. (This may also be called a *random urine specimen.*) The patient urinates into a specimen container.
- **First void urine specimens** must be collected when the patient first urinates (*voids*) in the morning. These specimens are more concentrated than specimens collected later in the day.
- **Clean-catch urine specimens** are collected in such a way that contamination of the specimen is reduced. The patient cleans the genital area before collecting the specimen and collects only the middle part of the urine voided. This is also called a *midstream* urine specimen.
- **24-hour urine specimens** are collected to analyze all of the urine produced over a full day/night period.

Because very small children are not able to control their urine flow, specimens from infants and toddlers are collected in bags that have adhesive-lined openings and fit over the child's genitals. The bag is removed after the child voids (Fig. 11-3).

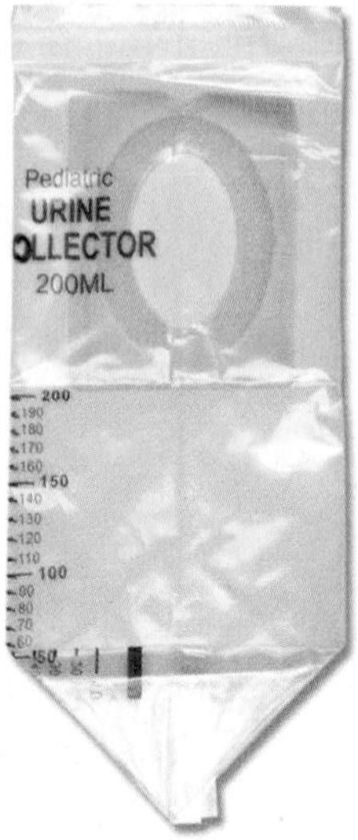

***Fig. 11-3.** The adhesive on this collection bag keeps it in place so a specimen can be collected whenever the child urinates.* (© MEDLINE 2020)

When a patient is unable to urinate normally, specimens are collected differently. A **catheter**, or a very thin tube, can be inserted into the bladder through the urethra to extract urine, or a specimen can be taken from a catheter that is already in place. Another collection method, **suprapubic aspiration**, involves insertion of a needle directly into the bladder through the patient's abdomen. This procedure is generally performed by a physician or nurse. It is used when a patient cannot be catheterized or when the specimen must not contain external microbes. The process of urination and collection can introduce contamination, even when performed with care. Catheter and suprapubic specimens will not be collected by PBTs, but PBTs may handle or transport them.

Depending on the tests that will be conducted, special handling requirements may apply. If urine will be cultured, the specimen should be taken to the laboratory immediately. If this is not possible, it must be refrigerated or transferred to tubes containing a chemical preservative. Urine specimens should generally be tested within one to two hours of collection or refrigerated if testing is delayed. Some should be protected from light. If a specimen will be tested for the presence of drugs of abuse, measures must be taken to ensure that the specimen is not tampered with (guidelines later in this learning objective). Phlebotomists should follow all facility procedures for collecting and processing specimens.

Phlebotomists are often patients' primary point of contact at an outpatient laboratory. In addition to drawing blood, PBTs will frequently instruct patients in the collection of urine specimens if urine tests are ordered. When a urine specimen is being collected at the laboratory, the phlebotomist must remember these guidelines:

Guidelines: On-Site Urine Specimen Collection

- Verify that the patient has met any requirements for the tests ordered. Glucose is sometimes monitored in **postprandial**, or after-meal, urine specimens. These specimens are collected two hours after the patient has eaten.
- Provide instructions for the patient regarding proper collection procedures and where to place the urine specimen after collection.
- Remember that some patients will find providing a urine specimen embarrassing or uncomfortable. Be empathetic, tactful, and professional.
- Wear gloves when you handle urine specimens. If urine is transferred or handled outside sealed containers, follow facility policy regarding PPE. Face masks and goggles, or face shields, may be required.
- **Label the specimen container itself (never the lid)** in front of the patient. Write the date/

time of collection and your initials on the label. Ask the patient to confirm that the identifying information on the label is complete and accurate.

- **G** Give the patient a specimen container appropriate to the test(s) ordered. Culture and sensitivity specimens are collected in sterile containers (Fig. 11-4).

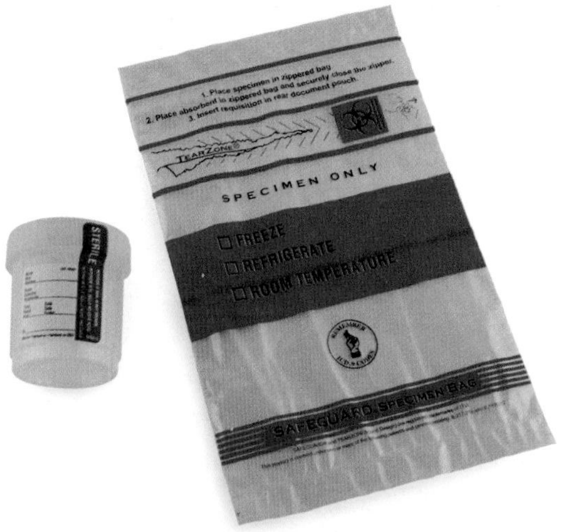

Fig. 11-4. *Specimen containers for some urine tests are sterile. All urine specimens are transported in biohazard bags.*

- **G** Instruct the patient not to touch the inside of the specimen container or lid.
- **G** Emphasize that feces, toilet paper, and water will contaminate a urine specimen and must not be included.
- **G** Ask the patient to make sure the container is at least half full to ensure an adequate amount for testing.
- **G** Transport specimens for testing as soon as possible.
- **G** Follow any facility protocol for refrigerating or preserving specimens that cannot be tested promptly.

Note: Patient identification steps are included here as a reminder. If blood and urine specimens are both collected during a single patient interaction, the patient does not need to be identified a second time.

Collecting a clean-catch (midstream) urine specimen

Equipment: specimen container and lid, specimen label, specimen bag for transport, cleansing wipes, gloves, pen

1. Greet the patient. Identify yourself by name and title.
2. Identify the patient using two unique identifiers. Usually this means asking the patient to state and spell his/her first and last names and to state his/her full date of birth. Check the information provided against the patient's wristband if wristbands are used at your facility.
3. Explain the procedure to the patient. Allow the patient to ask questions, but refer questions regarding the purpose or interpretation of tests to the ordering doctor.
4. Label the specimen container in front of the patient, initialing and noting the time and date of collection. Ask the patient to confirm that the identifying information on the label is correct. Depending on facility protocol, a biohazard bag may also be given to the patient for transporting the completed specimen out of the bathroom.
5. Give the patient the wipes required (2 for males; 3 for females), or direct him or her where to find the wipes if they are stored in the bathroom. Instruct the patient to collect the specimen according to the steps below (instructions are often printed and posted in the bathroom as well):
   - Open the collection container. Do not touch the inside of the container or lid. Place the lid facing upward to prevent contamination.
   - Wash hands before beginning.
   - Spread and clean the labia using the wipes provided. First use a clean wipe to clean down one side using a single

stroke, front to back. Then use another clean wipe to clean down the other side using a single stroke. Use one more clean wipe to wipe down the middle, making sure to clean the urethral opening. Men should clean the tip of the penis; uncircumcised men should retract the foreskin before cleaning. Move outward from the urethral opening in a circular motion and then repeat with a fresh wipe.

- Urinate a small amount into the toilet or urinal and then stop before urination is complete. Women should continue to hold the labia open while urinating.
- Place the container under the urine stream (taking care not to touch container to the genital area) and resume urinating.
- Fill the container at least half full. Stop urinating and remove the container.
- Finish urinating into the toilet or urinal.
- Place the lid firmly on the specimen container. Do not touch the inside of the specimen container or lid.
- Wipe off the outside of the container with a paper towel and discard the towel.
- Place the specimen either in the biohazard bag provided or in a designated drop location (e.g., cabinet in the bathroom that also opens to the outside for collection).
- Wash hands.
- Deliver the specimen to the technician if a drop location is not used.

6. Don gloves.
7. Take the urine specimen from the patient or retrieve it from the drop location.
8. Thank the patient and tell the patient he/she may leave and will receive results from the ordering practitioner.
9. Place the specimen and the requisition or any required paperwork in the appropriate transport bag or container.
10. Remove gloves and wash your hands.

When drug testing is performed on urine, additional steps are often required. Facilities that conduct drug testing train employees in their required procedures. These are general guidelines:

Guidelines: Collecting Urine Specimens for Drug Testing

- G Identify the patient (photo ID verification is generally required).
- G Do not allow the patient to take anything into the bathroom with him, or to wear a coat or jacket into the bathroom. Request to inspect the contents of the patient's pockets if required by facility policy.
- G Turn off or block water flow to the faucet and/or toilet. The patient must be given a way to clean his hands, but most drug testing protocols require that water be turned off to prevent possible dilution of the specimen. Often patients wash their hands at a sink outside the bathroom just before entering to provide the specimen.
- G Add coloring to the toilet water if required. This is also intended to prevent specimen dilution.
- G Tell the patient not to flush the toilet after specimen collection.
- G Test the temperature of the specimen immediately after collection (within four minutes for federal programs).
- G In many cases the specimen is collected in one container and then divided into a **split specimen**. To create a split specimen, pour at least 30 mL of urine into one specimen container and 15 mL into a second

container. Pour the split specimen in front of the patient. The larger specimen is used to conduct the initial drug testing and the smaller specimen may be tested to confirm a positive result.

- **G** Apply any required seals to the completed specimen in front of the patient. In most cases the patient will need to initial the seals.
- **G** Complete the "collector" portion of any necessary paperwork to accompany the specimen (e.g., the Federal Drug Testing Custody and Control Form).

The composition of urine changes throughout the day. Urine is sometimes collected over 24 hours in order to acquire a more complete specimen. These urine collections are performed as part of several different tests, many of which relate to kidney function. Patients are given equipment that will allow them to collect the specimen at home. The exact equipment may vary, but it will always include a large specimen container, usually with a 3-liter capacity (Fig. 11-5).

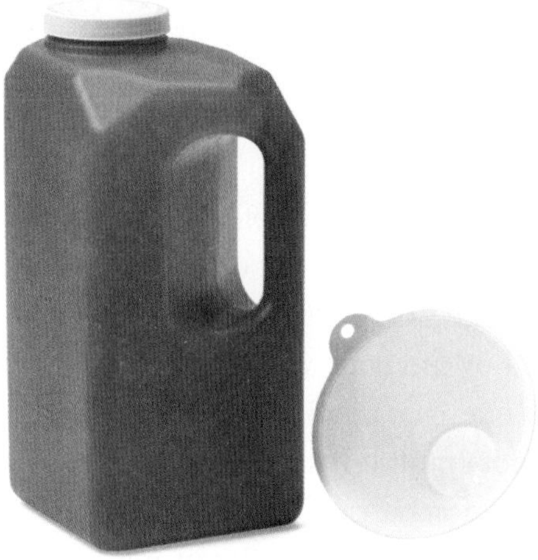

Fig. 11-5. *Since most people produce between one and two liters of urine per day, specimen containers for 24-hour urine collection are usually large enough to hold three liters.* (© MEDLINE 2020)

The urine is not collected directly in this large container, however, and so a *hat*, or collection container that can be fitted onto a toilet, and a funnel are also generally included (Fig. 11-6). The urine is collected in the hat and then poured carefully into the collection container. Instructions often include keeping the specimen cool. Facilities may provide a foam cooler to be filled with ice or ice slurry, or another type of outer container to help keep the specimen at the desired temperature. Alternately, patients may be instructed to keep the specimen refrigerated.

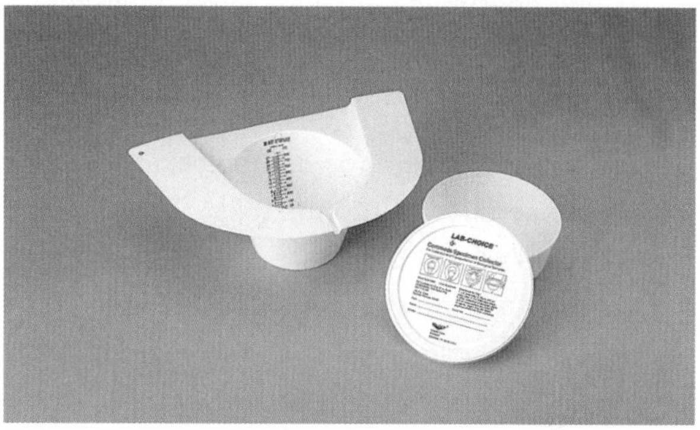

Fig. 11-6. *A hat is a container that can be placed under the toilet seat to collect a specimen.*

Depending on the test(s) that will be performed on a 24-hour urine specimen, the container may have chemical additives placed inside before it is given to the patient. These additives preserve particular substances in the urine, and they may be toxic or caustic (capable of damaging the skin). Phlebotomy technicians should warn patients to prevent splashing when transferring urine into the containers. PBTs should handle the additives carefully and wear proper PPE as required. Containers with additives must be marked to indicate the chemical(s) they contain. Facilities have stickers or another marking system for this purpose.

Some tests require both a 24-hour urine specimen and a blood specimen. An example is *creatinine clearance,* which measures how much of a particular waste product is present in the urine. The timing of the blood specimen will vary by facility. Ideally it is collected midway through the urine collection, but this is not always possible.

Although facilities usually provide written instructions for 24-hour urine testing, phlebotomy technicians must give clear verbal instructions to patients. They should follow these guidelines when assisting with the collection of a 24-hour urine collection:

Guidelines: 24-Hour Urine Specimens

- G Give the patient all of the equipment required for collecting and returning the specimen (3-liter specimen container with lid, hat for toilet and/or other collection receptacle, funnel, and cooler if used at your facility).
- G Instruct the patient to void the next morning's first urine directly into the toilet. This is not collected as part of the specimen. It allows the test to begin with an empty bladder. The time of the void is noted as the beginning of the 24-hour period. The time may be written on a label affixed to the specimen container or noted on an accompanying document. Follow facility procedures in instructing the patient where to note the time.
- G Tell the patient to collect *all* urine voided over the next 24 hours. Each time the patient urinates, the urine is collected in the hat or other container, and then added to the large specimen container. The lid should be replaced after each addition. The urine must be free of toilet paper and any other contaminants.
- G Instruct the patient to attempt to urinate first if she has to move her bowels as well. This reduces the possibility of fecal matter or toilet paper contaminating the urine specimen.
- G Direct the patient to void one last time at the end of the 24-hour period and to add this urine to the specimen container.
- G Remind the patient to attach the lid firmly to the completed specimen before returning it for analysis.
- G Instruct the patient to transport the specimen carefully, on the floor of her vehicle rather than on a seat. It should not be transported in the trunk, as the temperature of the trunk is not controlled. The specimen should be transported to the lab in a cooler if one was provided.
- G Don gloves before handling the urine specimen. Use other PPE as required by the facility (e.g., mask and goggles or face shield, along with gown or lab coat) if pouring or dividing the specimen.
- G Document the total urine volume before pouring or dividing.

Some tests routinely performed on urine specimens can be quickly and easily conducted using chemically treated strips dipped into the urine. This task may be part of a phlebotomist's duties. These strips, called **reagent strips**, or sometimes simply called *dipsticks* or *dip strips,* have different sections that change color when they react with urine. They can be used to test quickly for a number of substances or properties, including the following:

- **pH level.** This is measured on a scale from 0 to 14. The lower the number, the more acidic the fluid. The higher the number, the more alkaline (basic) the fluid. The normal pH for urine is 4.6–8.0. A pH imbalance may be due to medication, food, or illness.
- **Glucose and ketones.** These substances are associated with diabetes testing. Glucose is blood sugar, and it can appear in urine in some cases. Ketones are substances created by the body when fat is broken down for energy or fuel. This happens when there is not enough insulin to help the body use sugar for energy. When testing for glucose, a **double-voided specimen** may be required. This means that after an initial urine specimen is collected, the patient is encouraged to drink fluids and then a second specimen is collected approximately 30 minutes later. This may be ordered because urine that has been in the bladder for some time may not accurately reflect the amount of glucose present.

- **Blood.** Normal urine does not contain blood. Illness or disease can cause blood to appear in urine. Blood in urine may not be visible (it is considered hidden, or **occult**) but can be detected by testing.
- **Nitrite.** This is a substance often produced when a urinary tract infection is present.
- **Specific gravity.** This measurement is also called *urine density*. It determines the concentration of chemical particles in the urine. The test evaluates the body's water balance and urine concentration by showing how the density of the patient's urine compares to water.

The exact procedure and the tests performed may vary by facility. This procedure outlines the basic steps for using reagent strips to test urine:

Testing urine with reagent strips

Equipment: urine specimen as ordered, reagent strip, gloves, paper towel

1. Wash your hands.
2. Put on gloves.
3. Take a strip from the bottle and recap the bottle. Close it tightly.
4. Dip the strip into the specimen.
5. Follow the manufacturer's instructions for when to remove the strip from the specimen. Remove the strip at the correct time.
6. Follow the manufacturer's instructions for how long to wait after removing the strip. After the proper time has passed, compare the strip with the color chart on the bottle. Do not touch the bottle with the strip (Fig. 11-7).
7. Read the results.
8. Store the strips. Discard used items. Discard the specimen according to facility policy if further tests are not ordered.

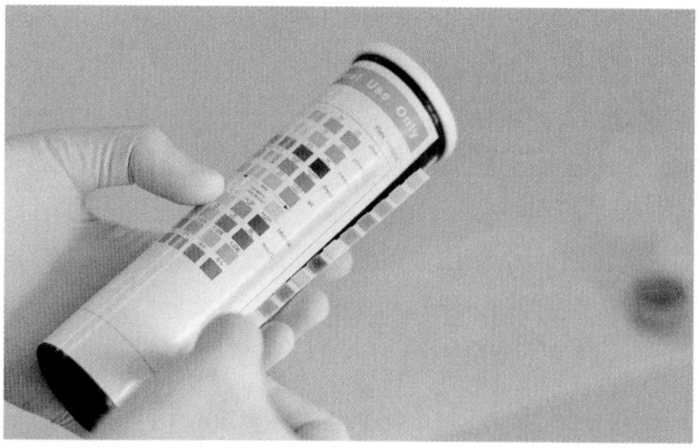

Fig. 11-7. *Reagent strips change color when they react with urine. The color is then compared to a color chart to determine the level of each chemical factor.*

9. Remove and discard gloves.
10. Wash your hands.
11. Document the procedure using facility guidelines.

Reagent strips may also be used to test urine for single analytes. Urine pregnancy tests, for example, test for the presence of hCG, a hormone associated with pregnancy. Some facilities use analyzing machines to perform similar tests on urine. If a PBT is expected to perform these tests, she will be trained to do so.

3. Describe tests performed on stool and instructions for handling a stool specimen

Waste eliminated from the body through the digestive tract is called **stool** or *feces*. It is a semisolid material made up of water, solid waste material, bacteria, and mucus. Stool specimens are sometimes collected so that the stool can be tested for blood, pathogens, fat (an indication that nutrients are not being absorbed properly), and for other things, such as worms or amoebas. In most cases, a patient will be instructed to collect a stool specimen at home following guidelines specific to the test ordered. Phlebotomists should always wear gloves when handling stool specimen containers.

Worms and amoebas can be detected by means of an **ova and parasites** test. Patients will be directed to collect a stool sample at home. The sample must be brought to the lab within two hours of collection or must be collected or stored in containers with a chemical preservative. Often multiple specimens are collected to guarantee an accurate diagnosis.

Fecal occult blood testing is another common test performed on stool. This test can detect blood in the stool, which indicates bleeding in the digestive tract. Bleeding may be caused by colon cancer, and fecal occult blood testing is often used as part of routine colon cancer screening. There are two processes commonly used to test stool for blood: the *fecal immunochemical test* (*FIT*) and the *stool guaiac test* (Fig. 11-8). The two types of tests have different requirements for preparation and collection.

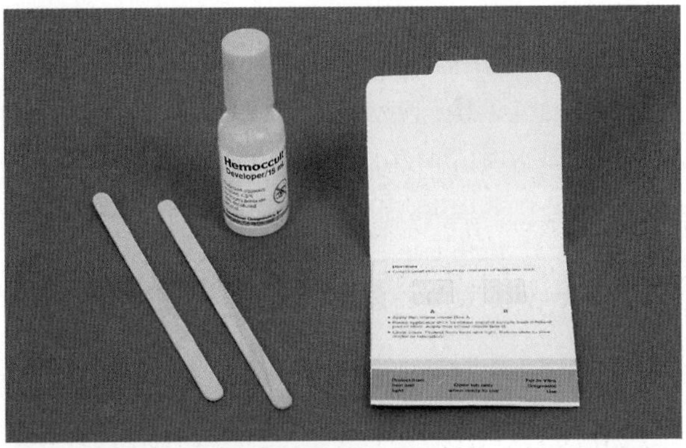

Fig. 11-8. *This is one type of stool guaiac test used to determine if occult blood is present.*

FIT tests vary by manufacturer but may require that feces be collected in a clean receptacle and then a small portion added to a tube containing a chemical solution. The tube is then sealed and taken to the laboratory for testing. This test is sensitive enough to determine whether any blood present is from the lower part of the digestive tract, so fewer special measures are required for patient preparation. The guaiac test involves smearing feces onto one or more windows on a test card. One smear is applied after each bowel movement. Then the card is sealed and delivered to the lab for testing. A chemical reagent is added to the smears in each window to detect the presence of blood. Because the test cannot distinguish the source of any blood in the specimen, it is important to limit sources of possible interference.

These are general guidelines for patient instruction regarding occult blood testing:

Guidelines: Fecal Occult Blood Testing

- **G** Ensure that the patient receives written instructions to take home, as well as verbal instructions.
- **G** Instruct the patient to wash hands thoroughly before and after collecting or handling specimens.
- **G** For guaiac testing, manufacturer instructions may vary, but some foods and medications are usually limited before and during the test due to possible distortion of test results:
  - Red meat (beef, lamb, blood sausage)
  - Raw fruits and vegetables
  - Horseradish
  - Vitamin C supplements
  - Aspirin and ibuprofen
- **G** For both types of testing, instruct the patient to collect stool in a clean, dry container. Toilet water, toilet paper, and urine cannot be included with the stool.
- **G** Demonstrate the use of the test card or other collection equipment. Tongue blades or other devices may be used to remove stool from the clean receptacle where it was collected and place it on the guaiac test window or in the FIT specimen tube. Instruct the patient based on facility protocol.
- **G** Describe how and when the patient should return the completed test. In the case of guaiac testing, an envelope is usually provided for mailing the sealed test card back to the laboratory.

For other types of stool testing, phlebotomy technicians should follow facility procedures for providing patient instructions. Some tests require that all stool be collected over a certain period (e.g., 72 hours). Others require only a certain amount of stool. When providing specimen containers and instructions to patients, it is always important to emphasize that toilet water, toilet paper, and urine can contaminate the specimen and invalidate test results. Professionalism and sensitivity are essential when communicating instructions about stool specimens.

4. Demonstrate how to obtain a throat culture and discuss other swabbing procedures

Several lab tests are performed on specimens taken by rubbing a swab over some part of a patient's body. The swabs may vary. Different synthetic fibers are used to make the soft, collecting portion of the swab stick, and the stick may be rigid or flexible, made of wood or some other substance. Some swabs, once a specimen has been collected, are stored in a vial with an **ampule**, or small container of liquid, that must be crushed to release a fluid designed to preserve the specimen. Some swabs have long sticks that must be broken off before storing the swab in its vial.

The swabbing procedure most likely to be performed by a phlebotomy technician is a **throat culture**. During a throat culture, the patient's tonsils and the back of his throat are rubbed with a specialized swab, and the microorganisms are then encouraged to grow. Bacteria called *Streptococcus pyogenes* are the cause of the illness known commonly as **strep throat** and can be detected by throat culture. Since most sore throats are caused by viruses, a throat culture is ordered when a doctor suspects that a patient has strep throat.

When performing throat cultures, phlebotomy technicians should remember these guidelines:

Guidelines: Throat Culture

G This test can be frightening or uncomfortable for patients. Be gentle and reassuring.

G Strep throat is most common among young patients (aged 5–15). Adjust your language and approach to the age of the patient. Lower yourself to the patient's level when speaking. Answer any questions patiently and with age-appropriate vocabulary.

G Allow children to sit in a parent's or guardian's lap during the procedure if they wish to do so.

G Do not touch the patient's *uvula*, the structure hanging down in the back of the throat. This can cause a gag reflex in the patient. Be aware that some patients will have a gag reflex triggered even if the uvula is avoided.

G Gently supporting the back of the patient's head during the procedure can help steady him until the procedure is over.

Note: Patient identification steps are included here as a reminder. If a blood specimen and throat culture are both collected during a single patient interaction, the patient does not need to be identified a second time.

Obtaining a throat culture

Equipment: culture kit including swab and vial, tongue depressor, gloves (and other PPE as required), specimen label, pen

1. Greet the patient. Identify yourself by name and title.

2. Identify the patient using two unique identifiers. Usually this means asking the patient to state and spell his first and last names and state his full date of birth. (For pediatric patients, a parent/guardian performs this step on the child's behalf, and the name of this person and her relationship to the child is documented.) Check the information

provided against the requisition form and against the patient's wristband if wristbands are used at your facility.

3. Explain the procedure to the patient. Allow the patient (and parent/guardian) to ask questions.
4. Gather the required equipment.
5. Wash (or sanitize) your hands. Don gloves and other PPE as required.
6. Remove the swab from its packaging (Fig. 11-9).

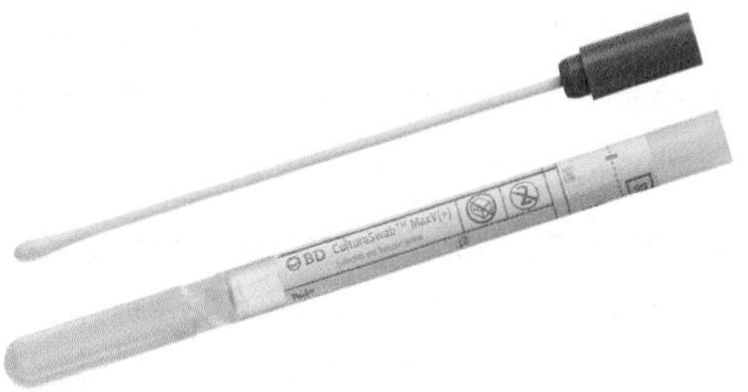

Fig. 11-9. *The swab should be removed from its packaging right before performing the procedure.* (PHOTO COURTESY AND © BECTON, DICKINSON AND COMPANY)

7. Ask the patient to tilt his head back slightly, open his mouth, and say "Ahhhh."
8. Use the tongue depressor to hold the tongue down and out of the way (Fig. 11-10). Insert the swab in the patient's mouth and rub it along both of the patient's tonsils and the back of the throat, avoiding the uvula. Be sure to swab any areas of the throat or tonsils that are white or blistered.

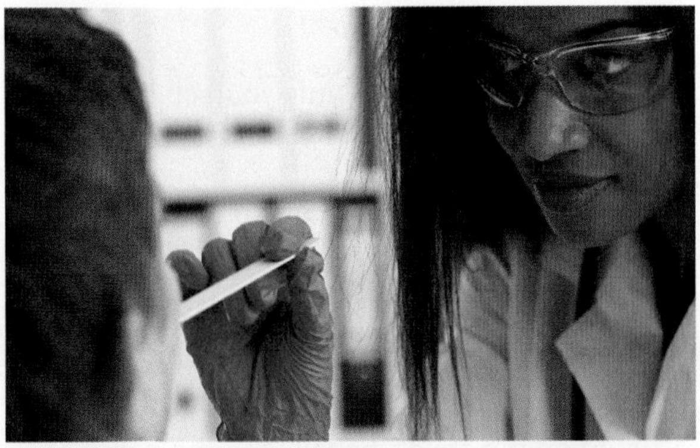

Fig. 11-10. *A tongue depressor can make it easier to reach the patient's tonsils and throat quickly and efficiently.*

9. Remove the swab and tongue depressor and allow the patient to close his mouth.
10. Place the swab in its transport vial/tube. It may be necessary to break off the swab stick and/or break a culture medium ampule before sealing the tube.
11. Label the tube in front of the patient, initialing and noting the time and date of the swab. Ask the patient (or parent/guardian) to confirm that the identifying information on the label is correct. Place the sealed tube and the requisition or any required paperwork in the appropriate transport bag or container. Properly discard any waste.
12. Thank the patient (and parent/guardian, as appropriate) and tell him he may leave and will receive results from the ordering practitioner.
13. Remove gloves and wash your hands.
14. Document the procedure according to facility policy.

Although a throat culture is the swabbing procedure a phlebotomist is most likely to perform, other types of swabbed specimens may also be collected:

- A **buccal swab** involves swabbing the inside of a patient's cheek. This might be done to test for illness (e.g., mumps) or to collect cells for DNA analysis.
- A **nasal swab** is performed by swabbing the nostrils. This type of swab may be used to test for various respiratory viruses or for the presence of particular bacteria (e.g., methicillin-resistant *Staphylococcus aureus*, or MRSA, a common healthcare-associated infection).
- **Nasopharyngeal swabs** are similar to nasal swabs but are collected further back in the nasal cavity, where it turns toward the throat. The swab is inserted until resistance is felt, and then rotated and removed.

Nasopharyngeal swabs may be tested for respiratory viruses, including influenza.

Many of the tests completed on nasal or nasopharyngeal swabs may also be conducted on *nasopharyngeal aspirate*. Collecting nasopharyngeal aspirate involves introducing sterile saline solution into the nasal cavity and then collecting the liquid for analysis. This procedure is not normally performed by PBTs.

5. Describe guidelines for the collection and handling of other nonblood specimens

Depending on the healthcare setting, a phlebotomist may assist in collecting or handling several other types of nonblood specimens. These guidelines refer to some of the most common specimens:

Guidelines: Managing the Collection of Other Nonblood Specimens

G **Breath testing.** A type of bacteria called *Helicobacter pylori* is associated with ulcers, or sores in the digestive tract. The presence of this bacteria can be detected by testing a patient's breath. Patients breathe into a bag and the breath is held in the bag for testing. The patient is then given a liquid to drink that contains a chemical called *urea*. The breath is collected again after a set time has passed. Patients are often asked not to take antibiotics or certain over-the-counter medications for two to four weeks before this test and are asked not to eat or drink anything (including water) for an hour before the test. Verify that patients have followed these instructions when this test is ordered.

G **Hair or fingernail specimens.** Hair and fingernails may be analyzed to determine exposure to or ingestion of specific chemicals. This type of analysis is rare, however, as blood and urine tests more accurately reflect the amount of exposure. Hair may also be tested for DNA. When DNA testing is performed on hair, the root must be included in the specimen. Other types of tests on hair do not necessarily require the root. If collection of these specimens is ordered, follow facility guidelines for collection procedures and handling.

G **Saliva specimens. Saliva** is a fluid secreted in the mouth, and it may be collected to test hormone levels, drug levels (of both therapeutic drugs and drugs of abuse), and/or antibodies. Collection methods vary. Saliva may be spit into tubes containing various additives or collected using an absorbent medium. Follow facility protocol.

G **Semen specimens. Semen** (also called *seminal fluid*) is the fluid associated with the male reproductive system. It contains the male reproductive cells, called *sperm*, suspended in fluids excreted by the glands of the reproductive system. Semen specimens may be collected in the course of fertility testing or to verify that a vasectomy, or operation to prevent the release of sperm, was effective. Men providing a semen specimen will generally be given a specimen container and instructions for collecting the specimen at home or, in some cases, at the laboratory. Instructions generally include a 2- to 5-day period of refraining from sexual activity prior to collecting the specimen. Emphasize to patients that specimens must not be collected in a condom. Condoms are usually treated with lubricants and/or spermicides that can contaminate or destroy the specimen. After collection, semen specimens must be kept close to body temperature, protected from direct light, and delivered to the laboratory within an hour. Make sure these specimens are delivered for testing promptly.

G **Sputum specimens. Sputum** is mucus from the respiratory tract. It is thicker than saliva and is coughed up rather than spit out. It may be tested to detect the presence of pneumonia or tuberculosis. Always wear appropriate PPE during the collection of sputum, as it may contain harmful pathogens. Gloves and an N95 respirator are required. The patient may first rinse his mouth with water, and then is encouraged to cough deeply and spit the resulting sputum into a specimen container. If necessary, the sputum may be loosened by the administration of inhaled medications. Sputum samples are collected most easily first thing in the morning.

Quality Counts

Aside from reception staff, PBTs are often the only healthcare workers a patient interacts with directly in an outpatient laboratory. In addition to drawing blood, they may collect, handle, or instruct patients on the collection of a wide variety of nonblood specimens. In all cases the PBT should remember to follow her scope of practice. Any questions regarding the purpose of a test or the possible outcomes should be referred to the healthcare professional who ordered the test. The job of the PBT is to collect and handle specimens with strict attention to facility procedures and quality standards, and to provide friendly, professional customer service to the patient.

Chapter Review

Multiple Choice

1. Specimens that are *aspirated* are often collected with a
   (A) Swab
   (B) Needle
   (C) Bag
   (D) Sponge

2. ____________________ fluid is found surrounding the lungs.
   (A) Pericardial
   (B) Synovial
   (C) Peritoneal
   (D) Pleural

3. Normal urine may be described as
   (A) Dark yellow, clear, and free of visible solids
   (B) Pale yellow, cloudy, and free of visible solids
   (C) Any shade of yellow, clear, and containing only very small solids
   (D) Pale yellow, clear, and free of visible solids

4. What must be checked promptly after collecting a urine specimen for drug testing?
   (A) The patient's identification
   (B) The temperature of the specimen
   (C) The patient's pockets
   (D) That the sink in the bathroom is not wet

5. What part of the urine specimen collection equipment should be labeled?
   (A) The inner lid of the specimen container
   (B) The outer lid of the specimen container
   (C) The specimen container itself
   (D) The biohazard bag into which the specimen is placed

6. Blood that is hidden in urine or stool is called
   (A) Invisible blood
   (B) Transparent blood
   (C) Elusive blood
   (D) Occult blood

7. The test performed on stool to detect amoebas or worms is called a(n) ____________________ test.
   (A) Ova and parasites
   (B) Postprandial
   (C) Fecal occult blood
   (D) Glucose tolerance

8. A throat culture is used to detect the presence of ____________________ on the patient's tonsils or in the back of the throat.
   (A) Bacteria called *Streptococcus pyogenes*
   (B) A cold virus
   (C) A fungal infection
   (D) Antibodies

9. A nasopharyngeal swab involves taking a specimen from the back of a patient's
   (A) Nasal cavity
   (B) Cheek
   (C) Ear
   (D) Head

10. Seminal fluid should never be collected in a
    (A) Bathroom
    (B) Condom
    (C) Sterile container
    (D) Cold room

11. Which of the following is true about sputum specimens?
    (A) They are identical to saliva specimens.
    (B) They are only collected in the late afternoon.
    (C) They require the patient to cough mucus up from the lungs.
    (D) They are sterile.

Glossary

24-hour urine specimen: urine specimen collected by adding all urine produced over a full day/night period.

ABO blood group system: system of classifying blood type based on the presence or absence of A and B antigens on a person's red blood cells.

abuse: purposeful mistreatment that causes physical, mental, or emotional pain or injury to someone.

accession number: a number printed on all specimen labels and documents associated with a particular requisition.

accredit: officially approve through a specific process.

acquired immunodeficiency syndrome (AIDS): the final stage of HIV infection, in which infections, tumors, and central nervous system symptoms appear due to a weakened immune system that is unable to fight infection.

acute: as related to illness, short-term and requiring immediate care.

additive: in phlebotomy, a chemical agent that affects how blood can be processed and tested.

admit: to check a patient in to a medical facility for inpatient care.

advance directive: legal document that allows people to decide what kind of medical care they wish to have in the event they are unable to make those decisions themselves.

aerobic bottle: in phlebotomy, a receptacle for the portion of a blood culture specimen to be tested for aerobic (oxygen-requiring) microorganisms.

aerosolize: to disperse a substance through the air in such a way that it might be inhaled.

aliquot: a small amount of a larger specimen.

American Hospital Association (AHA): a non-profit membership organization concerned with providing information to the healthcare industry and the public regarding healthcare issues and trends.

ampule: small container of liquid in a swab vial.

anaerobic bottle: in phlebotomy, a receptacle for the portion of a blood culture specimen to be tested for anaerobic (non-oxygen-requiring) microorganisms.

analyte: a substance measured or studied in a diagnostic test.

anemia: a condition in which a person has either too few red blood cells or too little hemoglobin in the blood.

antecubital fossa: the area inside the elbow.

antibody: a protein made by the body to protect against foreign substances.

anticoagulant: a substance that stops blood from clotting.

antigen: a substance that can prompt an immune response.

aortic valve: the heart valve located between the left ventricle and the aorta.

arterial blood: blood in the arteries; oxygenated and marked by a bright red color.

arterialize: in phlebotomy, to make capillary blood more closely resemble arterial blood by warming a capillary puncture site.

arteriovenous (AV) fistula: a connection between a vein and an artery.

artery: a blood vessel that carries oxygenated blood away from the heart.

ASAP: as soon as possible.

aspirate: to draw by suction.

assault: the use of words or actions to cause another person to feel fearful of being harmed.

atrium: one of the two upper chambers of the heart (plural *atria*).

atrioventricular junction: part of the electrical conduction system of the heart; located between the atrioventricular node and the bundle of His.

atrioventricular node: part of the electrical conduction system of the heart; located at the bottom of the right atrium.

basal state: a rested state in which no food or beverage except water has been consumed in the last 12 hours and no strenuous exercise has been performed.

basilic vein: one of the veins present in the antecubital area; may be used for venipuncture, but considered to be the vein of last resort due to its proximity to nerves and an artery.

basophil: a type of white blood cell.

battery: the intentional touching of another person without permission.

B cell: a type of lymphocyte that produces antibodies.

benzalkonium chloride: an antiseptic sometimes used in medical settings.

bevel: the angled opening of a phlebotomy needle.

bicuspid valve: the heart valve located between the left atrium and the left ventricle; also called the *mitral valve.*

bilirubin: a substance in the blood associated with liver function.

blood bank: a facility or department within a facility concerned with collecting and preparing blood for transfusion.

bloodborne pathogen: microorganism found in human blood, body fluid, draining wounds, and mucous membranes that can cause infection and disease in humans.

blood culture: a test for the presence of bacterial or fungal pathogens in the blood.

blood type: designation based on the presence or absence of specific antigens on a person's red blood cells; A, B, AB, and O are the most common blood types.

Bloodborne Pathogens Standard: federal law that requires that healthcare facilities protect employees from bloodborne health hazards.

buccal swab: collection of a specimen from inside a patient's mouth.

buffy coat: the middle layer of an anticoagulated blood specimen that has been spun in a centrifuge; contains white blood cells and platelets.

bundle branches: part of the electrical conduction system of the heart; they divide from the bundle of His and carry the electrical impulse to the walls of the ventricles.

bundle of His: part of the electrical conduction system of the heart; located in the upper part of the septum dividing the ventricles.

calcaneus: the heel bone.

capillary: the smallest blood vessels; they carry oxygen and nutrients to and remove carbon dioxide and wastes from cells throughout the body.

capillary bed: area where exchanges of oxygen and carbon dioxide, and nutrients and waste products, take place.

capillary blood: blood in the capillaries; contains both arterial and venous blood and its color is somwhere betweeen bright and deep red.

capillary puncture: the puncture of a patient's skin for the purpose of collecting a blood specimen from the capillaries beneath the puncture site; also called *dermal puncture.*

capillary tube: a small, thin, straw-like tube for collecting blood from a capillary puncture site.

cardiac conduction system: the pathway of electrical impulses that controls the heart's pumping action.

catheter: a thin tube inserted into the body to drain or inject fluids.

causative agent: a pathogenic microorganism that causes disease.

cell: basic structural unit of the body that divides, develops, and dies, renewing tissues and organs.

Centers for Disease Control and Prevention (CDC): a federal government agency that issues guidelines to protect and improve the health of individuals and communities.

Centers for Medicare & Medicaid Services (CMS): a federal agency within the US Department of Health and Human Services that is responsible for Medicare and Medicaid, among many other responsibilities.

central nervous system (CNS): the part of the nervous system that is composed of the brain and spinal cord.

centrifuge: a machine commonly used to separate substances within liquids through rapid spinning.

cephalic vein: one of the veins present in the antecubital fossa; may be used for venipuncture.

certification: a process used in healthcare to ensure skills are mastered for particular positions.

chain of command: the line of authority at a facility.

chain of custody: documentation of the exact path an item (e.g., a blood specimen) takes from its origin to its destination; provides legal proof that the item is not changed or tampered with.

chain of infection: a way of describing how disease is transmitted from one human being to another.

chemistry: in a clinical laboratory, the department concerned with analyzing specimens for the presence of particular chemicals.

chlorhexidine gluconate: an antiseptic often used to prepare a venipuncture site for blood culture collection.

civil law: branch of law dealing with disputes between individuals.

clean: in health care, a condition in which objects are not contaminated with pathogens.

clean-catch urine specimen: urine specimen collected in such a way that contamination of the specimen is reduced.

CLIA waived test: a diagnostic test determined by CLIA to be simple, easy to perform, and involving little risk of error; phlebotomists can often perform these tests.

cliché: phrase that is used over and over again and does not really mean anything.

clinical experience: experience working with patients in a healthcare facility.

Clinical & Laboratory Standards Institute (CLSI): a nonprofit organization that develops standards of practice for laboratories worldwide.

clinical laboratory: facility that collects and analyzes specimens from patients in order to provide doctors and other healthcare professionals with information.

Clinical Laboratory Improvement Amendments (CLIA): federal regulations regarding the staffing and operation of clinical laboratories.

clotting factor: blood protein involved in the process of blood clotting.

coagulation: the process of blood clotting.

coagulation cascade: the series of changes in the body to prevent blood loss while also avoiding unnecessary and dangerous excessive clotting.

cognitive: related to the ability to think and process information.

communication: the process of exchanging information with others by sending and receiving messages.

complete blood count (CBC): a common blood test used to determine the number of red blood cells, white blood cells, and platelets in a patient's blood; *CBC with differential* specifies how many of each type of white blood cell is present.

confidentiality: the legal and ethical principal of keeping information private.

conscientious: careful; guided by a sense of what is important and right.

consent: in health care, acknowledgement of agreement to treatment or to a procedure.

constrict: to narrow.

continuing education: in health care, education intended to keep healthcare workers up-to-date on changes in medicine that affect their jobs; it may address new equipment, new procedures, or policy changes, or provide a review of important topics.

criminal law: branch of law dealing with offenses considered to harm all of society.

critical value: range for diagnostic testing results that requires intervention and must be reported immediately.

culture: in medicine, to cause any microorganisms present to multiply.

culture and sensitivity test: test performed on urine to identify microorganisms present and to aid in antibiotic selection.

cyanotic: blue or gray, in reference to skin and/or nail bed color.

cytology: in a clinical laboratory, the department concerned with the examination of the structure and function of cells in specimens.

developmental disability: disability that is present at birth or emerges during childhood or early adulthood that restricts physical and/or mental ability.

diabetes: a condition in which the pancreas produces too little insulin or does not properly use insulin.

diagnose: to make a medical determination of illness.

dilate: to widen.

direct contact: a way of transmitting pathogens through touching the infected person or his secretions.

dirty: in health care, a condition in which objects have been contaminated with pathogens.

discard tube: a tube that will not be tested, drawn to ensure additives from one tube do not carry over to the next.

discharge: to release a patient from a medical facility.

disinfection: a process that destroys most, but not all, pathogens; it reduces the pathogen count to a level that is considered not infectious.

documentation: in health care, the creation of a record of care given to a patient.

doff: to remove.

don: to put on.

do-not-resuscitate (DNR): a medical order that instructs medical professionals not to perform cardiopulmonary resuscitation (CPR) in the event of cardiac or respiratory arrest.

double-voided specimen: urine specimen in which two samples are collected; one is collected initially, then another collected approximately a half-hour later.

durable power of attorney for health care: a signed, dated, and witnessed legal document that appoints someone else to make the medical decisions for a person in the event he or she becomes unable to do so.

edema: swelling.

EDTA: anticoagulant additive used in blood collection tubes; most commonly in tubes with lavender stoppers.

electrolyte: a substance that affects the flow of nutrients and the removal of waste products in the blood.

empathy: identifying with the feelings of others.

engineering controls: features incorporated in medical devices to make their use less hazardous.

enzyme: a substance in the body that speeds up a specific reaction.

eosinophil: a type of white blood cell.

ergonomics: the science of designing equipment, areas, and work tasks to make them safer and to suit the worker's abilities.

erythrocyte: a red blood cell; contains the protein (hemoglobin) that carries oxygen in the blood.

ethanol: the intoxicating ingredient in alcoholic beverages.

ethics: the knowledge of right and wrong.

evacuated tube system: a needle, holder, and vacuum tube used together to collect blood specimens by venipuncture.

exposure control plan: a plan designed to eliminate or reduce employee exposure to infectious material.

express consent: consent that is actively, consciously acknowledged.

facility: a place where health care is delivered or administered; may be a hospital, doctor's office, clinical laboratory, treatment center, etc.

fasting: in medicine, the requirement to not eat or drink anything but water for a specified amount of time, usually 8–12 hours, prior to a test or procedure.

fecal occult blood testing: a test used to detect bleeding in the digestive tract; part of routine colon cancer screening.

fibrin: a protein that cannot be dissolved; forms a mesh with platelets to stop bleeding when injury occurs.

fibrinogen: a protein associated with blood clotting; fibrinogen is turned into fibrin when injury occurs, creating a mesh with platelets to stop bleeding.

fibrinolysis: the breaking down of fibrin as an injury heals.

first void urine specimen: urine specimen collected when a patient first urinates in the morning.

flammable: able to catch fire easily.

formed elements: the solid portion of blood.

gauge: indication of the size of a phlebotomy needle; higher gauge numbers correspond to thinner needles.

geriatrics: a branch of medicine dealing with elderly patients.

gestational diabetes: a form of diabetes associated with pregnancy.

glucose: natural sugar.

glucose challenge test: initial form of glucose testing performed in pregnant women to screen for gestational diabetes; patients whose results are high take the full glucose tolerance test.

glucose tolerance test: a test for diabetes or gestational diabetes that measures fasting blood glucose and then measures changes to blood glucose after ingestion of a sweet beverage.

glycolysis: deterioration of glucose (blood sugar); happens quickly in a blood specimen if it is not collected in a tube containing sodium fluoride.

graft: a place where a person's vein has been redirected to a surgically implanted vein.

granulocyte: a category of short-lived white blood cell including eosinophils and basophils.

hand hygiene: washing hands with either plain or antiseptic soap and water and using alcohol-based hand rubs.

Hazard Communication Standard: OSHA's system of identifying potential hazards in the workplace.

healthcare-associated infection (HAI): an infection acquired in a healthcare setting during the delivery of medical care.

Health Insurance Portability and Accountability Act (HIPAA): a federal law that requires health information be kept private and secure and that organizations take special steps to protect this information.

heating block: a rack designed to hold tubes in an upright position while maintaining a specific temperature.

hematology: in a clinical laboratory, the department concerned with analyzing specimens to study properties, diseases, or disorders of the blood.

hematoma: injury caused by leaked blood beneath the skin.

hemoconcentration: a buildup of blood cells (solid components) relative to the liquid components of the blood.

hemoglobin: an oxygen-carrying protein in red blood cells.

hemolysis: destruction of red blood cells.

hemophilia: a disorder that can cause excessive bleeding.

hemostasis: the stopping of a flow of blood.

hemostatic plug: the mesh of fibrin and activated platelets formed at an injury site.

heparin: anticoagulant, often used as an additive in blood collection tubes; usually in tubes with green stoppers.

hepatitis: inflammation of the liver caused by certain viruses and other factors, such as alcohol abuse, some medications, and trauma.

homeostasis: the condition in which all of the body's systems are balanced and are working together to maintain internal stability.

hormone: a chemical substance created by the body that controls body functions.

hub: the threaded area at the base of a phlebotomy needle that can be screwed into a holder or syringe.

human immunodeficiency virus (HIV): the virus that attacks the body's immune system and gradually disables it; eventually can cause AIDS.

iatrogenic anemia: a type of anemia caused by excessive removal of a patient's blood (e.g., by phlebotomy); especially common in infants and patients in intensive care wards.

ice slurry: a mixture of crushed ice and water.

icteric: description of a plasma or serum specimen that is markedly yellow due to high bilirubin levels.

immunology: in a clinical laboratory, the department concerned with analyzing specimens to study the body's response to disease.

impairment: a loss of function or ability.

implied consent: the assumption that a person agrees to treatment or to a procedure; allows medical treatment to be provided in emergency situations, for example, even if the patient is not able to express consent.

incident: an accident, problem, or unexpected event during the course of care that is not part of the normal routine in a healthcare facility.

indirect contact: a way of transmitting pathogens from touching an object contaminated by the infected person.

infection: the state resulting from pathogens invading the body and multiplying.

infection prevention: the set of methods practiced in healthcare facilities to prevent and control the spread of disease.

infectious: contagious.

inferior vena cava: large vein that carries blood to the heart from the legs and trunk.

informed consent: in health care, acknowledgement of agreement to treatment or to a procedure that is given after receiving information regarding risks and benefits; informed consent must usually be documented before treatment begins.

inpatient: a type of medical care provided to patients who stay at a facility overnight.

integrity: having high quality and reliability.

integument: a natural protective covering.

invasive procedure: a procedure that involves inserting a foreign object into a patient's body.

iodine tincture: solution of iodine, usually in ethyl alcohol, used as an antiseptic.

isolate: to keep something separate or by itself.

isopropyl alcohol: an antiseptic commonly used to clean venipuncture and capillary puncture sites.

jaundice: an excess of bilirubin in the blood.

joint: the place at which two bones meet.

Joint Commission: an independent, nonprofit organization that evaluates and accredits healthcare organizations.

laboratory information system (LIS): computer system integrating every part of the laboratory testing process, from orders through analysis and reports.

lancet: a sharp instrument used to make small incisions, as in capillary puncture procedures.

law: a rule established to help people live peacefully together and to ensure order and safety.

leukocyte: white blood cell; capable of producing antibodies and destroying pathogens.

liability: a legal term that means someone can be held responsible for harming someone.

licensure: a legally required process that must be completed to practice a profession.

lipemic: description of a plasma or serum specimen that looks cloudy or milky due to fats in a patient's recent meal(s).

living will: a type of advance directive that outlines specific medical care a person wants, or does not want, in case he becomes unable to make those decisions.

localized infection: an infection that is limited to a specific location in the body and has local symptoms.

long-term care facility: a center that provides skilled care 24 hours a day to residents who live there.

lumen: the hollow space inside a phlebotomy needle.

lymph: a clear yellowish fluid tha[illegible]ries disease-fighting cells called lymphocyt[illegible]

lymphedema: a condition caused by faulty lymphatic draining; a risk if phlebotomy is performed on an arm on the same side as a previous mastectomy.

lymphocyte: a type of white blood cell that plays a role in boosting the body's immune system.

mandated reporter: person who is legally required to report suspected or observed abuse or neglect due to regular contact with vulnerable populations.

median cephalic vein: one of the veins present in the antecubital area.

median cubital vein: well-anchored vein in the middle of the antecubital fossa; first priority site for venipuncture.

medical asepsis: measures used to reduce and prevent the spread of pathogens.

medical social worker: employee at a healthcare facility who deals with patients' social, emotional, and financial needs.

megakaryocyte: a cell produced in the bone marrow that fragments into platelets.

metabolism: physical and chemical processes by which substances are broken down or transformed into energy or products for use by the body.

microbiology: in a clinical laboratory, the department concerned with the study of bacteria, viruses, fungi, and other microorganisms.

microclotting: formation of small clots within a blood specimen.

microcollection tube: a tube for collecting very small blood specimens, with volumes usually ranging between 125 and 600 microliters (μL); generally used for capillary puncture collections.

microorganism: living things so small they can only be seen under a microscope.

minor: a person less than 18 years of age.

mode of transmission: the way a pathogen travels.

monocyte: the largest of the white blood cells; matures into macrophages, which "eat" invading organisms.

mucous membranes: the membranes that line body cavities that open to the outside of the body, such as the linings of the mouth, nose, eyes, rectum, and genitals.

multidrug-resistant organisms (MDROs): microorganisms, mostly bacteria, that are resistant to one or more antimicrobial agents that are commonly used for treatment.

multisample needle: a double-sided needle used in phlebotomy; one side pierces the patient's skin and the other punctures the stoppers of collection tubes.

muscle: group of tissues that provides movement of body parts, protection of organs, and creation of body heat.

nasal swab: collection of a specimen from inside a patient's nostrils.

nasopharyngeal swab: collection of a specimen from the back of the nasal cavity.

negligence: an action, or the failure to act or provide the proper care, that results in unintended injury to a person.

neutrophil: a type of white blood cell that is the body's first defense against illness.

nonspecific immunity: a type of immunity that protects the body from disease in general.

nonverbal communication: communication without using words.

objective: based on what a person sees, hears, touches, or smells.

occult: hidden (e.g., blood in stool).

Occupational Safety and Health Administration (OSHA): a federal government agency that makes rules to protect workers from hazards on the job.

order of draw: the standard sequence in which collection tubes are filled during a blood draw.

organ: structural unit in the human body that performs a specific function.

osteomyelitis: a bone infection that can be caused if a lancet used for finger stick or heel stick strikes the bone.

outpatient: a type of medical care that does not require an overnight stay.

ova and parasites: a test performed on stool to detect the presence of worms or amoebas.

palpate: to examine the body using the fingers or hands.

panel: in phlebotomy, a group of tests either with related analytes or related to a unifying condition or organ.

pathogen: microorganism that is capable of causing infection and disease.

pathology: in a clinical laboratory, the department concerned with the study of the causes and effects of disease.

payer: a person or organization paying for health care.

peak: in relation to measuring medication levels, the point at which the medication is at its highest level in the bloodstream.

pediatrics: a branch of medicine dealing with people under the age of 18.

peripheral blood smear: a way of preparing blood for viewing under a microscope.

peripheral nervous system (PNS): part of the nervous system made up of the nerves that extend throughout the body.

personal: having to do with life outside a job.

personal protective equipment (PPE): equipment that helps protect employees from serious workplace injuries or illnesses resulting from contact with workplace hazards.

petechiae: a condition in which small, flat red or purple dots appear on the skin as a result of leaking capillaries.

phenylketonuria (PKU): a rare condition that can cause brain damage if left untreated; newborns are tested for this and other metabolic disorders.

phlebitis: inflammation of superficial veins.

phobia: a strong fear, usually inexplicable or illogical.

pipette: a narrow tube, often with a suction bulb, used to remove liquid from a specimen.

plantar surface: the sole of the foot.

plasma: the liquid portion of blood.

plasma separator tube (PST): a blood collection tube containing an anticoagulant and a gel designed to separate the liquid and solid components of blood after centrifugation.

plasmin: enzyme that plays a vital role in breaking apart fibrin as an injury heals.

pneumatic tube system: a type of automated specimen transport system used in some healthcare facilities.

point-of-care test: a diagnostic test performed near or in the presence of the patient; many are CLIA waived.

policy: a course of action that should be taken every time a certain situation occurs.

population: in health care, a particular and distinct group of patients.

portal of entry: any body opening on an uninfected person that allows pathogens to enter.

portal of exit: any body opening on an infected person that allows pathogens to leave.

postprandial: after a meal.

povidone-iodine: an antiseptic commonly used in medical settings.

preanalytical errors: errors in diagnostic testing that occur prior to the actual analysis of a specimen (e.g., use of the wrong collection tube).

primary hemostasis: the first stage of hemostasis, concluding with the formation of a platelet plug.

procedure: a method, or way, of doing something.

professional: having to do with work or a job.

professionalism: behaving properly when on the job.

protected health information: a person's private health information, which includes name, address, telephone number, social security number, email address, and medical record number.

provider: a person or organization that provides health care, including doctors, nurses, clinics, and agencies.

PT/INR: blood testing to determine a patient's prothrombin time and international normalized ratio, measures of blood clotting.

pulmonary circuit: the circulation of blood between the heart and the lungs.

pulmonary embolism: a blood clot in the lungs; potentially deadly disorder.

pulmonary valve: the heart valve located between the right ventricle and the pulmonary artery.

Purkinje fibers: part of the electrical conduction system of the heart; they divide from the bundle branches.

QNS: laboratory marking for *quantity not sufficient*; indicates a specimen that is too small to allow ordered tests to be performed.

quality assurance: in health care, ensuring that care is being provided according to facility policy and procedures, with results to meet expectations.

quality control: in health care, processes put into place to document that standards are being met.

quality improvement: in health care, practices that seek to make care better in a way that can be measured.

reagent strip: a strip used to test urine for presence or levels of various analytes; also called *dipstick* or *dip strip*.

reference laboratory: a facility that primarily analyzes specimens sent from other locations.

requisition: an order for diagnostic tests to be completed.

reservoir: a place where a pathogen lives and multiplies.

respiration: the process of inhaling air into the lungs and exhaling air out of the lungs.

Rh factor: a protein that may be present on a person's red blood cells.

Rh negative: designation for people who do not have Rh factor on their red blood cells.

Rh positive: designation for people who have Rh factor on their red blood cells.

routine: in phlebotomy, a designation indicating that a test is not urgent.

routine urine specimen: a urine specimen that can be collected at any time; also called a *random* urine specimen.

Safety Data Sheet (SDS): document describing the composition and possible hazards of chemicals in the workplace.

saliva: fluid secreted in the mouth.

scope of practice: the range of tasks a healthcare worker is allowed to perform according to state or federal law or to facility policy.

secondary hemostasis: the second stage of hemostasis, concluding with the formation of the hemostatic plug.

semen: the sperm-containing fluid associated with the male reproductive system; also called *seminal fluid*.

septum: in cardiology, the wall dividing the right and left sides of the heart.

serology: the study of blood serum.

serum: the liquid portion of blood that has been allowed to clot; it is distinct from plasma and does not contain fibrinogen.

serum separator tube (SST): a blood collection tube containing a clot activator and a gel designed to separate the liquid and solid components of blood after centrifugation.

sharps: needles, lancets, or other sharp objects.

sinoatrial node: part of the electrical conduction system of the heart; acts as the primary pacemaker of the heart.

sodium citrate: anticoagulant additive used in blood collection tubes; usually in tubes with light blue stoppers.

specific immunity: a type of immunity that protects the body against a particular disease that is invading the body at a given time.

specimen: a portion or sample of something larger, collected for study or analysis.

split specimen: a specimen that is divided into more than one container to allow for repeat testing.

sputum: mucus coughed up from the respiratory tract.

Standard Precautions: a method of infection prevention in which all blood, body fluids, non-intact skin, and mucous membranes are treated as if they were infected with an infectious disease.

stat: in medical facilities, a designation of urgency.

stat serum tube: a blood collection tube containing a fast-acting clot activator for quicker testing; usually has an orange stopper.

stem cell: a cell that can become any type of cell.

sterilization: cleaning measure that destroys all microorganisms, including pathogens.

stool: solid waste eliminated through the digestive tract; also called *feces.*

strep throat: an illness caused by the bacterium *Streptococcus pyogenes.*

stress: a state of being overwhelmed by mental or emotional demands.

stressor: something that causes stress.

superior vena cava: large vein that carries blood from the arms, head, and neck to the heart.

suprapubic aspiration: method of collecting a urine specimen in which a needle is inserted directly into the bladder through the patient's abdomen.

surgical asepsis: the state of being completely free of all microorganisms; also called *sterile technique.*

susceptible host: an uninfected person who could become sick.

swab: pad of synthetic material at the end of a stick or wire.

syncope: loss of consciousness; also called *fainting.*

syringe: a tubular device with a plunger that, when pulled, acts to draw in fluid (e.g., blood).

syringe transfer device: a device similar to a tube holder, used to safely transfer blood from a syringe into evacuated tubes.

systemic circuit: the circulation of blood between the heart and the rest of the body (except the lungs).

systemic infection: an infection that travels through the bloodstream and is spread throughout the body, causing general symptoms.

tactful: showing sensitivity and having a sense of what is appropriate when dealing with others.

T cell: a type of lymphocyte that can give chemical signals to regulate immune response or fight infected cells directly.

throat culture: a diagnostic test in which a patient's throat is swabbed and the specimen analyzed for the presence of bacteria.

thrombin: an enzyme in plasma that controls platelet response.

thrombocyte: part of the formed elements of blood; plays a role in blood clotting; also called *platelet.*

thrombophilia: a disorder that can cause excessive clotting.

thrombosis: the formation of a clot within a blood vessel.

thrombus: a clot formed within a blood vessel.

timed draw: a blood draw that must happen at a specific time, often depending upon when the patient last took a medication.

tissue: group of cells that perform a similar task.

tort: a violation of civil law (e.g., negligence).

tourniquet: in phlebotomy, a band that temporarily restricts the return of venous blood below the area where it is applied, making veins easier to locate and access.

transfusion: a transfer of blood from one person to the bloodstream of another.

transmission: passage or transfer.

Transmission-Based Precautions: a method of infection prevention used when caring for persons who are infected or may be infected with certain infectious diseases.

tricuspid valve: the heart valve located between the right atrium and the right ventricle.

trough: in relation to measuring medication levels, the point at which the medication is at its lowest level in the bloodstream.

tunica adventitia: the outer layer of veins or arteries.

tunica intima: the inner layer of veins or arteries.

tunica media: the middle layer of veins or arteries.

urinalysis: the visual, microscopic, and chemical testing of urine specimens.

vasoconstriction: reaction to injury in a blood vessel causing narrowing of muscular tissue at the site of the injury.

vein: a blood vessel that carries blood toward the heart.

venipuncture: the puncture of a vein with a hollow needle for the purpose of extracting a blood specimen.

venous blood: blood in the veins; it is deoxygenated and marked by a dark, deep red color.

ventricles: the two lower chambers of the heart.

verbal communication: communication involving the use of spoken or written words or sounds.

whole blood specimen: an anticoagulated blood specimen that has not been separated into solid and liquid components by spinning in a centrifuge.

winged collection set: a phlebotomy needle with flaps at the base, attached to a length of tubing, which may be used either with a tube holder or a syringe; commonly called a *butterfly needle.*

Bibliography

American Association for Clinical Chemistry. "Lab Tests Online." https://labtestsonline.org/.

American Society for Clinical Pathology (ASCP). *BOC Study Guide: Phlebotomy Certification Examinations; Phlebotomy Technician (PBT), Donor Phlebotomy Technician (DPT)*. 2nd ed. Chicago: ASCP Press, 2019.

BD Diagnostics. "Capillary Blood Collection: Best Practices." *Lab Notes* 20, no. 1, 2009.

Centers for Disease Control and Prevention (CDC). "Protecting Healthcare Personnel." https://www.cdc.gov/HAI/prevent/ppe.html.

Centers for Medicare & Medicaid Services. "Clinical Laboratory Improvement Amendments (CLIA)." https://www.cms.gov/Regulations-and-Guidance/Legislation/CLIA.

Clinical and Laboratory Standards Institute (CLSI). *GP41: Collection of Diagnostic Venous Blood Specimens*. 7th ed. Wayne, PA: CLSI, 2017.

Clinical and Laboratory Standards Institute (CLSI). *GP42-A6: Procedures and Devices for the Collection of Diagnostic Capillary Blood Specimens; Approved Standard*. 6th ed. Wayne, PA: CLSI, 2008.

Ernst, Dennis J., and Catherine Ernst. *The Lab Draw Answer Book: Answers to Hundreds of the Most Frequently Asked Questions on Collecting Blood Samples for Laboratory Testing*. 2nd ed. Corydon, IN: Center for Phlebotomy Education, 2017.

LabCorp. "Blood Specimens: Chemistry and Hematology." https://www.labcorp.com/resource/blood-specimens-chemistry-and-hematology.

National Accrediting Agency for Clinical Laboratory Sciences (NAACLS). *NAACLS Standards Compliance Guide*. https://www.naacls.org/docs/standardscomplianceguide.pdf. NAACLS, 2013.

National Center for Competency Testing (NCCT). *NCCT Interactive Review System: Phlebotomy Technician*. https://www.ncctinc.com/certifications/pt. Overland Park, KS: 2015.

National Healthcareer Association (NHA). *Certified Phlebotomy Technician (CPT) Online Study Guide 2.0*. https://www.nhanow.com/certifications/phlebotomy-technician. Assessment Technologies Institute, 2017.

Occupational Safety and Health Administration (OSHA). "Bloodborne Pathogens and Needlestick Prevention." https://www.osha.gov/SLTC/bloodbornepathogens/standards.html.

Occupational Safety and Health Administration (OSHA). *Laboratory Safety Guidance*. https://www.osha.gov/Publications/laboratory/OSHA3404laboratory-safety-guidance.pdf. OSHA, 2011.

World Health Organization (WHO). *WHO guidelines on drawing blood: Best practices in phlebotomy*. Geneva, Switzerland: WHO Press, 2010.

Index